Interventional Oncology

Interventional Oncology

Edited by

Aaron Rohr, Zachary S. Collins, Brandon Custer, Alan Reeves, Steven Lemons, Adam Alli and E. John Madarang

Cambridge Scholars Publishing

Interventional Oncology

Edited by Aaron Rohr, Zachary S. Collins, Brandon Custer, Alan Reeves, Steven Lemons, Adam Alli and E. John Madarang

This book first published 2023

Cambridge Scholars Publishing

Lady Stephenson Library, Newcastle upon Tyne, NE6 2PA, UK

British Library Cataloguing in Publication Data
A catalogue record for this book is available from the British Library

ISBN (10): 1-5275-2898-7
ISBN (13): 978-1-5275-2898-7

TABLE OF CONTENTS

CHAPTER 1

HISTORICAL INTRODUCTION OF INTERVENTIONAL ONCOLOGY

AARON ROHR MD, MS, JOLEY BEELER MD

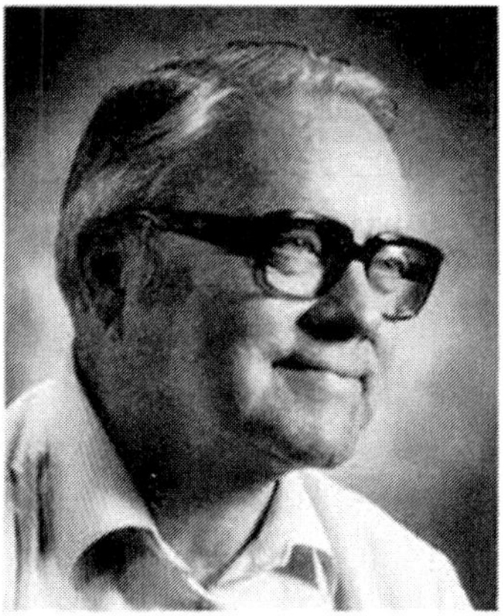

Dr. Sven-Ivar Seldinger

Interventional radiology (IR) is a relatively new, constantly evolving specialty. The first successful angiography in the human body was performed in 1923, though early angiography was performed by surgeons via direct cutdown. In 1953, Swedish doctor Sven-Ivar Seldinger (Reprinted from Sven-Ivar Seldinger: Biography and Bibliography, American Journal of Roentgenology, January 1984, Volume 142: 4-4. 10.2213/ajr.142.1.4, Copyright© 1984, copyright owner as specified in the American Journal of Roentgenology) introduced his Seldinger technique, which laid down the foundation of interventional radiology. The first angioplasty was performed by Dr. Charles Dotter in 1964, paving the way for therapeutic interventional radiology procedures (1). Since then, the field of interventional radiology has evolved rapidly from a diagnostic model to a robust clinical specialty with the ability to perform minimally invasive therapies involving nearly every organ system.

In the mid-1980s, IR continued to garner appreciation as a clinical specialty. As more therapies were discovered, an important subsidiary of IR emerged: interventional oncology.

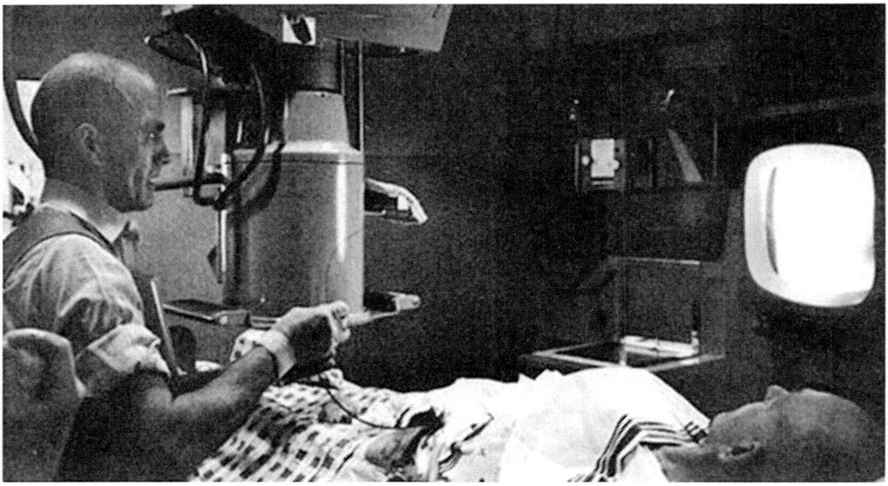

Dr. Charles Dotter in the angiography suite

Cancer is the second leading cause of death worldwide (2), and there has been a growing demand for faster, safer, and more individualized therapies. Traditional oncologic care, such as surgical resection of tumors, is often not possible due to size/location of tumor burden, and many oncologic patients are not surgical candidates. Interventional oncology, a technology-driven and minimally invasive subspecialty, emerged as a unique solution to these challenges. In addition to oncologic diagnosis via image guided tissue sampling, interventional oncology focuses on treatment and symptom palliation, primarily via transcatheter arterial embolization/therapies and percutaneous ablations. Alongside medical, surgical, and radiation oncology, interventional oncology is now considered the fourth pillar of modern oncology care. Several innovations throughout the second half of the 20th century facilitated the advancement of interventional oncology.

Transarterial embolization (TAE)

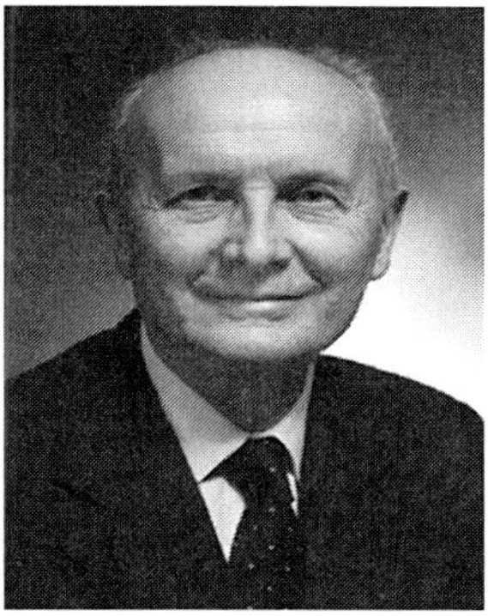

Dr. Josef Rosch

The groundwork for modern trans-arterial embolization (TAE) of tumors was implemented in the 1960-70s. The first attempt at tumor embolization to induce ischemic tumor necrosis was performed intraoperatively via hepatic artery ligation in 1966 (3), though the effect was transient due to development of collateral vessels. TAE was first attempted by Rosch et al for duodenal bleeding in 1972 (4). In 1974, the first successful TAE for liver tumors was performed (5), and this procedure has been adapted for devascularization of tumors in other organs, including renal cell carcinoma and bone tumors (6, 7).

Transarterial chemoembolization (TACE)

In the late 1970s, intrahepatic arterial injection of chemotherapeutic agents was employed for the treatment of HCC (8, 9). By the early 1980s, the combination of intrahepatic arterial injection of chemotherapy followed by TAE was found to be far more effective than TAE or chemotherapy alone (10), and the foundation for trans-arterial chemoembolization (TACE) was established. This basic approach has continued to undergo advancements to maximize oncologic tumoricidal intervention. More complex chemotherapeutic agents have been employed, individualized to cancer type. In the late 1980s, lipiodol, an iodized oil used as a lymphangiographic dye, was found to remain selectively within the neovascular and extravascular spaces of liver tumors when injected into the hepatic artery (11). Lipiodol began to be used not only as an embolic material but also as a carrier of chemotherapeutic agents. Even more recently, in the early 2000s, TACE has been performed utilizing drug-eluting beads (DEBs)—non-resorbable PVA-based microspheres that can be loaded with various chemotherapeutic agents (12, 13). In 2002-2003, publication of 2 randomized controlled trials established TACE as standard of care for patients with unresectable HCC (14, 15).

Transarterial radioembolization (TARE)

Trans-arterial radioembolization (TARE) has evolved alongside TACE, utilizing similar arterial embolization techniques with the administration of particles loaded with a radionuclide (yttrium-90) to selectively target high levels of ionizing radiation to tumors within the liver. Embolization with yttrium-90 (90Y) microspheres has been investigated for cancer treatment in animal models since the 1960s (16, 17), demonstrating promise in hepatic applications (18). Human trials followed, with TARE demonstrating safety and efficacy in the treatment of liver metastases and unresectable HCC in the 1990s (19-21). The two currently available radioembolization delivery methods, Y90 incorporated into a glass matrix (22) and 90Y-doped resin (23), were approved by the FDA in 1999 and 2002, respectively.

Thermal Ablations

Image-guided percutaneous tumor ablation focally destroys tumors by inducing irreversible cellular injury by the direct application of chemical (i.e., nonenergy) or thermal/nonthermal (i.e., energy-based) therapies (24). Early tumor ablations utilized percutaneous chemical injection to treat hepatic tumors. Ethanol was the first ablation agent used in the 1980s (25, 26), and shortly after acetic acid was utilized with increased efficacy (27). However, chemical ablation therapy is limited by the difficulty in achieving uniform diffusion throughout a larger tumor volume (28).

Energy-based, thermal ablations were then introduced, with the ability to destroy tumors by increasing or decreasing temperatures to induce irreversible cellular injury. There are three main modalities for thermal ablation—radiofrequency ablation, microwave ablation, and cryoablation—with the modality selected based on tumor size, location, and operator preference.

Radiofrequency length sound waves have long been known to heat tissue, first described in 1891 and leading to the creation of the intraoperative electrocautery Bovie knife in 1928 (29). Initial utilization of radiofrequency for percutaneous ablation of hepatic tumor in animal models was described using a modified Bovie knife with an insulated needle in 1990 (30, 31). Radiofrequency ablation (RFA) was trialed in humans in the 1990s and was shown to be superior to chemical ablation with respect to local recurrence and overall survival in hepatocellular carcinoma (32). RFA has been generalized to tumors in other locations such as renal, lung, bone (33-35), and more recently in thyroid tumors (36).

Microwave ablation (MWA) utilizes electromagnetic energy at specific frequencies to heat tissue. The evolution of MWA in the early 2000s has permitted several advantages over RFA, including more efficient heating, better penetration through tissue with higher impedance, and less susceptibility to the heat sink effect (37, 38).

Cryotherapy induces cell death by disrupting cellular membranes through alternately freezing and thawing, though early cryotherapy systems were large and limited to open operative use (39). Technological advances in the 1990s resulted in smaller cryoprobes and the ability to use cryotherapy percutaneously, which have been demonstrated safe and effective for use in kidney and lung tumors (40, 41).

Energy-based, non-thermal techniques, such as irreversible electroporation and histotripsy, are the newest developments in ablation and will be discussed in the new innovations chapter.

Collectively, these advancements have established interventional oncology as an essential pillar within oncologic care over time (Fig. 1). While the benefits of interventional oncology are many—shorter recovery, treatments on an outpatient basis freeing up hospital beds, intra-arterial chemotherapy increases potency and removes harsh systemic side effects—oncology is a field that relies heavily on data. To that end, mounting evidence and major clinical trials have demonstrated the efficacy of interventional oncology treatment and even incorporated interventional therapies into accepted clinical guidelines. The ensuing chapters are intended to help illuminate, in detail, current therapies provided by IR for oncologic treatment.

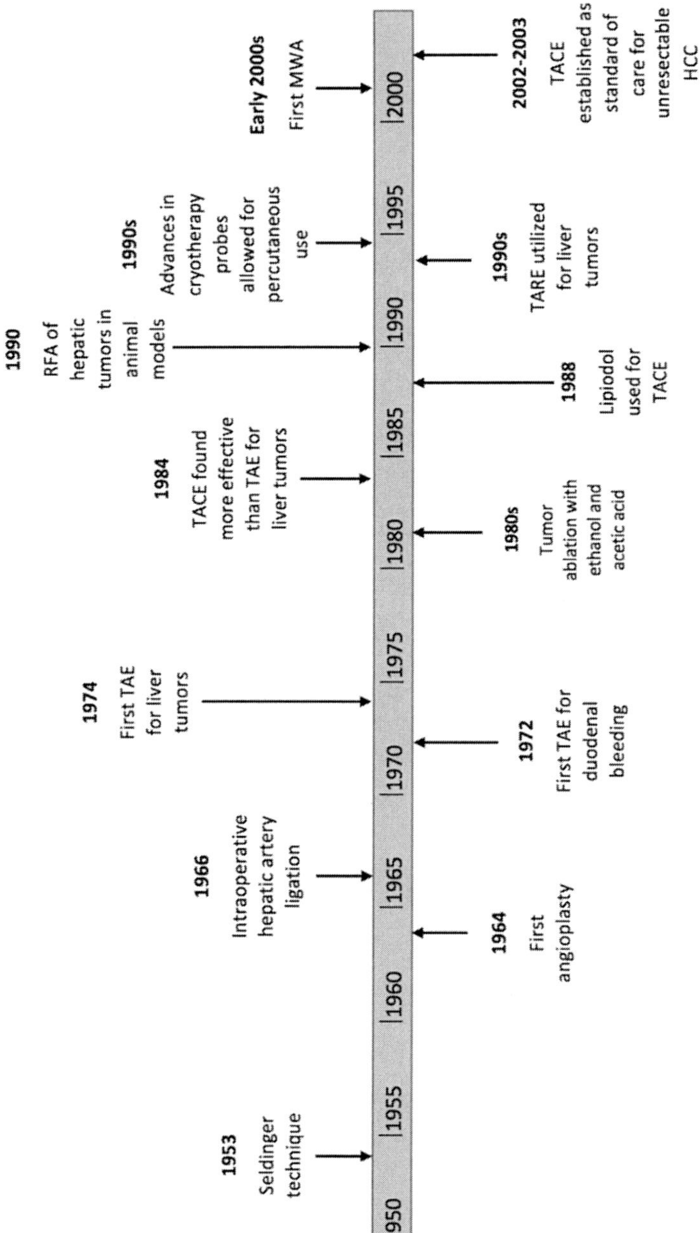
1950
1955
1960
1965
1970
1975
1980
1985
1990
1995
2000
1953
Seldinger technique
1966
Intraoperative hepatic artery ligation
1974
First TAE for liver tumors
1984
TACE found more effective than TAE for liver tumors
1990
RFA of hepatic tumors in animal models
1990s
Advances in cryotherapy probes allowed for percutaneous use
Early 2000s
First MWA
1964
First angioplasty
1972
First TAE for duodenal bleeding
1980s
Tumor ablation with ethanol and acetic acid
1988
Lipiodol used for TACE
1990s
TARE utilized for liver tumors
2002-2003
TACE established as standard of care for unresectable HCC

References

1. Tang Z, Jia A, Li L, Li C. [Brief history of interventional radiology]. Zhonghua Yi Shi Za Zhi. 2014 May;44(3):158-65. Chinese. PMID: 25208839.
2. Hulvat MC. Cancer Incidence and Trends. Surg Clin North Am. 2020 Jun;100(3):469-481. doi: 10.1016/j.suc.2020.01.002. Epub 2020 Mar 27. PMID: 32402294.
3. Mori W, Masuda M, Miyanaga T. Hepatic artery ligation and tumor necrosis in the liver. Surgery. 1966 Mar;59(3):359-63. PMID: 5906225.
4. Rösch J, Dotter CT, Brown MJ. Selective arterial embolization. A new method for control of acute gastrointestinal bleeding. Radiology. 1972 Feb;102(2):303-6. doi: 10.1148/102.2.303. PMID: 4536688.
5. Doyon D, Mouzon A, Jourde AM, Regensberg C, Frileux C. L'embolisation artérielle hépatique dans les tumeurs malignes du foie [Hepatic, arterial embolization in patients with malignant liver tumours (author's transl)]. Ann Radiol (Paris). 1974 Oct;17(6):593-603. French. PMID: 4142843.
6. Ellman BA, Parkhill BJ, Curry TS 3rd, Marcus PB, Peters PC. Ablation of renal tumors with absolute ethanol: a new technique. Radiology. 1981 Dec;141(3):619-26. doi: 10.1148/radiology.141.3.7302214. PMID: 7302214.
7. Chuang VP, Soo CS, Wallace S, Benjamin RS. Arterial occlusion: management of giant cell tumor and aneurysmal bone cyst. AJR Am J Roentgenol. 1981 Jun;136(6):1127-30. doi: 10.2214/ajr.136.6.1127. PMID: 6786025.
8. Friedman MA, Volberding PA, Cassidy MJ, Resser KJ, Wasserman TH, Phillips TL. Therapy for hepatocellular cancer with intrahepatic arterial adriamycin and 5-fluorouracil combined with whole-liver irradiation: a Northern California Oncology Group Study. Cancer Treat Rep. 1979 Nov-Dec;63(11-12):1885-8. PMID: 230895.
9. Misra NC, Jaiswal MS, Singh RV, Das B. Intrahepatic arterial infusion of combination of mitomycin-C and 5-fluorouracil in treatment of primary and metastatic liver carcinoma. Cancer. 1977 Apr;39(4):1425-9. doi: 10.1002/1097-0142(197704)39:4<1425::aid-cncr2820390411>3.0.co;2-k. PMID: 192431.
10. Ando K. Evaluation of conservative therapeutic modalities for hepatocellular carcinoma--analysis of 206 cases. Gastroenterol Jpn. 1984 Oct;19(5):436-46. doi: 10.1007/BF02807256. PMID: 6097497.

11. Nakajo M, Kobayashi H, Shimabukuro K, Shirono K, Sakata H, Taguchi M, Uchiyama N, Sonoda T, Shinohara S. Biodistribution and in vivo kinetics of iodine-131 lipiodol infused via the hepatic artery of patients with hepatic cancer. J Nucl Med. 1988 Jun;29(6):1066-77. Erratum in: J Nucl Med 1988 Nov;29(11):1879. PMID: 2836573.
12. Morise Z, Sugioka A, Kato R, Fujita J, Hoshimoto S, Kato T. Transarterial chemoembolization with degradable starch microspheres, irinotecan, and mitomycin-C in patients with liver metastases. J Gastrointest Surg. 2006 Feb;10(2):249-58. doi: 10.1016/j.gassur.2005.08.004. PMID: 16455458.
13. Varela M, Real MI, Burrel M, Forner A, Sala M, Brunet M, Ayuso C, Castells L, Montañá X, Llovet JM, Bruix J. Chemoembolization of hepatocellular carcinoma with drug eluting beads: efficacy and doxorubicin pharmacokinetics. J Hepatol. 2007 Mar;46(3):474-81. doi: 10.1016/j.jhep.2006.10.020. Epub 2006 Nov 29. PMID: 17239480.
14. Lo CM, Ngan H, Tso WK, Liu CL, Lam CM, Poon RT, Fan ST, Wong J. Randomized controlled trial of transarterial lipiodol chemoembolization for unresectable hepatocellular carcinoma. Hepatology. 2002 May;35(5):1164-71. doi: 10.1053/jhep.2002.33156. PMID: 11981766.
15. Llovet JM, Bruix J. Systematic review of randomized trials for unresectable hepatocellular carcinoma: Chemoembolization improves survival. Hepatology. 2003 Feb;37(2):429-42. doi: 10.1053/jhep.2003.50047. PMID: 12540794.
16. Flynn WJ. Il trattamento delle metastasi polmonari mediante microsfere di yttrio 90 [The treatment of pulmonary metastases with microspheres of yttrium 90]. Minerva Med. 1967 Dec 12;58(99):4498-500. Italian. PMID: 5625456.
17. GREENE WM. EMBOLIZATION OF DOG PROSTATES WITH YTTRIUM-90 MICROSPHERES. J Urol. 1963 Oct;90:451-7. doi: 10.1016/s0022-5347(17)64436-7. PMID: 14063380.
18. Wollner I, Knutsen C, Smith P, Prieskorn D, Chrisp C, Andrews J, Juni J, Warber S, Klevering J, Crudup J, et al. Effects of hepatic arterial yttrium 90 glass microspheres in dogs. Cancer. 1988 Apr 1;61(7):1336-44. doi: 10.1002/1097-0142(19880401)61:7<1336::aid-cncr2820610711>3.0.co;2-k. PMID: 3345490.
19. Gray B, Van Hazel G, Hope M, Burton M, Moroz P, Anderson J, Gebski V. Randomised trial of SIR-Spheres plus chemotherapy vs. chemotherapy alone for treating patients with liver metastases from primary large bowel cancer. Ann Oncol. 2001 Dec;12(12):1711-20. doi: 10.1023/a:1013569329846. PMID: 11843249.

20. Salem R, Lewandowski RJ, Atassi B, Gordon SC, Gates VL, Barakat O, Sergie Z, Wong CY, Thurston KG. Treatment of unresectable hepatocellular carcinoma with use of 90Y microspheres (TheraSphere): safety, tumor response, and survival. J Vasc Interv Radiol. 2005 Dec;16(12):1627-39. doi: 10.1097/01.RVI.0000184594.01661.81. PMID: 16371529.
21. Stubbs RS, Cannan RJ, Mitchell AW. Selective internal radiation therapy with 90yttrium microspheres for extensive colorectal liver metastases. J Gastrointest Surg. 2001 May-Jun;5(3):294-302. doi: 10.1016/s1091-255x(01)80051-2. PMID: 11360053.
22. TheraSphere [US package insert]. Rev. 11ed. Ottawa, ON:Nordion (Canada) Inc.; 2011.
23. SIR-Spheres [US package insert]. SIR-TeX Medical Limited. Australia; 2011.
24. Ahmed M, Solbiati L, Brace CL, Breen DJ, Callstrom MR, Charboneau JW, Chen MH, Choi BI, de Baère T, Dodd GD 3rd, Dupuy DE, Gervais DA, Gianfelice D, Gillams AR, Lee FT Jr, Leen E, Lencioni R, Littrup PJ, Livraghi T, Lu DS, McGahan JP, Meloni MF, Nikolic B, Pereira PL, Liang P, Rhim H, Rose SC, Salem R, Sofocleous CT, Solomon SB, Soulen MC, Tanaka M, Vogl TJ, Wood BJ, Goldberg SN; International Working Group on Image-guided Tumor Ablation; Interventional Oncology Sans Frontières Expert Panel; Technology Assessment Committee of the Society of Interventional Radiology,; Standard of Practice Committee of the Cardiovascular and Interventional Radiological Society of Europe. Image-guided tumor ablation: standardization of terminology and reporting criteria--a 10-year update. Radiology. 2014 Oct;273(1):241-60. doi: 10.1148/radiol.14132958. Epub 2014 Jun 13. PMID: 24927329; PMCID: PMC4263618.
25. Kawano M. An experimental study of percutaneous absolute ethanol injection therapy for small hepatocellular carcinoma: effects of absolute ethanol on the healthy canine liver. Gastroenterol Jpn. 1989 Dec;24(6):663-9. doi: 10.1007/BF02774165. PMID: 2606302.
26. Shiina S, Tagawa K, Unuma T, Takanashi R, Yoshiura K, Komatsu Y, Hata Y, Niwa Y, Shiratori Y, Terano A, et al. Percutaneous ethanol injection therapy for hepatocellular carcinoma. A histopathologic study. Cancer. 1991 Oct 1;68(7):1524-30. doi: 10.1002/1097-0142 (19911001)68:7<1524::aid-cncr2820680711>3.0.co;2-o. PMID: 1654196.
27. Tsai WL, Cheng JS, Lai KH, Lin CP, Lo GH, Hsu PI, Yu HC, Lin CK, Chan HH, Chen WC, Chen TA, Li WL, Liang HL. Clinical trial: percutaneous acetic acid injection vs. percutaneous ethanol injection

for small hepatocellular carcinoma--a long-term follow-up study. Aliment Pharmacol Ther. 2008 Aug 1;28(3):304-11. doi: 10.1111/j.1365-2036.2008.03702.x. PMID: 19086330.
28. Ahmed M, Brace CL, Lee FT Jr, Goldberg SN. Principles of and advances in percutaneous ablation. Radiology. 2011 Feb;258(2):351-69. doi: 10.1148/radiol.10081634. PMID: 21273519; PMCID: PMC6939957.
29. McLEAN AJ. THE BOVIE ELECTROSURGICAL CURRENT GENERATOR: SOME UNDERLYING PRINCIPLES AND RESULTS. *Arch Surg.* 1929;18(4):1863–1873. doi:10.1001/archsurg.1929.01140130965064
30. Rossi S, Fornari F, Pathies C, Buscarini L. Thermal lesions induced by 480 KHz localized current field in guinea pig and pig liver. Tumori. 1990 Feb 28;76(1):54-7. PMID: 2181746.
31. McGahan JP, Browning PD, Brock JM, Tesluk H. Hepatic ablation using radiofrequency electrocautery. Invest Radiol. 1990 Mar;25(3): 267-70. doi: 10.1097/00004424-199003000-00011. PMID: 2185179.
32. Lin SM, Lin CJ, Lin CC, Hsu CW, Chen YC. Randomised controlled trial comparing percutaneous radiofrequency thermal ablation, percutaneous ethanol injection, and percutaneous acetic acid injection to treat hepatocellular carcinoma of 3 cm or less. Gut. 2005 Aug;54(8):1151-6. doi: 10.1136/gut.2004.045203. Erratum in: Gut. 2005 Oct;54(10):1508. PMID: 16009687; PMCID: PMC1774888.
33. Campbell S, Uzzo RG, Allaf ME, Bass EB, Cadeddu JA, Chang A, Clark PE, Davis BJ, Derweesh IH, Giambarresi L, Gervais DA, Hu SL, Lane BR, Leibovich BC, Pierorazio PM. Renal Mass and Localized Renal Cancer: AUA Guideline. J Urol. 2017 Sep;198(3):520-529. doi: 10.1016/j.juro.2017.04.100. Epub 2017 May 4. PMID: 28479239.
34. Dupuy DE, Fernando HC, Hillman S, Ng T, Tan AD, Sharma A, Rilling WS, Hong K, Putnam JB. Radiofrequency ablation of stage IA non-small cell lung cancer in medically inoperable patients: Results from the American College of Surgeons Oncology Group Z4033 (Alliance) trial. Cancer. 2015 Oct 1;121(19):3491-8. doi: 10.1002/cncr.29507. Epub 2015 Jun 19. PMID: 26096694; PMCID: PMC4578219.
35. Goetz MP, Callstrom MR, Charboneau JW, Farrell MA, Maus TP, Welch TJ, Wong GY, Sloan JA, Novotny PJ, Petersen IA, Beres RA, Regge D, Capanna R, Saker MB, Grönemeyer DH, Gevargez A, Ahrar K, Choti MA, de Baere TJ, Rubin J. Percutaneous image-guided radiofrequency ablation of painful metastases involving bone: a multicenter study. J Clin Oncol. 2004 Jan 15;22(2):300-6. doi: 10.1200/JCO.2004.03.097. PMID: 14722039.

36. Fuller CW, Nguyen SA, Lohia S, Gillespie MB. Radiofrequency ablation for treatment of benign thyroid nodules: systematic review. Laryngoscope. 2014 Jan;124(1):346-53. doi: 10.1002/lary.24406. Epub 2013 Oct 22. PMID: 24122763.
37. Wright AS, Sampson LA, Warner TF, Mahvi DM, Lee FT Jr. Radiofrequency versus microwave ablation in a hepatic porcine model. Radiology. 2005 Jul;236(1):132-9. doi: 10.1148/radiol.2361031249. PMID: 15987969.
38. Yang D, Converse MC, Mahvi DM, Webster JG. Measurement and analysis of tissue temperature during microwave liver ablation. IEEE Trans Biomed Eng. 2007 Jan;54(1):150-5. doi: 10.1109/TBME.2006.884647. PMID: 17260866.
39. Rubinsky B, Lee CY, Bastacky J, Onik G. The process of freezing and the mechanism of damage during hepatic cryosurgery. Cryobiology. 1990 Feb;27(1):85-97. doi: 10.1016/0011-2240(90)90055-9. PMID: 2311412.
40. Wang H, Littrup PJ, Duan Y, Zhang Y, Feng H, Nie Z. Thoracic masses treated with percutaneous cryotherapy: initial experience with more than 200 procedures. Radiology. 2005 Apr;235(1):289-98. doi: 10.1148/radiol.2351030747. PMID: 15798173.
41. Georgiades CS, Hong K, Bizzell C, Geschwind JF, Rodriguez R. Safety and efficacy of CT-guided percutaneous cryoablation for renal cell carcinoma. J Vasc Interv Radiol. 2008 Sep;19(9):1302-10. doi: 10.1016/j.jvir.2008.05.015. Epub 2008 Jul 11. PMID: 18725093.

CHAPTER 2

OVERVIEW OF PRIMARY HEPATIC MALIGNANCY

ADAM ALLI MD, LARRY MATHIAS MD, ADRIEN CAYE MSIV

At the time of writing, the World Health Organization's (WHO) international agency for research on cancer currently lists primary hepatic malignancy as the sixth most common cancer in the world amongst all age groups. However, primary liver cancer is noted to be the third most deadly malignancy behind lung and colorectal cancer.[1] Within the United States (US), primary hepatic malignancy falls off the list of the ten most common malignancies. Despite this it continues to be the sixth most common cause of mortality related to malignancy with death rates increasing significantly for both men and women.[2] While data is not available based on Tumor, Metastases, and Nodal (TMN) staging the American Cancer Society (ACS) estimates the 5-year mortality rate at 20% for all stages of liver cancer.[3]

Traditionally, primary liver cancer was predominantly attributed with either alcoholic or viral hepatitis, with hepatitis B (HBV) and hepatitis C (HCV) as the most likely infectious etiologies. However, the steadily rising rates of morbid obesity and development of effective treatments for viral hepatitis have allowed for a shift in the pendulum with primary liver cancer now more frequently directly attributable to non-alcoholic fatty liver disease (NAFLD). In many developed nations such as the US, the increasing incidence of non-alcoholic steatohepatitis (NASH) is noted to coincide with the rising rates of hepatocellular carcinoma (HCC). There is now direct evidence correlating NASH as the most rapidly growing cause of HCC amongst liver transplant patients.[4] Overall, both increasing rates of primary hepatic carcinoma alongside an overall poor prognosis have made primary hepatic malignancy the fastest growing cause of cancer related death within the US.[4]

While certainly variants of primary hepatic malignancy do exist (e.g., mixed hepatocholangiocarcinoma), the two most common types of primary liver cancer, hepatocellular carcinoma (HCC), and intrahepatic cholangiocarcinoma (ICC) will be the focus of this discussion.

Hepatocellular Carcinoma

Most malignancies are noted to arise in setting of pathologically normal tissues. However, HCC is somewhat novel in that it often arises in the setting of chronic hepatic parenchyma change. Most causes of HCC result in chronic hepatic inflammation, which overtime leads to the development of hepatic fibrosis and cirrhosis. This milieu creates an environment ideal for hepatocarcinogenesis, which is comprised of aberrant hepatocyte regeneration. Often considered the first step in hepatocarcinogenesis, dysplastic foci are microscopic foci of hepatocytes with cytologic changes measuring less than 1.0 mm pathologically.[5,6] As foci begin to accumulate and chronic inflammatory change progresses, the gates begin to open for the development of nodularity, which should be considered as a spectrum rather than a continuum. The spectrum of hepatic nodularity begins with regenerative nodularity, leading to dysplastic nodularity and ultimately culminating in the development of HCC; with shifts in hepatocyte function and blood supply/neovascularity central to this pathway.[6]

Regenerative nodules, also called siderotic or iron-laden nodules retain their normal hepatocyte function.[7] However, as dysplasia is allowed to continue within a background of chronic hepatic injury, regenerative nodularity is ultimately allowed to progress to dysplastic nodularity which are the true premalignant lesions. Dysplastic nodules can be further differentiated into low grade or high-grade nodules, with the presence of cytologic atypia as the defining factor of high-grade nodularity.[8] Additionally, high-grade nodules contribute the greatest risk to the development of HCC. Ultimately, the defining point of what separates dysplastic nodularity from true HCC is the presence of stromal invasion pathologically, which when present allows for a confident diagnosis of HCC. It should be noted that while this pathway is thought of as a spectrum, histologically defined steps could be skipped.

The second prong of the hepatocarcinogenic pathway is neovascularity and shift in the physiologically normal hepatocyte blood supply.[5,9] It is widely accepted that normal hepatocyte blood supply predominantly arises from the portal venous system rather than the hepatic arteries.[10] Overall, this can be generalized as portal venous supply accounting for approximately 2/3rd of blood supply to the liver, with the hepatic arteries supplying the additional

1/3rd. However, as carcinogenesis progresses, atypical hepatocytes induce neovascularity and angiogenesis resulting in a shift from portal venous, to predominantly hepatic arterial supply. Due to the marked increase in neovascular arterial supply related to angiogenesis, early dysplastic nodules actually are theorized to have less overall blood supply related to surrounding hepatic parenchyma. As neovascular blood supply becomes more predominant, the physiologic hepatic arteries are observed to degenerate initially accounting for the overall drop in blood supply. This is then thought to allow for up-regulation of vascular endothelial growth factor (VEGF) which paves the way for even further angiogenesis resulting in the loss of the portal veins. As a reduction of portal venous supply occurs, full-scall neovascularity predominates resulting in dominant inflow to the aberrant hepatocytes to arise from the neovascularized arteries. Thus, overt HCC does not have vascular supply arising from portal veins (paired blood supply), but rather is solely supplied only by abnormal hepatic arteries (unpaired blood supply).[10]

HCC is rare in patients without a history of liver disease with 80-90% of cases arising in patients with a history of hepatic cirrhosis.[11] The most common risk factors for the development of HCC include NASH/NAFLD, viral hepatitis (most commonly HBV and HCV) and alcohol. Exposure to foods containing aflatoxin and exposure to chemical carcinogens also noted to contribute to the risk of HCC development. When taken separately, each risk factor certainly contributes an increased risk for the development of HCC with obesity and NAFLD independently conferring a 2.1 times increased risk for the development of HCC.[12] However, when multiple risk factors are encountered in combination, as is a common occurrence, a synergistic effect can be noted. Take for example the synergistic effect of heavy alcohol intake in patients with untreated HCV, which essentially doubles the risk for the development of HCC.[11]

Screening for Hepatocellular Carcinoma

The prognosis of HCC largely depends upon tumor stage at diagnosis. As previously discussed, if HCC is encountered at a late and/or progressed stage it is commonly associated with a dismal prognosis. Additionally, there is a propensity of patients with HCC to not present with symptoms beyond those associated with chronic or end stage liver disease until it has become incurable. Furthermore, if caught early, life-prolonging and potentially curable treatments may be offered to patients. Given the propensity of HCC to arise in patients with high risk factors, certain actions are commonly both recommended and implemented in the form of screening for HCC to allow for both early detection and treatment. The recommendation for screening is based largely a study demonstrating mortality reduction of 37% when high risk patients were screened every six months with a combination of alpha-fetoprotein analysis and dedicated liver ultrasound.[11] High-risk groups are currently categorized as: patients with cirrhosis (Child-Pugh Class A and B or awaiting liver transplant in Class C); patients with chronic HCV and advanced hepatic fibrosis; patients with porphyria; non-cirrhotic patients with HBV and High-risk groups are currently categorized as: patients with cirrhosis (Child-Pugh Class A and B or awaiting liver transplant in Class C); patients with chronic HCV and advanced hepatic fibrosis; patients with porphyria; non-cirrhotic patients with HBV and active hepatitis (transaminitis); patients with a family history of HCC; those of African descent, African Americans, and Asian males over 40 and females over 50 years old.[12,13] Interestingly, there is no current recommendation for screening patients with NASH until the progression to cirrhosis. However, the caveat to these recommendations is that surveillance is currently limited to high-risk patients who would be candidates for treatment if cancer were found at an early stage.

When screening is initiated in high-risk patients, at its most basic it is comprised of limited abdominal ultrasound focused at the liver every 6 months. While ultrasound alone is the most basic recommendation (sensitivity in detecting early stage HCC = 78%), there is evidence to support that the addition of alpha-fetoprotein (AFP) to a bi-annual screening regiment which has been shown to increase sensitivity to 97%.[14,15] Additionally, some practices opt to perform CT or MRI every 6 months as a form of screening in patients given the low sensitivity of HCC detection in ultrasound alone.[14] This is even more prevalent in patients whom have a body habitus or fatty hepatic parenchyma consistency, which would prevent adequate visualization of small suspicious lesions by ultrasound. However, current recommendations are that cross sectional imaging, although more sensitive in the detection of early stage HCC should not routinely be pursued. Furthermore contrast enhanced ultrasound as a screening modality remains under investigation; and AFP analysis alone as a method of screening is not recommended as elevated AFP levels may be caused by various factors, including cases of viral hepatitis.[14]

When a hepatic nodule is ultimately detected by screening, the possibility of HCC should always be questioned and further work-up immediately initiated as indicated.[9] In cases when the nodule measures less than 1.0 cm, a repeat ultrasound in 3 months should be obtained to evaluate for interval growth. If the nodule remains stable, follow up sonography should then be repeated in three months for further assessment. If stability can be demonstrated over two years, regular 6-month follow up screening can then be resumed. However, in a situation where a nodule either enlarges or is initially discovered measuring greater than 1.0 cm, it is considered suspicious for HCC and immediate work-up with a CT or MRI utilizing a liver mass protocol (dynamic phase contrast enhancement) should then ensue.[9]

When a screening test shows signs promising for the diagnosis of HCC, further workup with dynamic contrast enhanced imaging should be pursued.[16, 17] Utilizing extravascular contrast agents, changes in the aforementioned physiologic arterial flow occurring in HCC as opposed to the surrounding physiological normal hepatic parenchyma allows for HCC to be diagnosed based solely upon imaging characteristics. After pre-contrast enhanced thin slice CT or T1-weighted MR images through the abdomen centered upon the liver, post-contrast enhanced T1-weighted images or thin slice CT image acquisition is repeated in conjunction with contrast bolus timing to ensure portal venous phase, and delayed phase images are then obtained. Commonly iodinated contrast is administered at a rate of 4-6 mL/second for CT, whereas gadolinium agents are administered at 2 mL/second for MRI. A saline chaser of the intravenous tubing/line is then performed to ensure residual contrast is cleared. Ultimately, the hallmark features of HCC include hyperenhancement ("wash-in") on arterial phase imaging, followed by "wash-out" on portal venous or delayed phase images.

Imaging of Hepatocellular Carcinoma

Characteristically, and as would be expected, when utilizing extracellular contrast agents HCC preferentially enhances on arterial phases of image acquisition which is characterized by peak contrast bolus within the anatomic hepatic arteries. Of note, arterial phase can be further divided into early and late hepatic arterial phase, the later of which is characterized by the presence of contrast within both the hepatic arteries and the hepatic veins.[18, 19] Conversely, while the hepatic arteries will be opacified in the early hepatic arterial phase, contrast will not yet have reached the hepatic veins. The importance of this difference becomes apparent when considering in the early hepatic arterial phase, hypervascular HCC may be subtle or missed altogether. Imaging should therefore be performed utilizing contrast bolus tracking given the importance of imaging the liver at late hepatic arterial phase, with many centers currently omitting the acquisition of early hepatic arterial phase altogether. The physiology of HCC enhancement on arterial phase occurs on imaging due to HCC's unpaired blood supply from aberrant hepatic arteries as previously discussed. Additionally, only further contributing to its apparent arterial enhancement is the dilution of contrast medium within the surrounding hepatic parenchyma due to the preferential vascular supply to hepatic parenchyma by the portal venous supply, which will have a low contrast burden by design. Therefore, by convention, progressed HCC should be observed to hyperenhance on arterial images; whereas both regenerative and dysplastic nodules, as well as early stage HCC may demonstrate a hypo-enhancing or iso-enhancing appearance given the paired hepatic arterial and portal venous blood supply at this stage of disease.

While hyper-enhancement is characteristic of HCC, other entities may demonstrate a similar appearance. These include small benign flash-filling hemangiomas, focal nodular hyperplasia, atypical cases of focal or confluent fibrosis, and areas of atypical regenerative or dysplastic nodularity.[16,17] Alterations in enhancement characteristics visible only during arterial phase images caused by the duality of hepatic blood supply can also be encountered, with transient hepatic attenuation differences (THAD) and transient hepatic intensity differences (THID) commonly encountered in CT and MRI respectively.[18,19] While these entities may be seen in patients without underlying hepatic dysfunction, these findings may also be noted in patients with cirrhosis or chronic hepatitis where a large majority of wedge shaped and sub-capsular foci of enhancement measuring less than 2.0 cm are typically non-neoplastic. Additionally, non-hepatocellular neoplasms such as hypervascular metastases and small ICCs can also demonstrate a similar appearance of brisk arterial enhancement.[19] Due to the ability of different hepatic lesions to demonstrate similar appearance, care should be taken to compare any encountered suspicious lesion seen on an arterial phase sequence to their delayed contrast enhanced counterparts.

Following the evaluation of arterial phase imaging, attention should then be turned to portal venous phase which is characterized by peak contrast bolus within the portal veins, and commonly occurs at 60-70 seconds status post initial bolus administration; whereas delayed phase images are obtained arbitrarily at 3-5 minutes.[16, 17] These two phases are critical to evaluate in order to detect key features diagnostic of HCC. The first and most likely encountered imaging feature is loss of mass attenuation on CT, or signal intensity on MRI, when compared with the surrounding normal hepatic parenchyma. This finding is colloquially referred to as "wash-out" and is defined as reduction in enhancement relative to surrounding hepatic parenchyma from an arterial to portal venous/delayed phase. The mechanism of this finding is poorly understood, with several currently suggested etiologies including increased early venous drainage of contrast from the tumor (coined true wash-out), progressive enhancement of background hepatic parenchyma, reduced portal venous vascular supply, lesion hypercellularity with corresponding reduction in extracellular volume, and intrinsic hypoattenuation/hypointensity. This "washout" may be more conspicuous in the delayed compared with the portal venous phase, and in some lesions, "washout" may be depicted only in the delayed phase.[23, 24] The rate at which the tumor appears to washout may also be important as certain studies suggest the presence of washout on portal venous phase imaging likely predicts a higher grade of HCC and higher grade of microvascular invasion than washout only encountered on delayed phase images.[25-27]

Similar to the finding of arterial phase hyperenhancement, the presence of washout alone is not specific for HCC as this appearance may also be encountered within cirrhotic and dysplastic nodularity.[16,17] Furthermore, washout may also be encountered in areas of hepatic parenchymal distortion and enhancing fibrosis thus contributing to the perception of washout.[28] Therefore, given the possible appearance of washout within entities other than HCC, it has been suggested that washout alone should not be utilized in the diagnosis of HCC unless additional findings are present.

Another imaging feature of HCC is the presence of an enhancing capsule surrounding the hepatic mass on portal, and delayed phase images. This appears as a smooth rim of peripheral hyperenhancement with the degree of enhancement continuously increasing after the administration of contrast.[16, 17] This finding may be more likely to be encountered on delayed phase images rather than portal venous phase. The cause for this progressive enhancement has been attributed to slow flow within the vessels supplying the capsule, as well as contrast retention within the extravascular tissues of the capsule itself.[17, 22] The significance of this finding is realized when considering that capsules are not present in regenerative or dysplastic nodules, or even early stage HCC; rather, when a capsule is present it is highly suggestive of an advanced HCC. However, while the presence of an enhancing capsule on imaging certainly correlates with the presence of a capsule on pathologic analysis, there is evidence to suggest that only one out of four nodules with capsules detected on imaging will possess a true capsule at pathologic analysis and in some instances the radiographic capsule actually corresponds with a pseudocapsule. Regardless, because precursor lesions (cirrhotic and dysplastic nodules) do not demonstrate progressive peripheral enhancement, the presence of a progressively enhancing capsule on imaging has been shown to be a strong predictor of, and hallmark for the presence of HCC. Some investigators have discovered that the presence of a progressively enhancing capsule on imaging is incredibly valuable in that it permits the diagnosis of HCC in the absence of contrast washout.[22]

The integrity of a capsule associated with HCC should be carefully inspected when encountered, as findings of capsule disruption are highly suggestive of tumor infiltration.[17] This finding may imply the presence of microinvasion into the surrounding hepatic parenchyma, or possibly even macroinvasion. While microinvasion may only be diagnosed pathologically, imaging features specific for the presence of macroinvasion include direct extension of tumor into adjacent vessel. This is common occurrence and imaging feature of HCC and portends a poor prognosis. This manifests as expansile thrombus within an occluded hepatic or portal vein immediately adjacent HCC, which many times can be visualized as a tangle of enhancing neovessels within the vein. Expansion of a thrombosed main portal vein to 23 mm or more is also highly suggestive of intraluminal thrombus, however this finding should be used with caution as bland thrombus may also result in portal venous expansion.[17]

One of the unique features of HCC is its ability to be diagnosed with a degree of certainty by imaging alone. While each aforementioned unique feature may be associated with other entities (other than the presence of a progressive enhancing capsule) and thus may not be suggestive of HCC in isolation; when collectively encountered are diagnostic of HCC with near 100% specificity.[17] When a lesion is visualized demonstrating brisk enhancement on arterial phase, "wash-out" on either portal venous or delayed phase and is associated with a progressively enhancing capsule; the diagnosis of HCC can be confidently made. However, while these imaging findings together are highly specific for the presence of HCC, they have relatively low sensitivity given that they are often only seen together in large advanced HCC and not in early stage HCC, progressed HCC small in size and infiltrative HCC. Therefore ancillary features present on MRI and CT to a lesser extent, are visualized alongside hallmark feature can help to increase the certainty of and can further assist in the characterization of nodules. These can be further divided into features supportive of the diagnosis of HCC, versus supportive of the presence of malignancy. Imaging features suggestive of HCC include the presence of intralesional fat, corona enhancement (transient zone or rim, "corona" of enhancement around a hypervascular HCC when then fades into background becoming isointense on subsequent phases), nodule-in-nodule appearance (the presence of a nodule within a larger mass) and mosaic architecture (mass of randomly distributed internal nodules or compartments differing in enhancement). Conversely, the presence of mild to moderately increased signal intensity of T2 weighted images, and restricted diffusion are suggestive of the presence of malignancy, but not specific for HCC. Despite low specificity, these sequences may be utilized to increase the conspicuity of intrahepatic lesions and thus contribute to the increased sensitivity in the diagnosis of HCC[17].

While the discussion to this point has been geared towards extracellular contrast agents in both CT and MRI, contrast geared towards the evaluation of tumor vascularity and hepatocyte function in the form of hepatobiliary is also available which targets organo anion transporters (OATP).[17] Two agents currently predominate the market, Multihance (Bracco Diagnostics, Princton, NJ) and Primovist/Eovist (Bayer Healthcare, Princeton, NJ); and while the exact cause of contrast accumulation is incompletely understood, the predominant interaction depends upon the degree of OATP expression.[29] When OATP expression is normal, hepatobiliary contrast agents are taken up allowing normal hepatocytes to appear isointense or hyperintense on hepatobiliary phase of imaging.[30,31] As hepatocarcinogenesis progresses, OATP expression decreases which in turn results in a decline in hepatobiliary contrast accumulation and expression. As hepatocarcinogenesis progresses, suspicious liver lesions or nodules demonstrating hypointensity on hepatobiliary phase should be considered suspicious due to the underexpression of OATP. Conversely, most cirrhotic nodules, low grade dysplastic nodules, and some high-grade dysplastic nodules are iso- to hyperintense due to preserved expression of OATP. Another benefit of hepatobiliary contrast agents is to further delineate vascular lesions, which demonstrate strong hyperenhancement on arterial phase images, but are not associated with any significant washout on delayed images. In these lesions there should be preservation of signal intensity on hepatobiliary phase given the preservation of OATP in these lesions thus helping to further differentiate these "pseudolesions" from true arterially enhancing HCC.[32,33] Understanding the interplay between lesion intensity on hepatobiliary phase related to OATP expression allows one to exploit this interaction for diagnostic benefit and further diagnose high-risk premalignant nodules and HCC with confidence.

Liver Imaging Reporting and Data System (LI-RADS)

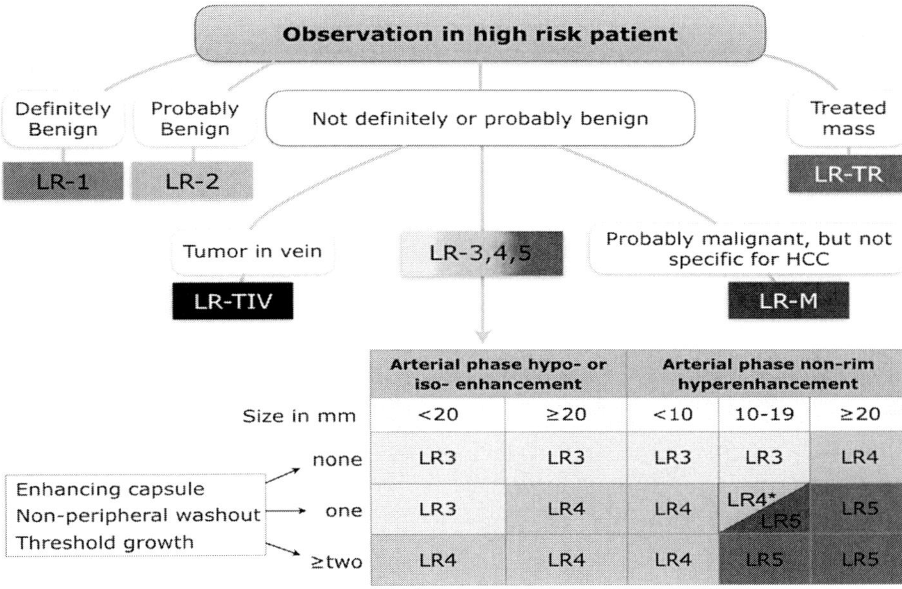

Figure 1.

As discussed, a wide spectrum of liver lesions (observation per LI-RADS terminology) may be encountered, all of which can demonstrate a breadth of findings on imaging. Given the variability of both imaging findings and style of reporting and interpretation amongst radiologists, the American College of Radiology (ACR) in conjunction with the American Association for the Study of Liver Disease (AASLD) developed LI-RADS (Figure 1).[42] While the first iteration was 2006, it has subsequently undergone multiple revisions and at the time of writing is in its 5th version with the 2018 adaption as the most recent publication. While the purpose of this chapter is not to delve into the depths of the LI-RADS manual, touching upon the algorithm is of the utmost importance given its propensity to guide both diagnosis and treatment of suspicious liver lesions in high-risk patients.

The LI-RADS reporting system grades liver lesions in high-risk patients on a scale from 1-5, with LI-RADS 1 encompassing benign lesions and category 5 being characterized as HCC. The two categories of most importance within this spectrum in regards to the treatment of HCC are categories 4 and

5; with approximately 80% of LI-RADS 4 observations being HCC, and 98% of LI-RADS 5 observations being HCC. Of important note, all LI-RADS 5 lesions are HCC; however, not all HCC can be categorized as LI-RADS 5 due to the variability of HCC on imaging. The goal is for LI-RADS 5 to have a strong positive predictive value in the diagnosis of HCC and therefore only observations meeting strict criteria to be labeled as such. This strong positive predictive value allows healthcare professionals to often forego biopsy and proceed straight to treatment in the case of LI-RADS 5 lesions, and LI-RADS 4 lesions to a lesser extent after multidisciplinary discussion. While multidisciplinary discussion is recommended for LI-RADS 5 observations as well, this is for the purpose of guiding treatment. Finally, while a LI-RADS 5 observation does not require biopsy prior to treatment, it may often times be performed for the purpose of molecular characterization or for clinical trial requirement.[121]

Additional LI-RADS categories worth mentioning include LI-RADS TIV (tumor in vein), and LI-RADS M (probably or definitely malignant, not HCC specific). LI-RADS M is defined as high probability or 100% certainty of the presence of malignancy, but in the absence of features of HCC. Imaging features consistent with LI-RADS M include: the presence of a targetoid mass with dynamic enhancement, restricted diffusion or increased signal intensity on post-arterial phase sequences; or the presence of a non-targetoid mass without tumor expansion into a vein (indicative of LI-RADS LIV - discussed below), and associated with an infiltrative appearance, restricted diffusion, necrosis or ischemia, or other features suggestive of malignancy. LI-RADS TIV should only be reported when there is 100% certainty that macroinvasion of HCC has occurred and enhancing soft tissue is present within vein, regardless of visualization of a parenchymal mass. When this finding is present LI-RADS TIV can be reported with certainty. However, if there are only findings suggestive of tumor in vein such as an occluded vein next to a parenchymal mass, ill-defined venous walls, presence of intravenous restricted diffusion, or heterogeneous enhancement not related to artifact; caution should be utilized to not over diagnose LI-RADS TIV.[121]

If there ever exists any uncertainty about the presence of HCC (LI-RADS 5), malignancy (LI-RADS M) or tumor in vein (LI-RADS LIV); than the LI-RADS category should be downgraded to preserve the high positive predictive value. Take into consideration a hepatic observation meeting many, but not all of the criteria necessary to diagnose a LI-RADS 5 observation. If uncertainty regarding the presence of HCC is present or additional differential considerations are possible, the LI-RADS 4 designation should be assigned rather than LI-RADS 5. Similarly any uncertainty regarding the presence of tumor in vein should deter one from assigning a LI-RADS TIV and the LI-RADS 5 (if applicable) or LI-RADS M should be assigned. It should then come as no surprise that if uncertainty exists regarding the presence of malignancy (LI-RADS M), the designation should not be assigned to an observation and rather the appropriate designation be utilized to guide follow-up.[121]

Staging Hepatocellular Carcinoma

In general terms, staging of malignancy is geared towards determining the overall tumor burden by accounting for the size and number of tumors, and presence of metastases; with the goal of to predict overall prognosis and to guide treatment. Unlike many other cancers which may be found incidentally in otherwise healthy patients, HCC commonly arises in patients with underlying chronic liver disease necessitating special consideration given this added variable affecting overall prognosis and treatment consideration.[12,13,35-38] Systems are heavily reliant upon anatomic considerations including the TNM (Tumor-Node-Metastases), American Joint Committee on Cancer (AJCC) and International Union Against Cancer (UICC) systems, although adequacy to predict tumor extension is considered poor in these patients. Having taken this variable into consideration, multiple different staging systems have been developed in order to best stratify patients into an appropriate prognostic and treatment categories.

Table 1.

Tumor Size *Largest cross sectional area of tumor relative to largest cross sectional area of liver	>50% = + <50% = −
Ascites	Clinically detectable = + Clinically undetectable = −
Serum albumin	< 3 g/dL = + > 3 g/dL = −
Serum bilirubin	> 3 g/dL = + < 3 g/dL = −

The system to first successfully combine the degree of hepatic dysfunction alongside anatomic considerations was the Okuda system.[39] Developed in 1984, this system took into consideration tumor volume (> or ≤ 50% of total liver volume) and hepatic function utilizing three main factors (bilirubin, albumin and the presence of ascites). Given its success in combining anatomy with functional status, the system was widely utilized for over 2 decades. The system is composed of four categories (tumor size, presence of ascites, serum albumin and serum bilirubin), with each category assigned a positive or negative based upon the presence of absence of each risk factor (Table 1). Staging of the Okuda system occurs in three grades based upon the absence of any positive scores (Grade 0), presence of one or two positives (Grade 1) and presence of three of four positives (Grade 2). Ultimately, one of the downfalls of the system is its inability to account for early stage HCC given is inability to further differentiate tumor less than half the size of the liver parenchyma as noted within Table 1. This oversight of the Okuda system has allowed for newer systems, most notably the Barcelona Clinic Liver Cancer (BCLC) staging system, to have been developed and realize wide use given their ability to account for and categorize smaller lesions far below 50% of total liver volume.

Most HCC staging now occurs by the BCLC system, which has become the predominant system given not only its strong predictive power for determining patient survival, but also its ability to guide treatment strategies. Currently, it is the only system that accounts for the presence of liver disease and constitutional systems in addition to tumor extension allowing it to select early stage patients who could benefit from curative therapies.[40] Staging within the BCLC system occurs on a spectrum of 0, A, B, C or D; with 0 encompassing very early stage HCC and D essentially representing patients with end stage disease. Factors included within the staging criteria include: performance status, Child-Pugh Score and radiologic characteristics of the tumor (Table 2).[41, 42] Of important note, while radiologic characteristics are taken into account for stages 0 – C, stage D is strictly a clinical diagnosis and does not have imaging contributions.

Performance status (PS) is typically graded along the lines of the Eastern Cooperative Oncology Group (ECOG) scale, which is designed to determine functional status throughout the time of disease based upon a patients' ability to perform everyday tasks and activity.[42] The grading system occurs on a scale of 0–5 with a grade of 0 encompassing patients who have no restrictions, are fully active, and are able to carry out activities of daily living (ADL) without any assistance; and a grade of 5 signifying patients who are deceased. Grade 1 signifies patients who are restricted in strenuous activity, but otherwise able to carry out other ADL without restriction. Grade 2 signifies patients who are ambulatory and capable of self-care for more than 50% of waking hours. Grade 3 signifies patients who are capable of only limited self care, and/or confined to a bed or chair for more than 50% of waking hours. Grade 4 encompasses patients who are completely disabled and are totally confined to a bed or chair. PS/ECOG score is considered by many to be the best predictor of outcome with treatments only occurring in patients with a score of 0 – 2. In general, with symptomatic treatment being the only available treatment option in patients determined to have a score of 3 or above.

Table 2

Barcelona radiologic characteristics of HCC	
Very early stage - Stage 0	• Solitary lesion measuring less than 2.0 cm
Early stage - Stage A	• Solitary lesion greater than 2.0 cm • Early multifocal disease characterized by up to 3 lesions measuring less than 3.0 cm

Intermediate Stage - Stage B	• Presence of multifocal disease:
	  • More than one lesion with at least one over 3.0 cm
	  • More than 3 lesions regardless of their size

Advanced Stage - Stage C	• Characterized by the presence of vascular invasion, nodal disease and/or metastatic disease
End stage - Stage D	• Is a clinical stage, does not have a radiologic component

Child-Pugh is a scoring system designed to grade the severity of liver disease in patients inclusive of cirrhosis and occurs on a range from A, B or C with an increasing score (from A to C) signifying worsening hepatic function (Figure 2).[41, 42] This range helps determine which patients have a higher opportunity for "liver mortality" due to reduced hepatic reserve and thus can assist in deciding which patients will have higher risk for morbidity after liver resection and how much liver parenchyma may be resected. Ultimately, a Child-Pugh score of A indicates a 5% perioperative mortality and a patient who would be able to have up to half of their liver resected. A score of B indicates a 10-15% mortality risk and allows for no more than

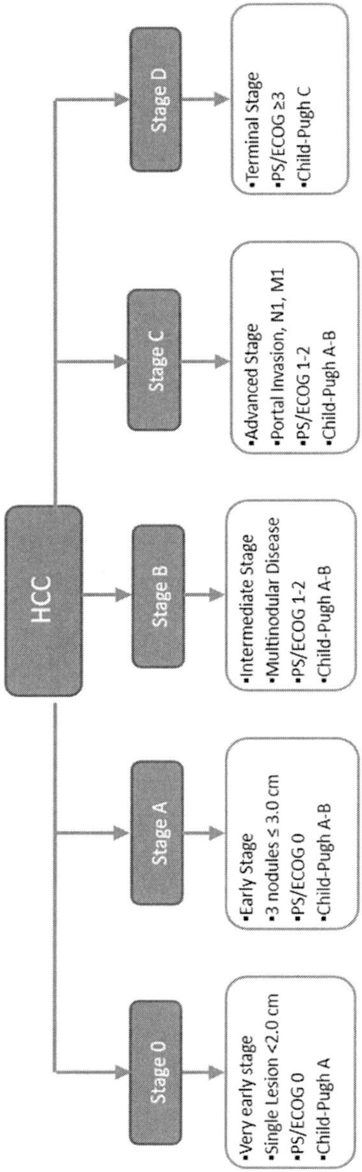
HCC
Stage 0
Stage A
Stage B
Stage C
Stage D
▪Very early stage
▪Single Lesion <2.0 cm
▪PS/ECOG 0
▪Child-Pugh A
▪Early Stage
▪3 nodules ≤ 3.0 cm
▪PS/ECOG 0
▪Child-Pugh A-B
▪Intermediate Stage
▪Multinodular Disease
▪PS/ECOG 1-2
▪Child-Pugh A-B
▪Advanced Stage
▪Portal Invasion, N1, M1
▪PS/ECOG 1-2
▪Child-Pugh A-B
▪Terminal Stage
▪PS/ECOG ≥3
▪Child-Pugh C

Figure 2.

25% of liver parenchyma resection; whereas a score of C indicates a greater than 25% mortality risk and contraindicates any hepatic resection. There are five components of the score which include: total bilirubin, serum albumin, international normalized ratio (INR), presence of ascites and presence of encephalopathy with each category given a sub-score from one to three depending on its severity. For example, as would be expected as the albumin decreases (signifying reduced capacity of hepatic protein synthesis), the Child-Pugh score will increase. Ultimately, treatment for HCC is only considered in patients with a Child-Pugh grade of A or B. Child-Pugh C signifies such reduced hepatic function and hepatic reserve that treatment, other than symptomatic relief, can often not be offered patients other than in rare circumstances.

After classifying a patients' imaging findings, PST/ECOG and Child-Pugh score a patient can be stratified within a BCLC classification (21) in order to best guide therapy and treatment based upon a patients' Stage.[41, 42, 43]

Treatment of Hepatocellular Carcinoma

Given the specific discussions provided in subsequent chapters, the purpose of this section is not to provide an all-inclusive discussion regarding the methods available to combat HCC, but rather to provide an overview of the various treatments available. As with all malignancies, treatment of HCC is geared towards mortality reduction while maintaining optimal quality of life. Additionally, it should be noted that treatment of HCC should be provided within a multispecialty setting from a multidisciplinary approach in order to provide state of art care for optimal outcome.

Similar to the treatment for most diseases, the treatment of HCC is variable based both upon stage and extent of disease and the desires of the patient (Figure 3) taking into account the aforementioned PS/ECOG function, and the Child-Pugh score. As would be expected, the treatment for HCC when discovered earlier in time and thus lower in stage varies markedly from disease found late within the process and at advanced stage. Of note, patients with terminal or BCLC stage D disease are deemed ineligible to receive curative, locoregional or often times systemic treatment depending upon the specifications of that case. Therefore, treatment in patients with PS/ECOG grades of 3 or above, and Child-Pugh scores of C is contraindicated.[40-43]

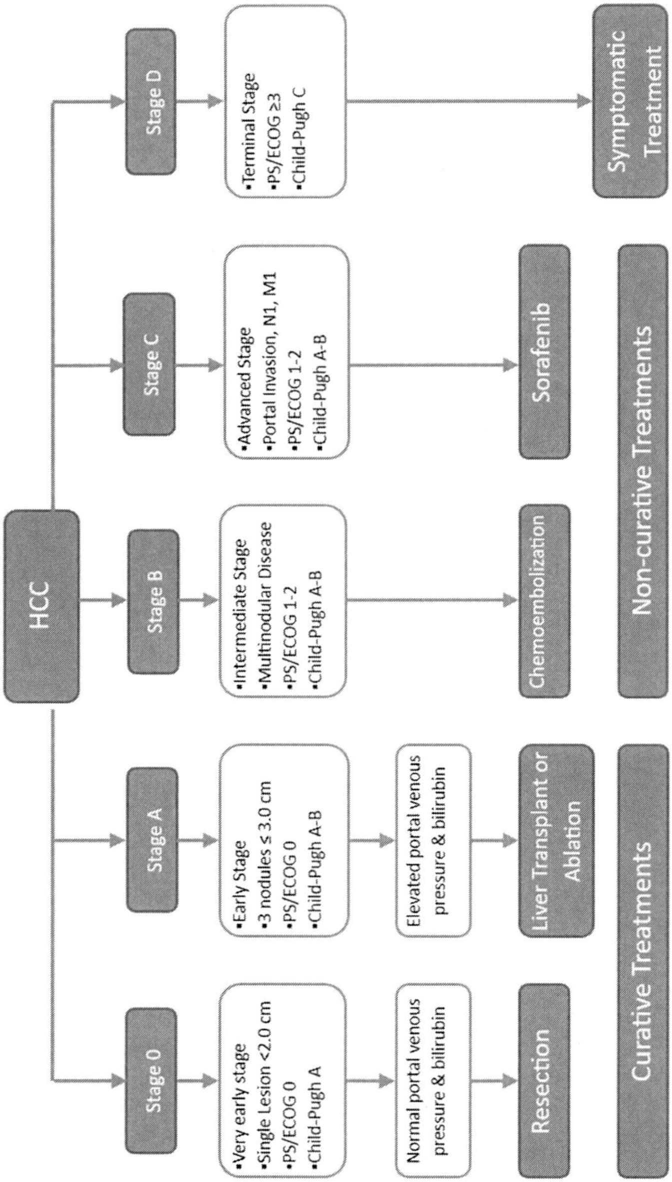
HCC
Stage 0
Stage A
Stage B
Stage C
Stage D
▪Very early stage
▪Single Lesion <2.0 cm
▪PS/ECOG 0
▪Child-Pugh A
▪Early Stage
▪3 nodules ≤ 3.0 cm
▪PS/ECOG 0
▪Child-Pugh A-B
▪Intermediate Stage
▪Multinodular Disease
▪PS/ECOG 1-2
▪Child-Pugh A-B
▪Advanced Stage
▪Portal Invasion, N1, M1
▪PS/ECOG 1-2
▪Child-Pugh A-B
▪Terminal Stage
▪PS/ECOG ≥3
▪Child-Pugh C
Normal portal venous pressure & bilirubin
Elevated portal venous pressure & bilirubin
Resection
Liver Transplant or Ablation
Chemoembolization
Sorafenib
Symptomatic Treatment
Curative Treatments
Non-curative Treatments

Figure 3.

While many different and effective treatments exist and are continuously being developed, there are three treatments for HCC that are considered curative: surgical resection, liver transplant and ablation. However, these interventions are traditionally reserved for HCC in BCLC stage 0 or A; with treatment success of BCLC stage 0 patients at an almost 100% success rate due to tumor size and location.

Liver transplantation can be considered curative given its ability to both address cirrhotic liver acting as the underlying disease process and the malignancy contained within the hepatic parenchyma.[44] Since its induction the Milan criteria has served as a guideline for determining which patients are suitable for hepatic transplant in patients with HCC occurring in the setting of cirrhosis.[45] Simply put, the guidelines state that a patient is a candidate for transplantation if they have either:

1. A single tumor with a diameter less than or equal to 5.0 cm or up to three tumors each with diameter less than or equal to 3.0 cm
2. Absence of extra-hepatic involvement
3. Absence of major vessel involvement

If all of these factors are met than a patient can be deemed a candidate for transplantation, and again generally speaking this occurs in patients with BCLC grade 0 or A. However, in 2009 the Milan criteria was expanded by the developers to the so-called "New Milan Criteria" which states a patient is a candidate for transplant if: the diameter of the largest tumor (in cm) plus the total normal of discrete tumors is less than 7.[46] Evidence of portal venous invasion or extrahepatic metastases are factors for exclusion for each criteria. In certain circumstances transplantation may still occur given specific circumstances associated with a case. For example, patients initially outside of the Milan window for transplant may undergo locoregional treatments as a method of bridging to transplantation. Essentially, treatment may be directed at decreasing either tumor burden or size in order to bring a patient into the criteria window allowing for transplantation to occur in a patient who would otherwise not have been eligible.

Although liver resection or transplantation remain the most desirable options for early stage (BCLC 0 and A) HCC treatment, it is estimated that approximately 80% of patients would not be surgical candidates.[46] Percutaneous ablation is therefore an additional option for curative intent in patients with early stage HCC deemed ineligible to undergo hepatic transplantation for any reason and would not be candidate for surgical resection.[47] Potentially curative results can be realized with ablation for small (3.0 cm) and even medium sized (3.0-3.5 cm) lesions. Additionally, as previously discussed ablation can "bridge" patients to orthotopic liver transplant by decreasing tumor burden and prolonging time to transplant. Ablation comes in many different flavors, including: ethanol injection, radiofrequency ablation (RFA), microwave ablation (MWA) and cryoablation. While various comparative studies between the different treatment methods have been performed it often times falls to the discretion of the performing physician which method will be utilized with MWA commonly being the treatment method most utilized for hepatic malignancies. It would also be prudent to mention newer ablation modalities such as high intensity focus ultrasound ablation (HIFU) and histotripsy (HistoSonics ®), which find themselves on the horizon for potential treatment. These do not require percutaneous access required for treatment, which is performed entirely external to the patient.

When the aforementioned curative treatments are no longer an option either due to tumor size, presence of vascular invasion or reduction in patients PS/ECOG, non-curative transarterial embolization can then be considered. The primary indication for transarterial chemoembolization (TACE) is the treatment of unresectable HCC, specifically intermediate stage/BCLC stage A; although TACE may be offered and is effective in patients with BCLC stage B and even stage C. In fact, TACE continues to be the gold standard (level 1 evidence) in the treatment of unresectable HCC prompting its inclusion in all HCC guidelines.[48-51] At it's most basic, this procedure comes in two separate forms and involves selective embolization of the hepatic arterial supply to tumor resulting in necrosis and tumor death given the aforementioned propensity of HCC to derive its blood supply from the hepatic arteries rather than the portal system as the disease process progresses. While the predominant effect of TACE remains its arterial embolic effect, chemotherapy is added into the embolic agent in order to increase the potency of embolic agent and further assist in the treatment of the malignancy. The available selections for TACE chemotherapy agents are cisplatin, doxycycline or mitomycin (Irinotecan can also be used in cases of colorectal metastatic disease) or any combination of the three depending upon the availability of cisplatin. Caution should be taken for the use of TACE patients with portal venous thrombus or invasion by tumor as many consider this finding to be a relative, if not absolute contraindication to TACE. This is due to the fact that in patients with portal venous obstruction, the blood supply to the liver is already compromised. Therefore if arterial embolization were to occur in patients with already limited hepatic reserve, the risk for hepatic infarction of fulminant hepatic failure is felt to be too great. While some studies do exist showing the safety of TACE in this patient population, physicians should be prudent to err on the side of caution in patients whose residual hepatic function is deemed tenuous.[52] TACE may be undertaken multiple times with the optimal frequency of TACE administration not known. Despite this, studies have shown a significant increase in survival in groups only undergoing TACE when necessary.[53, 54]

The first form of TACE is coined "conventional TACE (cTACE)" and is comprised of arterial embolization utilizing a combination of chemotherapy, Ethiodol/lipiodol (derivative from poppy seed oil), and an embolic agent (historically gelfoam, now most commonly microbeads). Conversely, the second and newer form of TACE is termed "Drug Eluting Bead-TACE" (DEB) which combines the microbead embolization agent with the selected chemotherapeutic agent and eliminates the use of lipiodol allowing for a sustained delivery of chemotherapy over a prolonged time. Various studies have been performed to evaluate the success rates of cTACE vs DEB-TACE and ultimately DEB-TACE has not been shown to be consistently superior to cTACE in terms of survival, however DEB-TACE has shown to be associated with reduction in post-procedural discomfort and thereby hospitalization time.[51] Despite this, lipiodol continues to play a vital role in HCC treatment given the affinity HCC has for the substance and is radiopaque nature.

It is worth mentioning transarterial embolization (TAE), which is also referred to as bland embolization. This treatment option works in the same manner as TACE, however does not have the assistance of concurrent chemotherapy administration and rather utilizes embolic microspheres with or without lipiodol as a stand-alone treatment. Additionally, as is the case with TACE, the use of TAE in patients with portal venous invasion is limited given the similar mechanism of treatment, that being arterial occlusion resulting in tumor necrosis. Various studies have shown conflicting results regarding the efficacy of TACE over TAE.[55, 56] Given these findings some there have been mixed recommendations for TACE over TAE; however it is generally accepted, as is the case at our institution that TACE is the preferred treatment for intermediate stage – Stage B HCC rather than TAE.[57, 58]

Another embolic technique valuable in the battle against HCC is radioembolization in the form of Yttrium-90 (Y-90). Y-90 is a pure beta admitter with the admitted beta particles traveling an average of 2.5 mm in tissue, and up to a maximum of 10 mm.[59] This allows for the administered radioembolic microparticles to travel to the distal arterioles of the targeted tissue where they deliver large doses of radiation directly to the targeted tumor thereby inducing radiation necrosis. These particles come in two forms: SIR-spheres (Sirtex Medical, Lane Cove, Australia) which are resin microspheres and Theraspheres (MDS Nordion, Kanata, ON, Canada), which are glass microspheres. Ideal candidates for treatment with Y-90 include patients who would meet criteria for TACE (BCLC 2 and 3).[60] However, Y-90 therapy can also be offered to patients with hepatic metastatic disease in whom surgical resection is not an option. Furthermore, in patients with widespread but liver predominant metastatic disease, Y-90 has also shown to be of benefit. Unlike TACE, Y-90 can also be extended to patients with HCC who have portal venous thrombosis given the lack of hepatic arterial occlusion and preservation of forward arterial flow, which occurs with the treatment.[61]

Sorafenib (Nexavar, Bayer HealthCare Pharmaceuticals–Onyx Pharmaceuticals) is an additional systemic treatment option in the form of molecular targeted therapy which is available for patients determined to have advanced stage HCC, and is the standard of care for patients with BLCL stage C having been shown to improve overall survival in this patient population by nearly 3 months.[62] This medication works to inhibit tumor proliferation and angiogenesis, and increases the rate of apoptosis through inhibition of Raf-1, B-Raf, vascular endothelial growth factor receptors (VEGFRs), and platelet-derived growth factor receptor β (PDGFR-β). Of great benefit is that this already effective treatment can be given concurrently with TACE and while data is somewhat mixed, there is increased overall survival in patients receiving both treatments at 6 months and one year versus placeboe.[63-66] While concern has been expressed about the benefit of Sorafenib post-TACE given the effective of arterial occlusion which in theory may limit delivery of the drug, data does exist showing both its safety and effectiveness.[67]

Ultimately, in patients with advanced disease chemotherapy and immunotherapy may comprise the final considerations for treatment. While a detailed conversation is beyond the scope and focus of this book, brief discussion is warranted. Unfortunately, no single systemic treatment has been deemed superior to another as only moderate efficacy and benefit of cytotoxic chemotherapy in patients with advanced HCC, and the duration of chemotherapy effect is limited.[68] When considering systemic treatment, hepatic reserve and thus side effect profile need to be considered given the already reduced ability of patient tolerance and short life span in this population. Treatment should therefore commonly be chosen based upon the hepatic reserve and level of fitness tolerance, although treatment options do exist in limited capacity for patients with exhausted reserve.

Immunotherapy is certainly an additional option for the treatment of advanced HCC, however the treatment modality is somewhat novel for HCC when compared to other malignancies.[69] While treatment regimens are available in the United States, the benefit of first line immunotherapy remains uncertain given the environment HCC develops. Cirrhosis having been show to decrease the therapeutic effect of these agents. However, strong interest in the pursuit of immunotherapy as a potential treatment option continuously being researched.

Hepatocellular Carcinoma Follow Up

After treatment for HCC is initiated, response to therapy needs to be evaluated in order to ensure adequacy of treatment and necessity for further treatment. As previously alluded to, AFP levels can be evaluated in the initial diagnosis of HCC; however, blood AFP levels also serve as a useful marker to assess response to treatment of HCC. Studies have shown that an adequate response to treatment should be shown as a greater than 50% reduction in AFP from pre- to post-treatment.[70, 71] Conversely, less than 50% reduction in AFP from pre-intervention to post-treatment has been shown to correlate with a poorer prognosis, and thereby poor response to treatment. Therefore regular AFP follow up can be performed as a method to detect failure of treatment and/or early recurrence of HCC.

The mainstay of assessing HCC treatment response comes in the form of imaging.[72] After an initial diagnose of HCC is completed and treatment is initiated, serial imaging studies can be performed to assess response to treatment, and recurrence if curative treatment is achieved. While useful in screening for HCC, ultrasound is not recommended in the follow up of HCC once treatment is initiated. Conversely, investigation into contrast-enhanced ultrasound (CEUS) has been performed as a potential modality for follow-up given its widespread availability. While artifact related to lipiodol may result in obscuration of arterial enhancement on CT, this factor does not come into play with ultrasound. Some reports are available showing CEUS to be more sensitive than contrast enhanced CT for detection of small residual foci post-TACE.[73] CEUS is not currently approved for regular follow up in the US and thus is rarely performed. Rather, CT and MRI are the mainstays in the diagnosis of HCC and assessing the response to treatment. Worth mentioning is the fact that one of the benefits MRI has over CT is a lack of beam hardening artifact associated with lipiodol, which may result in obscuration of small areas of residual enhancement. Lesions having undergone microwave ablation or TACE may undergo coagulation necrosis making evaluation for residual enhancement difficult and necessitating the use of subtraction techniques for follow up. Ultimately the greatest factor, regardless of method utilized, is the timing of image acquisition to allow for earlier detection of subtle residual neoplasm. Recurrence of malignancy post-treatment occurs 6.5 times more likely within the first year and thus the frequency of imaging follow up is needs to be more frequent during this time span.[74] Recommendations vary and many follow up regiments are at the discretion of the medical care team with initial follow ups often occurring every 3 months during the first year, 6 months during the second year and annually thereafter. However it has been offered that while this method traditionally has worked in patients determined to be low risk for recurrence, it may be ineffective in patients deemed high risk for recurrence. As a conservative measure, the Journal of Vascular and Interventional Radiology has published recommendations that the optimal follow up schedule in high risk patients occur eight times within the first two years (imaging acquisition at 2, 4, 6, 8, 11, 14, 18 and 24 months) to help balance costs associated with imaging against diagnostic delay[74].

Cholangiocarcinoma

Introduction

Cholangiocarcinoma is the most common biliary malignancy, and in particular intrahepatic cholangiocarcinoma (ICC) is the second most common primary hepatic malignancy, constituting 3% of all gastrointestinal malignancies. [76-77] Biliary cancers may be found anywhere along the biliary tree and when arising within the confines of the hepatic parenchyma are termed intrahepatic bile-duct cancer/ICC.[78] Additionally, a specific subtype of ICC occurs at the bifurcation of the bile ducts receiving the eponym of a Klatskin tumor, which is named after Dr. Gerald Klatskin who first described this subtype of hepatobiliary cancer in 1965.[79] Conversely when arising within the gallbladder, extrahepatic bile ducts or ampulla of Vater it is considered extrahepatic bile-duct cancer which is more common in occurrence than intrahepatic disease, accounting for 80-90% of cholangiocarcinomas.[80] Extrahepatic cholangiocarcinoma can also be further divided into perihilar and distal extrahepatic based upon locations.[81] Perihilar cholangiocarcinoma usually indicates a extrahepatic mass occurring just distal to the origin of the cystic duct, whereas distal extrahepatic occurs between the origin of the cystic duct a the ampulla. While classically the division of perihilar and distal extrahepatic cholangiocarcinoma occurs at the level of the cystic duct, it can have variable locations of insertions along the biliary tree and it is not uncommon for a tumor determined to be perihilar in location to have a component, which is intrahepatic. In terms of incidence, perihilar is the most common location for cholangiocarcinoma to occur, followed by distal extrahepatic disease and lastly intrahepatic cholangiocarcinoma.[82]

The overwhelming majority of patients with cholangiocarcinoma are noted to develop symptoms when presenting at advanced stage of disease. The classic symptom of cholangiocarcinoma is painless jaundice; however commonly cholangiocarcinoma presents with nonspecific symptoms such as abdominal pain, fatigue, malaise, night sweats and cachexia. Ultimately the clinical presentation depends upon tumor size/stage, the location and growth pattern dependent upon which surrounding structures may be involved. In patients suspected to have a neoplastic process of the bile ducts, carbohydrate antigen 19-9 can be evaluated, however elevations of this antigen have been noted in patients with cholangitis and choledocholithiasis, which can confound findings. Historically the disease was commonly found within Japanese and Southeastern Asian population where there is a high prevalence of liver fluke (*Opisthorchis viverrini* and *Clonorchiasis sinensis*) infestations. However, the disease has steadily been on the rise in western countries over the last decade. Overall this malignancy is relatively an uncommon disease arising annually in approximately 1-2 out of every 100,00 individuals within the US, and representing approximately 5-20% of all hepatic malignancies with approximately 7,500 new diagnoses arising annually.[78, 83-87] Despite increasing prevalence, the disease carries a dismal prognosis with a 5 year survival of 10%. This is especially true in patients with unresectable disease where there is only a 5–8-month survival after initial diagnosis.[88-90] Given the typical advanced stage of disease at the time of diagnosis, about 30% of patients are eligible for surgical resection with patient survival rates remaining low even if resection is possible (20%-56% at 3 years).

Pathogenesis of Cholangiocarcinoma

In addition to the aforementioned risk factors, the development of cholangiocarcinoma includes cholelithiasis, primary sclerosing cholangitis, primary biliary cirrhosis, tobacco abuse, alcohol abuse, cirrhosis due to other causes, metabolic syndrome, biliary tract malformations (Caroli's Disease/Choledochocal cysts), toxins (thorotrast and dioxins), and biliary papillomatosis.[77, 84] genetic predispositions to cholangiocarcinoma exist with Lynch syndrome, BRCA 1 and BRCA 2 demonstrating a predisposition to the development of the malignancy. Many cases of cholangiocarcinoma are not found to be attributable to any risk factor and are felt to represent the spontaneous development of neoplasms.[91]

Both intrahepatic and extrahepatic cholangiocarcinomas most commonly are adenocarcinomas with most cases of cholangiocarcinoma felt to arise from malignant transformation of cholangiocytes.[92] It is possible that transformation of biliary epithelial cells within peribiliary glands and/or progenitor cells such as biliary stem cells may also contribute to its development. Regardless of cell line origin, it is accepted that chronic inflammation and cholestasis are key contributors to the pathogenesis of cholangiocarcinoma due to increased concentrations of cytokines, growth factors and bile acids which alters cell proliferation, apoptosis, senescence and cell cycle regulation.[80] This provides an environment promoting damage in tumor suppressor genes such as p53, proto-oncogenes, and DNA mismatch repair genes and proteins. As with other forms of malignancy, this milieu of inflammation and cholestasis set up an environment of stromal alteration and angiogenesis promoting carcinogenesis, thereby initiating a downward cycle ultimately resulting in the development of fulminant cholangiocarcinoma.[80]

Two major categories of premalignant biliary ductal lesions exist: biliary intraepithelial neoplasms (BIN) which can only be found on microscopic examination, and intraductal papillary neoplasms of the bile duct (IPNB) which is proliferation of atypical epithelium forming visible papillary lesions within the dilated bile duct.[94] While both of these lesions can develop into cholangiocarcinoma, BIN commonly develops into conventional tubular adenocarcinoma; whereas IPNB, which also includes a biliary papilloma and biliary papillomatosis, can result in either tubular adenocarcinoma or colloid (mucinous noncystic) carcinoma. Incidentally, biliary cystadenoma and cystadenocarcinoma may now be categorized as a cystic form of IPNB if there is biliary communication and absence of ovarian-like stroma, or as a mucinous cystic neoplasm if there is an absence of biliary communication but the presence of an ovarian-like stroma.[84]

Imaging of Cholangiocarcinoma

Radiographic assessment of cholangiocarcinoma commonly begins with diagnostic ultrasound (either transabdominal or endoscopic) in a patient with clinical and laboratory findings suggestive of the process.[93] Frequently biliary duct dilation concordant with the location of the mass will be visualized. However, not infrequently the causative mass may not be visualized. Regardless, ultrasound should only serve as an initial modality for investigation thereby prompting further workup with cross sectional imaging when concerning findings are realized.

CT is the most commonly performed modality in the workup of cholangiocarcinoma allowing full visualization of the tumor and allowing for treatment planning depending upon the findings of vascular invasion, pathologic lymphadenopathy and distant metastatic disease.[94] Similar to HCC, multiphase image acquisition is performed thereby allowing complete evaluation of the mass in terms of size and enhancement characteristics to occur as well as the relation of the primary tumor to adjacent vascular structures allowing for preoperative planning. Pre-contrast enhanced images are useful in detection of intraductal stones which are a risk factor for the development of cholangiocarcinoma. Arterial phase, portal venous phase and delayed phase (3-10 minute) imaging should also be acquired. Arterial and venous phases allow for assessment of vascular anatomy and the presence of vascular invasion; whereas prolonged/delayed imaging post-contrast administration is particularly useful for cholangiocarcinoma given its propensity for continuous delayed enhancement due to the abundant fibrous stromal proliferation associated with the tumor.

Contrast enhanced MRI has been increasingly performed for imaging of cholangiocarcinoma given its ability to provide both dynamic contrast enhanced images similar to CT and magnetic resonance cholangiopancreatography (MRCP). MRCP is a heavily T2 weighted sequence specifically tailored towards the visualization of the biliary and pancreatic ducts which despite requiring longer acquisition time, provides a non-invasive 3-dimensional view of the biliary tree. As opposed to endoscopic retrograde cholangiopancreatography (ERCP) which can lead to complications such as biliary sepsis and structuring, MRCP is relatively noninvasive. Additionally, ERCP may lead to incomplete biliary duct evaluation in patients with high grade biliary structuring of stenosis, which is alleviated by MRCP. Conversely ERCP allows for stent placement for the purpose of symptomatic relief and/or palliation, and also provides an opportunity for tissue procurement both at the time of acquisition. Similar to CT, dynamic enhanced image acquisition can be performed by MRI as well with similar progressive enhancement noted on delayed images, as is the case with CT. Additionally, MRI has the added benefit of diffusion weighted images which can aid in the detection of both intrahepatic, regional and distant metastatic disease.

Flourine-18 fluorodeoxyglucose (F-18 FDG) PET with concurrent CT (PET/CT) or MRI (PET/MRI) can be a valuable tool in the diagnosis and workup of cholangiocarcinoma in patients with potentially respectable tumors by evaluating for the presence of local and distant metastatic disease thereby assisting in tumor staging. PET/CT is also useful in tumor detection for lesions which may have not been visible by CT or MRI alone. PET/CT is valuable in the post treatment follow up of cholaniocarcinoma by evaluatieng both changes of size, and the avidity with which both the primary and any associated metastatic disease take up the radiotracer. Considering that MRI with MRCP are commonly performed in patients with cholangiocarcinoma as well as PET imaging, it stands to reason that PET/MRI may be performed thereby eliminating the need to undergo concurrent CT and leading to a more efficient workup. The clinical benefit of this modality has yet to be fully demonstrated and PET/MRI has not yet been widely accepted with further validation and clinical trials required prior to adapting this otherwise financially costly modality.

While CT and MRI are often sufficient to differentiate ICC from HCC, situations may arise where there is difficulty in determining which neoplastic process is present. For example, ICC less than 2.0 cm in size may mimic HCC because of the absence of appreciable progressive enhancement on delayed imaging due to size limitations, and in these cases, pathologic tissue sampling may be necessary to both guide diagnosis and treatment options.[81] For example, patients with an indeterminate lesion by imaging who are within Milan criteria for transplantation should have a biopsy performed. This is because patients who have ICC as opposed to HCC should not undergo liver transplantation resulting in dramatic changes to their treatment if the assumption was that they were presenting HCC.

Classification of Cholangiocarcinoma

Various classification schemes exist for intrahepatic (nodular, massive and diffuse) and extrahepatic (nodular/exophytic, sclerosing/infiltrative and polypoid/papillary) cholangiocarcinoma based upon both gross and radiographic appearance. When applied generally these terms are often misleading and can be somewhat vague resulting in confusion which can be alleviated simply by differentiated cholangiocarcinoma as: mass-forming (nodular), peri-ductal infiltrating (sclerosing), and intraductal-growing (papillary).[95-98]

Intrahepatic cholangiocarcinoma commonly forms a mass (mass-forming subtype) which grossly appears as a grey-white mass with a will defined undulated margin.[98] Size can widely vary, though the mass may be associated with exuberant desmoplasia, demonstrate central necrosis, fingerlike extensions along portal triads and rarely associated calcifications. When mass-like cholangiocarcinoma forms in an extrahepatic location, they are more often smaller ranging from 1-2 cm in size arising from within the mucosa and ultimately extending into lumen resulting in biliary obstruction. Mass-forming cholangiocarcinoma arises with the bile duct lumen and eventually penetrates the biliary tree wall allowing it to grow outward and insinuate between hepatocyte plates eventually invading small vessels resulting in portal vein thrombosis. Satellite nodularity is common with further tumor progression ultimately resulting in the coalescent of nodules into one large mass with irregular borders. On CT the mass appears as a homogenously low-attenuating mass on non-contrast enhanced scans. Arterial images will display a mass irregular peripheral enhancement and minimal, if any enhancement centrally due to necrosis initially. Progressive central enhancement is noted on delayed images depending upon the degree of central tumor fibrosis. The presence of hepatic capsular retraction and dilation of the bile ducts distal to the mass is also a diagnostic hallmark. Associated mass effect upon adjacent hepatic or portal veins is rare, however if present oftentimes leads to lobar or segmental atrophy of the liver.[95-98]

Peri-ductal infiltrating is the second subtype of cholangiocarcinoma. This is characterized by tumor growth along the bile duct walls, which results in concentric wall thickening and stenosis of the affected bile ducts thereby resulting in an elongated and spiculated appearance to the affected portions of the biliary tree. There is variation in the degree of stenosis as a result of this process ranging from mildly narrowed to complete obstruction with involved segments varying in length depending upon involvement. Due to this finding, the liver will present as bile stained and green in color due to biliary stasis and collapse of the gallbladder and extrahepatic bile ducts. Often times no sizeable or discreet mass will be identified, rather only diffuse thickening of the biliary ductal walls. Dense desmoplasia may result in compression or encasement of adjacent vessels and microscopic vascular invasion may be noted pathologically as well. Not infrequently both the intrahepatic and extrahepatic biliary ducts may be involved. Eventually, the tumor tends to spread along the Glissen sheath via the lymphatic vessels which allows for distal metastasis. Imaging of this subtype is similar to the previously described characteristics of cholangiocarcinoma, that being increasingly noticeable contrast enhancement visualized from arterial to delayed phase images.[95-98]

Finally, intraductal-growing or papillary subtype of cholangiocarcinoma is an adenocarcinoma of the bile ducts and a distinct entity characterized by the presence of intraluminal papillomas resulting in alternating stenosis and dilation of the biliary tree depending upon the degree of disease. This is a low grade tumor associated with innumerable papillary frond-like infoldings that are small in size, but large in number spreading along the superficial mucosal surface without invasion deep into the fibromuscular layer. Complete obstruction may occur if the masses are large enough in number or size or if enough mucin is produced by the masses to obstruct at an area of stenosis or at the ampulla due to inability to pass into the small bowel. Persistent production of mucin alongside the associated stenosis and/or occlusion can lead to a markedly dilated and somewhat aneurysmal appearance of the affected bile ducts. These papillary projections are often long and slender lending to their friable composition and resulting in sloughing off of cells into the biliary tree. Detached neoplastic cells are then able to disseminate throughout the biliary tree resulting in multifocal tumor deposits within either the intrahepatic or extrahepatic ducts. As cells begin to accumulate, intraluminal-floating masses may develop which can mimic biliary duct stones. The late stage of this disease is characterized by infiltration of the bile duct walls and rarely metastasis. Imaging often times shows segmental ductal ectasia with intermittent areas of narrowing, with or without the presence of a detectable mass. If visualized, the mass will appear hypoattenuating with irregular margins on pre-contrast images and will display progressive enhancement of portal venous and delayed phases.[95-98]

If a tumor is not found to align specifically with one of the previously mentioned criteria, that can be grouped into a fourth criteria termed "undefined."[81] Tumors with features of more than one of the previously mentioned criteria can be connected by a plus (+) sign and would therefore be defined as mass-forming + intraductal-growing.

The most important factor to consider is the timely diagnosis of cholangiocarcinoma allowing for effective treatment to be initiated. Differentiation of the specific subtype of cholangiocarcinoma can be helpful in guiding the type of treatment recommended, or method of surgical resection best suited for that specific patient. Determining the specific subtype of cholangiocarcinoma can also help in predicting prognosis based upon the fact that poor prognosis associated with the mass forming subtype, and an overall excellent prognosis is associated with the intraductal-growing subtype.

Staging Cholangiocarcinoma

As with HCC, the purpose of staging cholangiocarcinoma is to estimate the prognosis of the patient, guide therapy, and provide standards to objectively compare therapies. Staging cholangiocarcinoma is largely dependent upon the location of the primary malignancy and inaccurate staging can result in inappropriate treatment options that may either expose patients to excessive or inefficient treatment, both of which have risks of elevated morbidity of mortality.

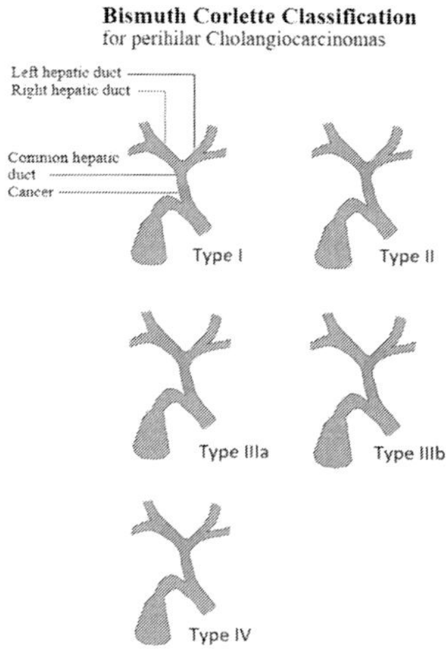

Figure 4.

While there are three potential staging systems for ICC (American Joint Committee on Cancer (AJCC)/Union for International Cancer Control (UICC), Liver Cancer Study Group of Japan (LCSGJ), and the National Cancer Center of Japan (NCCJ)), no one dominant system has been declared. Most recently, the AJCC/UICC released their 8th revised edition, however this revision has received mixed results due to its requirement for pathologic analysis thereby limited its ability to perform preoperative staging.[99-101] Despite that lack of an ideal staging system for ICC, the prognosis largely depends upon tumor size with tumors greater than 5.0 cm having an independent prognostic factor for survival. Lymph node metastasis, quantity of hepatic tumors or intrahepatic metastasis, and vascular invasion are additional considerations.[102-105]

One of the first systems available for the description of pCC was the Bismuth-Corlette system (Figure 4), which although helpful is not strictly a staging system, but rather provides a guide for surgical resection.[107-109] The Bismuth-Corlette system divides pCC into four separate categories based upon its extrahepatic location of malignancy, with recent changes taking into account vascular encasement, hepatic atrophy and value of remaining hepatic parenchyma.[109] The system does not take into account patients with biliary anomalies such as biliary tree trifurcations, accessory ducts or aberrant ducts. The Memorial Sloan-Kettering Cancer Center (MSKCC) is an additional system available to describe pCC based upon tumor location, extent of biliary tree involvement, portal venous invasion and hepatic lobar atrophy. It does have a history of improperly categorizing patients as having possible resectable disease preoperatively, who were then found to have non-resectable cancer intra-operatively. Staging of pCC is similar to ICC given the lack of a single dominant system; with the most commonly utilized staging system again being the TMN system specific to pCC as described in 8th edition of the AJCC/UICC. Staging of distal extrahepatic cholangiocarcinoma also falls in line with the TMN system of the AJCC/UICC due to a lack of any other available staging system. [107-109}

Table 3.

Bismuth Corlette Classification	
Type I	Distal to hepatic duct confluence
Type II	Extend to and involve the hepatic duct confluence
Type IIIa	Involve the hepatic duct confluence and proximal right hepatic duct
Type IIIb	Involve the hepatic duct confluence and proximal left hepatic duct
Type IV	Extend from the hepatic duct confluence bilaterally to the proximal hepatic ducts and segmental bile ducts
Type V	Junction of cystic duct and bile duct

Treatment of Cholangiocarcinoma

If possible, the treatment of choice for ICC and pCC are surgical resection, with the specific style of resection dependent upon the location of the tumor.[92, 110] Commonly partial hepatectomy, regional lymphadenectomy and Roux-en-Y hepaticojejunostomy are performed as a measure to ensure treatment. In cases where tumor is potentially resectable but the volume of the remnant hepatic parenchyma is deemed too small, resection can be achieved by portal vein embolization of the affected lobe resulting in compensatory hyperplasia of the contralateral unaffected lobe.

IPNB and BIN lesions are a precursor to distal cholangiocarcinoma, both of which are effectively treated by surgical resection with pancreaticoduodenectomy (Whipple procedure) thereby entailing a good long-term prognosis post resection. When negative margins are obtained and progression to distal cholangiocarcinoma occurs the 5-year survival decreases to 27%. The role of chemotherapy in patients with these lesions are limited, and only in patients who are not ideal surgical candidates should chemotherapy be considered.[92-110]

Liver transplantation in patients with cholangiocarcinoma has been considered and performed in the past, though with mixed results. The greatest benefit being realized in patients with the periductal-infiltrating subtype with one study showing a 5-year survival rate of 65%.[111] Potential curative measures in the periductal-infiltrating subtype is for patients to undergo both resection and neoadjuvant chemotherapy followed by hepatic transplant. Conversely, liver transplant has shown a lack of benefit in patients with the ICC and the mass-forming subtype with another study showing a recurrence rate of 70% 5-years post transplant.[112] Due to results such as these, ICC is considered a contraindication by many transplant centers due to historically poor results post transplant and high tumor recurrence rates.[113]

While the interventional radiologist plays a large role in the primary treatment of HCC, interventional radiology's role in cholangiocarcinoma is less clear given the preference for surgical management as the only potentially curative measure. Many of the following treatments only provide modest survival benefit through the provision of time when compared to the curative intent of surgical resection. Nevertheless, interventional radiology does have the opportunity to provide strong assistance in the treatment of patients with both resectable and unresectable cholangiocarcinoma as will be detailed below.

Similar to HCC, percutaneous ablation can be performed in patients with cholangiocarcinoma, especially in patients deemed to be unfit for surgical resection or with recurrence. Current guidelines recommend this locoregional therapy for intrahepatic-limited disease when resection is not an option. There also may be a benefit of ablation to bridge patients to resection in the form of neoadjuvant locoregional therapy. While some studies have shown ablation as a possible treatment option to compete with surgical resection given similar outcomes compared to surgery, the number of studies comparing ablation directly to resection is limited and the outcome of those available demonstrate heterogeneity.

As is the case in thermal ablation, the number of studies detailing the use of TACE and Y-90 radioembolization in the treatment of cholangiocarcinoma are limited. In regards to TACE specifically, there are studies detailing its use in patients with unresectable ICC, with some showing a benefit of adjuvant TACE alongside surgical resection, especially in patients with high risk of recurrence.[114-117] There is also data supporting the use of both Y-90 treatment and TACE to aid in conversion of non-surgical to surgical patients.[118, 120] TACE may also offer a survival benefit in patients with high risk for early intrahepatic recurrence. There is also evidence that TACE alone in non-surgical patients or patients seeking palliation can be safe and effective for when proper technique is utilized and that TACE may portend a survival benefit when compared with systemic chemotherapy in patients with liver only, or liver dominant extrahepatic disease.[119] Both TARE and TACE are generally well tolerated without the side effect profile associated with chemotherapy making either an attractive therapeutic option for palliation over systemic chemotherapy in order to alleviate symptoms and prolong life.

Systemic chemotherapy options are available as previously eluded to, however even the current standard chemotherapeutic agents (gemcitabine and cisplatin) have been shown to provide modest survival benefits prompting many to investigate more effective alternative treatments.[121] One such treatment has been termed "Hepatic Arterial Infusion (HAI)" of chemotherapy (floxuridine alone, or in combination with bevacizumab) which entails the concurrent administration of chemotherapeutic agents directly into the hepatic arterial system alongside systemic therapy. The benefit of this method is the ability to allow higher dose and concentrations of antineoplastic agents to be directed towards the hepatic disease due to the minimization of systemic side effects, while the systemic treatment is geared towards the treatment of regional metastatic lymphadenopathy or distal metastatic disease. There is a hope that HAI may improve resection rates in patients diagnosed at an advanced, unresectable stage.

References

1. International Agency for Research on Cancer, World Health Organization. Cancer today (https://gco.iarc.fr/today/home.).
2. Xu JQ. Trends in liver cancer mortality among adults aged 25 and over in the United States, 2000–2016. NCHS Data Brief, no 314. Hyattsville, MD: National Center for Health Statistics. 2018.
3. Howlader N, Noone AM, Krapcho M, et al (eds). SEER Cancer Statistics Review, 1975-2016, National Cancer Institute, Bethesda, MD, https://seer.cancer.gov/csr/1975_2016/, based on November 2018 SEER data submission, posted to the SEER website, April 2019.
4. Younossi, Z., Stepanova, M., Ong, J. P., Jacobson, I. M., Bugianesi, E., Duseja, A., et. al. (2019). Nonalcoholic Steatohepatitis Is the Fastest Growing Cause of Hepatocellular Carcinoma in Liver Transplant Candidates. *Clinical Gastroenterology and Hepatology, 17*(4), 630-637. doi:10.1016/j.cgh.2018.05.057
5. Dhanasekaran, R., Bandoh, S., & Roberts, L. R. (2016). Molecular pathogenesis of hepatocellular carcinoma and impact of therapeutic advances. *F1000Research*, *5*, F1000 Faculty Rev-879. https://doi.org/10.12688/f1000research.6946.1
6. Welzel, T. M., Graubard, B. I., Zeuzem, S., El-Serag, H. B., Davila, J. A., & McGlynn, K. A. (2011). Metabolic syndrome increases the risk of primary liver cancer in the United States: a study in the SEER-Medicare database. *Hepatology (Baltimore, Md.)*, *54*(2), 463–471. http://doi.org/10.1002/hep.24397
7. Halpert, R. D., & Boland, G. W. (2014). *Gastrointestinal Imaging: The Requisites*. Saunders.
8. Molecular pathogenesis of hepatocellular carcinoma and impact of therapeutic advances. (2016). Molecular pathogenesis of hepatocellular carcinoma and impact of therapeutic advances., *5*. http://doi.org/10.12688/f1000research.6946.1
9. McEvoy, S. H., McCarthy, C. J., Lavelle, L. P., Moran, D. E., Cantwell, C. P., Skehan, S. J., et al. (2013, October). Hepatocellular carcinoma: illustrated guide to systematic radiologic diagnosis and staging according to guidelines of the American Association for the Study of Liver Diseases. *RadioGraphics*. Radiological Society of North America. http://doi.org/10.1148/rg.336125104
10. Tajima T, Honda H, Taguchi K, et al. Sequential he- modynamic change in hepatocellular carcinoma and dysplastic nodules: CT angiography and patho- logic correlation. *AJR* 2002; 178:885–897

11. Zhang, B.-H., Yang, B.-H., & Tang, Z.-Y. (2004). Randomized controlled trial of screening for hepatocellular carcinoma. *Journal of Cancer Research and Clinical Oncology*, *130*(7), 417–422. http://doi.org/10.1007/s00432-004-0552-0
12. Diagnosis, Staging, and Management of Hepatocellular Carcinoma: 2018 Practice Guidance by the American Association for the Study of Liver Diseases. (2018, August). Diagnosis, Staging, and Management of Hepatocellular Carcinoma: 2018 Practice Guidance by the American Association for the Study of Liver Diseases. http://doi.org/10.1002/hep.29913
13. EASL Clinical Practice Guidelines: Management of hepatocellular carcinoma. (2018). EASL Clinical Practice Guidelines: Management of hepatocellular carcinoma., *69*(1), 182–236. http://doi.org/10.1016/j.jhep.2018.03.019
14. Surveillance Imaging and Alpha Fetoprotein for Early Detection of Hepatocellular Carcinoma in Patients With Cirrhosis: A Meta-analysis. (2018). Surveillance Imaging and Alpha Fetoprotein for Early Detection of Hepatocellular Carcinoma in Patients With Cirrhosis: A Meta-analysis., *154*(6), 1706–1718.e1. http://doi.org/10.1053/j.gastro.2018.01.064
15. Accuracy of ultrasonography, spiral CT, magnetic resonance, and alpha-fetoprotein in diagnosing hepatocellular carcinoma: a systematic review. (2006). Accuracy of ultrasonography, spiral CT, magnetic resonance, and alpha-fetoprotein in diagnosing hepatocellular carcinoma: a systematic review., *101*(3), 513–523. http://doi.org/10.1111/j.1572-0241.2006.00467.x
16. Choi, J.-Y., Lee, J.-M., & Sirlin, C. B. (2014). CT and MR imaging diagnosis and staging of hepatocellular carcinoma: part I. Development, growth, and spread: key pathologic and imaging aspects. *Radiology*, *272*(3), 635–654. http://doi.org/10.1148/radiol.14132361
17. Choi, J.-Y., Lee, J.-M., & Sirlin, C. B. (2014). CT and MR imaging diagnosis and staging of hepatocellular carcinoma: part II. Extracellular agents, hepatobiliary agents, and ancillary imaging features. *Radiology*, *273*(1), 30–50. http://doi.org/10.1148/radiol.14132362
18. Kim MJ, Choi JY, Lim JS, et al. Optimal scan window for detection of hypervascular hepatocellular carcinomas during MDCT examination. AJR Am J Roentgenol 2006; 187(1):198–206.
19. Ichikawa T, Kitamura T, Nakajima H, et al. Hypervascular hepatocellular carcinoma: can double arterial phase imaging with multidetector CT improve tumor depiction in the cirrhotic liver? AJR Am J Roentgen-ol 2002;179(3):751–758.

20. Colagrande, S., Centi, N., Galdiero, R., & Ragozzino, A. (2007). Transient hepatic intensity differences: part 1, Those associated with focal lesions. *AJR. American Journal of Roentgenology*, *188*(1), 154–159. http://doi.org/10.2214/AJR.05.1368
21. Colagrande, S., Centi, N., Galdiero, R., & Ragozzino, A. (2007). Transient hepatic intensity differences: part 2, Those not associated with focal lesions. *AJR. American Journal of Roentgenology*, *188*(1), 160–166. http://doi.org/10.2214/AJR.05.1367
22. Grazioli L, Olivetti L, Fugazzola C, et al. The pseudocapsule in hepatocellular carcinoma: correlation between dynamic MR imaging and pathology. Eur Radiol 1999;9(1):62–67.
23. Lim JH, Choi D, Kim SH, et al. Detection of hepatocellular carcinoma: value of adding de- layed phase imaging to dual-phase helical CT. AJR Am J Roentgenol 2002;179(1):67–73.
24. Monzawa S, Ichikawa T, Nakajima H, Kitanaka Y, Omata K, Araki T. Dynamic CT for detecting small hepatocellular carci- noma: usefulness of delayed phase imaging. AJR Am J Roentgenol 2007;188(1):147–153.
25. Enomoto S, Tamai H, Shingaki N, et al. As- sessment of hepatocellular carcinomas using conventional magnetic resonance imaging correlated with histological differentiation and a serum marker of poor prognosis. Hepatol Int 2011;5(2):730–737.
26. Okamoto D, Yoshimitsu K, Nishie A, et al. Enhancement pattern analysis of hypervas- cular hepatocellular carcinoma on dynamic MR imaging with histopathological cor- relation: validity of portal phase imaging for predicting tumor grade. Eur J Radiol 2012;81(6):1116–1121.
27. Griffin N, Addley H, Sala E, et al. Vascu- lar invasion in hepatocellular carcinoma: is there a correlation with MRI? Br J Radiol 2012;85 (1014):736–744.
28. Khan AS, Hussain HK, Johnson TD, Weadock WJ, Pelletier SJ, Marrero JA. Value of delayed hypointensity and delayed enhancing rim in magnetic resonance imag- ing diagnosis of small hepatocellular carci- noma in the cirrhotic liver. J Magn Reson Imaging 2010;32(2): 360–366.
29. Higaki A, Tamada T, Sone T, et al. Potential clinical factors affecting hepatobiliary enhancement at Gd-EOB-DTPA-enhanced MR imaging. Magn Reson Imaging 2012;30(5):689–693.
30. Narita M, Hatano E, Arizono S, et al. Expression of OATP1B3 determines uptake of Gd-EOB-DTPA in hepatocellular carcinoma. J Gastroenterol 2009;44(7):793–798.

31. Kitao A, Zen Y, Matsui O, et al. Hepatocellular carcinoma: signal intensity at gadoxetic acid-enhanced MR Imaging—correlation with molecular transporters and histopathologic features. Radiology 2010;256(3):817–826.
32. Park G, Kim YK, Kim CS, Yu HC, Hwang SB. Diagnostic efficacy of gadoxetic acid- enhanced MRI in the detection of hepa- tocellular carcinomas: comparison with gadopentetate dimeglumine. Br J Radiol 2010;83(996):1010–1016.
33. Sun HY, Lee JM, Shin CI, et al. Gadoxetic acid-enhanced magnetic resonance imaging for differentiating small hepatocellular car- cinomas (, or 5 2 cm in diameter) from arterial enhancing pseudolesions: special emphasis on hepatobiliary phase imaging. Invest Radiol 2010;45(2): 96–103.
34. American College of Radiology. Liver Imaging Reporting and Data System version 2018.1. http://www.acr.org/Quality-Safety/Resources/LIRADS/. Accessed October 12, 2021.
35. Maida, M., Orlando, E., Cammà, C., & Cabibbo, G. (2014). Staging systems of hepatocellular carcinoma: a review of literature. *World Journal of Gastroenterology*, *20*(15), 4141–4150. http://doi.org/10.3748/wjg.v20.i15.4141
36. Bruix J, Sherman M. Management of hepatocellular carcinoma. *Hepatology* 2005; 42: 1208-1236 [PMID: 16250051]
37. Cho, C. S. (2015). Prognostication systems as applied to primary and metastatic hepatic malignancies. *Surgical Oncology Clinics of North America*, *24*(1), 41–56. http://doi.org/10.1016/j.soc.2014.09.010
38. Ayuso, C., Rimola, J., Vilana, R., Burrel, M., Darnell, A., García-Criado, Á., et al. (2018). Diagnosis and staging of hepatocellular carcinoma (HCC): current guidelines. *European Journal of Radiology*, *101*, 72–81. http://doi.org/10.1016/j.ejrad.2018.01.025
39. Okuda K, Obata H, Nakajima Y, Ohtsuki T, Okazaki N, Ohnishi K. Prognosis of primary hepatocellular carcinoma. *Hepatology* 1984; 4: 3S-6S [PMID: 6319264]
40. Befeler AS, Di Bisceglie AM. Hepatocellular carcinoma: diagnosis and treatment. Gastroenterology 2002;122:1609 –1619.
41. Llovet JM, Brú C, Bruix J. Prognosis of hepatocellular carcinoma: the BCLC staging classification. Semin. Liver Dis. 1999;19 (03): 329-38. doi:10.1055/s-2007-1007122
42. Forner A, Reig ME, de Lope CR et-al. Current strategy for staging and treatment: the BCLC update and future prospects. Semin. Liver Dis. 2010;30 (01): 61-74. doi:10.1055/s-0030-1247133

43. Oken M, Creech R, Tormey D et al. Toxicity and response criteria of the Eastern Cooperative Oncology Group. Am J Clin Oncol. 1982;5(6): 649-55. PMID 7165009
44. Pavel, M. C., & Fuster, J. (2018). Expansion of the hepatocellular carcinoma Milan criteria in liver transplantation: Future directions. *World journal of gastroenterology*, *24*(32), 3626–3636. https://doi.org/10.3748/wjg.v24.i32.3626
45. Mazzaferro V, Regalia E, Doci R, Andreola S, Pulvirenti A, Bozzetti F, et al. *Liver transplantation for the treatment of small hepatocellular carcinomas in patients with cirrhosis.* N Engl J Med. 1996;334:693-9.
46. Mazzoferro V, Llovet JM, Miceli R, Bhoori S, Schiavo M, Mariani L, et al. *Predicting survival after liver transplantation in patients with hepatocellular carcinoma beyond the Milan criteria: a retrospective, exploratory analysis.* Lancet Oncol. 2009;10:35-43.
47. Petrowsky H, Busuttil RW. Resection or ablation of small hepatocellular carcinoma: what is the better treatment? J Hepatology 2008; 49:502–504.
48. Mcwilliams, J. P., Yamamoto, S., Raman, S. S., Loh, C. T., Lee, E. W., Liu, D. M., & Kee, S. T. (2010). Percutaneous Ablation of Hepatocellular Carcinoma: Current Status. *Journal of Vascular and Interventional Radiology, 21*(8), 204-213. doi:10.1016/j.jvir.2009.11.025
49. Llovet JM, Real MI, Montaña X, Planas R, Coll S, Aponte J, Ayuso C, Sala M, Muchart J, Solà R, Rodés J, Bruix J; Barcelona Liver Cancer Group. Arterial embolisation or chemoembolisation versus symptomatic treatment in patients with unresectable hepatocellular carcinoma: a randomised controlled trial. Lancet. 2002 May 18;359 (9319):1734-9. doi: 10.1016/S0140-6736(02)08649-X. PMID: 12049862.
50. Lo CM, Ngan H, Tso WK, Liu CL, Lam CM, Poon RT, Fan ST, Wong J. Randomized controlled trial of transarterial lipiodol chemoembolization for unresectable hepatocellular carcinoma. Hepatology. 2002 May;35(5):1164-71. doi: 10.1053/jhep.2002.33156. PMID: 11981766.
51. Cammà C, Schepis F, Orlando A, Albanese M, Shahied L, Trevisani F, Andreone P, Craxì A, Cottone M. Transarterial chemoembolization for unresectable hepatocellular carcinoma: meta-analysis of randomized controlled trials. Radiology. 2002 Jul;224(1):47-54. doi: 10.1148/radiol.2241011262. PMID: 12091661.
52. Kandarpa, K., Gexchwind, J.-F. H., Tsitskari, M., & Georgiades, C. S. (2016). Chapter 23: Hepatocellular Carcinoma: Chemoembolization. In

Handbook of Interventional Radiologic Procedures (pp. 351–358), Wolters Kluwer.

53. Ajit, Y., Sudarsan, H., Saumya, G., Abhishek, A., Navneet, R., Piyush, R., Anil, A., & Arun, G. (2014). Transarterial chemoembolization in unresectable hepatocellular carcinoma with portal vein thrombosis: a perspective on survival. *Oman medical journal*, *29*(6), 430–436. https://doi.org/10.5001/omj.2014.114
54. Ernst O, Sergent G, Mizrahi D, Delemazure O, Paris JC, L'Hermine. *Treatment of hepatocellular carcinoma by transcatheter arterial chemoembolization: Comparison of planned periodic chemoembolization and chemoembolization based on tumor response.* AJR Am J Roentgenol. 1999;172:59-64.
55. Elliott R, Ram S, Khanna V. Classification and Current Treatment of Hepatocellular Carcinoma. Am J Interv Radiol 2018, 2(8) 1-12.Kluger, M. D., Halazun, K. J., Barroso, R. T., Fox, A. N., Olsen, S. K., Madoff, D. C., et. al. (2014). Bland embolization versus chemoembolization of hepatocellular carcinoma before transplantation. *Liver Transplantation, 20*(5), 536-543. doi:10.1002/lt.23846
56. Tsochatzis EA, Fatourou E, O'Beirne J et-al. Transarterial chemoembolization and bland embolization for hepatocellular carcinoma. World J. Gastroenterol. 2014;20 (12): 3069-77. doi:10.3748/wjg.v20.i12.3069
57. Bruix J, Sherman M; for American Association for the Study of Liver Diseases. Management of hepatocellular carcinoma: an update. Hepatology 2011;53:1020-1022.
58. European Association for the Study of the Liver; European Organisation for Research and Treatment of Cancer. EASL-EORTC clinical practice guidelines: management of hepatocellular carcinoma. J Hepatol 2012;56:908-943.
59. Kandarpa, K., Lewandowski RJ, Salem, R. (2016). Chapter 24: Hepatic Malignancies: Radioembolization. In *Handbook of Interventional Radiologic Procedures* (pp. 359–366), Wolters Kluwer.
60. Salem, R., & Thurston, K. G. (2006). Radioembolization with 90Yttrium Microspheres: A State-of-the-Art Brachytherapy Treatment for Primary and Secondary Liver Malignancies. *Journal of Vascular and Interventional Radiology, 17*(8), 1251-1278. doi:10.1097/01.rvi.0000233785.75257.9a
61. Abouchaleh, N., Gabr, A., Ali, R., Asadi, Al, A., Mora, R. A., Kallini, J. R., et al. (2018). ^{90}Y Radioembolization for Locally Advanced Hepatocellular Carcinoma with Portal Vein Thrombosis: Long-Term Outcomes in a 185-Patient Cohort. *J Nucl Med*, *59*(7), 1042.

62. Llovet, J. M., Ricci, S., Mazzaferro, V., Hilgard, P., Gane, E., Blanc, J.-F., et al. (2008). Sorafenib in Advanced Hepatocellular Carcinoma. *The New England Journal of Medicine*, *359*(4), 378–390. http://doi.org/10.1056/NEJMoa0708857
63. Kirstein MM, Schweitzer N, Hinrichs JB, Marquardt J, Worns MA, Kloeckner R, et al. *Transarterial chemoembolization versus sorafenib in patients with hepatocellular carcinoma and extrahepatic disease.* United European Gastroenterol J. 2018;6:238-46.
64. Pinter M, Hucke F, Graziadei I, Vogel W, Maieron A, Königsberg R, et al. *Advanced-stage hepatocellular carcinoma: Transarterial chemoembolization versus sorafenib.* Radiology. 2012;263:590-9.
65. Cai R, Song RF, Pang PF, Yan Y, Liao Y, Zhou C, et al. *Transcatheter arterial chemoembolization plus sorafenib versus transcatheter arterial chemoembolization alone to treat advanced hepatocellular carcinoma: A meta-analysis.* BMC Cancer. 2017;17: 714.
66. Elliott R, Ram S, Khanna V. Classification and Current Treatment of Hepatocellular Carcinoma. Am J Interv Radiol 2018, 2(8) 1-12.
67. Ikeda, M., Mitsunaga, S., Shimizu, S., Ohno, I., Takahashi, H., Okuyama, H., et al. (2013). Efficacy of sorafenib in patients with hepatocellular carcinoma refractory to transcatheter arterial chemoembolization. *Journal of Gastroenterology, 49*(5), 932-940. doi:10.1007/s00535-013-0853-7
68. Stuart, K. (n.d.). Systemic treatment for advanced hepatocellular carcinoma. Retrieved January 19, 2022, from https://www.uptodate.com/contents/systemic-treatment-for-advanced-hepatocellular-carcinoma
69. Johnston, M. P., & Khakoo, S. I. (2019). Immunotherapy for hepatocellular carcinoma: Current and future. *World journal of gastroenterology*, *25*(24), 2977–2989. https://doi.org/10.3748/wjg.v25.i24.2977
70. Rungsakulkij, N., Suragul, W., Mingphruedhi, S., Tangtawee, P., Muangkaew, P., & Aeesoa, S. (2018). Prognostic role of alpha-fetoprotein response after hepatocellular carcinoma resection. *World journal of clinical cases*, *6*(6), 110–120. https://doi.org/10.12998/wjcc.v6.i6.110
71. Shen JY, Li C, Wen TF, Yan LN, Li B, Wang WT, Yang JY, Xu MQ. Alpha fetoprotein changes predict hepatocellular carcinoma survival beyond the Milan criteria after hepatectomy. *J Surg Res.* 2017;209: 102–111.

72. Yaghmai, V., Besa, C., Kim, E., Gatlin, J. L., Siddiqui, N. A., & Taouli, B. (2013). Imaging Assessment of Hepatocellular Carcinoma Response to Locoregional and Systemic Therapy. *American Journal of Roentgenology*, *201*(1), 80–96. http://doi.org/10.2214/AJR.13.10706
73. Kim HJ, Kim TK, Kim PN, et al. Assessment of the therapeutic response of hepatocellular carcinoma treated with trasncatheter arterial chemoembolization: comparision of contrast-enhanced sonography and 3-phase computed tomography. *J Ultrasound Med* 2006: 25:477-486
74. Boas FE, Do B, Louie JD, Kothary N, Hwang GL, Kuo WT, Hovsepian DM, Kantrowitz M, Sze DY. Optimal imaging surveillance schedules after liver-directed therapy for hepatocellular carcinoma. J Vasc Interv Radiol. 2015 Jan;26(1):69-73. doi: 10.1016/j.jvir.2014.09.013. Epub 2014 Nov 4. PMID: 25446423.
75. Banales J.M. Cardinale V. Carpino G. et al. Expert consensus document: Cholangiocarcinoma: current knowledge and future perspectives consensus statement from the European Network for the Study of Cholangiocarcinoma (ENS-CCA). *Nat Rev Gastroenterol Hepatol.* 2016; 13: 261-280
76. Tariq, N. U., McNamara, M. G., & Valle, J. W. (2019). Biliary tract cancers: current knowledge, clinical candidates and future challenges. *Cancer management and research*, *11*, 2623–2642. https://doi.org/10.2147/CMAR.S157092
77. De Groen, P. C., Gores, G. J., LaRusso, N. F., Gunderson, L. L., & Nagorney, D. M. (1999). Biliary tract cancers. *New England Journal of Medicine, 341*(18), 1368-1378. doi:10.1056/nejm199910283411807
78. Klatskin G. Adenocarcinoma of the hepatic duct at its bifurcation within the porta hepatis: an unusual tumor with distinctive clinical and pathological features. Am J Med1965;38:241-256
79. Blechacz, B., & Gores, G. J. (2008). Cholangiocarcinoma: advances in pathogenesis, diagnosis, and treatment. *Hepatology (Baltimore, Md.)*, *48*(1), 308–321. https://doi.org/10.1002/hep.22310
80. Blechacz, B., Komuta, M., Roskams, T., & Gores, G. J. (2011). Clinical diagnosis and staging of cholangiocarcinoma. *Nature reviews. Gastroenterology & hepatology*, *8*(9), 512–522. https://doi.org/10.1038/nrgastro.2011.131
81. Nakeeb A, Pitt HA, Sohn TA, et al. Cholangiocarcinoma: a spectrum of intrahepatic, perihilar, and distal tumors. Ann Surg 1996;224(4): 463–473; discussion 473–475.
82. Buettner, S., Braat, A. J., Margonis, G. A., Brown, D. B., Taylor, K. B., Borgmann, A. J., et. al. (2020). Yttrium-90 radioembolization in intrahepatic cholangiocarcinoma: A Multicenter retrospective analysis.

Journal of Vascular and Interventional Radiology, 31(7), 1035-1043. doi:10.1016/j.jvir.2020.02.008

83. Díaz-González, Á, Vilana, R., Bianchi, L., García-Criado, Á, Rimola, J., Rodríguez de Lope, C., et. al. (2020). Thermal ablation for intrahepatic cholangiocarcinoma in cirrhosis: Safety and efficacy in non-surgical patients. *Journal of Vascular and Interventional Radiology, 31*(5), 710-719. doi:10.1016/j.jvir.2019.06.014
84. Shin HR, Oh JK, Masuyer E, et al. Comparison of incidence of intrahepatic and extrahepatic cholangiocarcinoma–focus on East and South-Eastern Asia. Asian Pac J Cancer Prev 2010; 11:1159–1166.
85. Singal AK, Vauthey JN, Grady JJ, Stroehlein JR. Intra-hepatic cholangiocarcinoma–frequency and demographic patterns: thirty-year data from the M.D. Anderson Cancer Center. J Cancer Res Clin Oncol 2011; 137:1071–1078.
86. Everhart JE, Ruhl CE. Burden of digestive diseases in the United States Part III: liver, biliary tract, and pancreas. Gastroenterology 2009; 136: 1134–1144.
87. De Groen, P. C., Gores, G. J., LaRusso, N. F., Gunderson, L. L., & Nagorney, D. M. (1999). Biliary tract cancers. *New England Journal of Medicine, 341*(18), 1368-1378. doi:10.1056/nejm199910283411807
88. Chou FF, Sheen-Chen SM, Chen YS, Chen MC, Chen CL. Surgical treat- ment of cholangiocarcinoma. Hepato- gastroenterology 1997; 44:760–765.
89. Pitt HA, Grochow LB, Abrams RA. Cancer of the biliary tree, 5th ed. Phil- adelphia: Lippincott-Raven, 1997.
90. Tyson GL, El-Serag HB. Risk factors for cholangiocarcinoma. Hepatology 2011; 54:173–184.
91. Rizvi, S., & Gores, G. J. (2013). Pathogenesis, diagnosis, and management of Cholangiocarcinoma. *Gastroenterology, 145*(6), 1215-1229. doi:10.1053/j.gastro.2013.10.013
92. Olthof, S. C., Othman, A., Clasen, S., Schraml, C., Nikolaou, K., & Bongers, M. (2016). Imaging of Cholangiocarcinoma. *Visceral medicine*, *32*(6), 402–410. https://doi.org/10.1159/000453009
93. Joo, I., Lee, J. M., & Yoon, J. H. (2018). Imaging diagnosis of intrahepatic and perihilar cholangiocarcinoma: Recent advances and challenges. *Radiology, 288*(1), 7-13. doi:10.1148/radiol.2018171187
94. H Eggel (1901) Uber das primare Carcinoma der Leber *Beitr Pathol Anat Allg Pathol* **30** 506–604
95. T Rosai (1996) Ackerman's surgical pathology, 8th ed Mosby St Louis
96. K Weinbren SS Mutum (1983) Pathological aspects of cholangiocarcinoma *J Pathol* **139** 217–238

1:STN:280:BiyC3sfht1w%3D 6298394
97. Lim, J., Park, C. Pathology of cholangiocarcinoma. *Abdom Imaging* **29,** 540–547 (2004). https://doi.org/10.1007/s00261-004-0187-2
98. American Joint Committee on Cancer, American College of Surgeons. AJCC Cancer Staging Form Supplement, AJCC Cancer Staging Manual, Eighth Edition. 2018.
99. Lee AJ, Chun YS. Intrahepatic cholangiocarcinoma: the AJCC/UICC 8th edition updates. (2018) Chinese clinical oncology. 7 (5): 52. doi:10.21037/cco.2018.07.03
100. Kim Y, Moris DP, Zhang XF, Bagante F, Spolverato G, Schmidt C, Dilhoff M, Pawlik TM. Evaluation of the 8th edition American Joint Commission on Cancer (AJCC) staging system for patients with intrahepatic cholangiocarcinoma: A surveillance, epidemiology, and end results (SEER) analysis. (2017) Journal of surgical oncology. 116 (6): 643-650. doi:10.1002/jso.24720
101. Tamandl D, et al. Lymph node ratio after curative surgery for intrahepatic cholangiocarcinoma. *Br J Surg.* 2009;96:919–925.
102. Endo I, et al. Intrahepatic cholangiocarcinoma: rising frequency, improved survival, and determinants of outcome after resection. *Ann Surg.* 2008;248:84–96.
103. Shen WF, et al. Clinicopathological and prognostic analysis of 429 patients with intrahepatic cholangiocarcinoma. *World J Gastroenterol.* 2009;15:5976–5982.
104. Weber SM, et al. Intrahepatic cholangiocarcinoma: resectability, recurrence pattern, and outcomes. *J Am Coll Surg.* 2001;193:384–391.
105. Bismuth H, Corlette MB. Intrahepatic cholangioenteric anastomosis in carcinoma of the hilus of the liver. *Surg Gynecol Obstet.* 1975;140: 170–178.
106. Bismuth H, Nakache R, Diamond T. Management strategies in resection for hilar cholangiocarcinoma. *Ann Surg.* 1992;215:31–38.
107. Joo I, Lee JM, Yoon JH. Imaging Diagnosis of Intrahepatic and Perihilar Cholangiocarcinoma: Recent Advances and Challenges. (2018) Radiology. 288 (1): 7-13. doi:10.1148/radiol.2018171187
108. M.L. Deoliveira, R.D. Schulick, Y. Nimura, et al. New staging system and a registry for perihilar cholangiocarcinoma Hepatology, 53 (2011), pp. 1363-1371
109. Palmer WC, Patel T. Are common factors involved in the pathogenesis of primary liver cancers? A meta-analysis of risk factors for intrahepatic cholangiocarcinoma. J Hepatol 2012; 57:69–76.
110. Darwish Murad, W.R. Kim, D.M. Harnois, et al. Efficacy of neoadjuvant chemoradiation, followed by liver transplantation, for

perihilar cholangiocarcinoma at 12 US centers Gastroenterology, 143 (2012), pp. 88-98

111. G. Sapisochin, N. Fidelman, J.P. Roberts, et al. Mixed hepatocellular cholangiocarcinoma and intrahepatic cholangiocarcinoma in patients undergoing transplantation for hepatocellular carcinoma Liver Transpl, 17 (2011), pp. 934-942
112. Robles R, Figueras J, Turrion VS, et al. Spanish experience in liver transplantation for hilar and peripheral cholangiocarcinoma. Ann Surg 2004; 239:265–271.
113. Boehm LM, Jayakrishnan TT, Miura JT, Zacharias AJ, Johnston FM, Turaga KK, Gamblin TC: Comparative effectiveness of hepatic artery based therapies for unresectable intrahepatic cholangiocarcinoma. J Surg Oncol 2015;111:213–220.
114. Ray CE Jr, Edwards A, Smith MT, Leong S, Kondo K, Gipson M, Rochon PJ, Gupta R, Messersmith W, Pur- cell T, Durham J: Metaanalysis of survival, complications, and imaging response following chemotherapy- based transarterial therapy in patients with unresectable intrahepatic cholangiocarcinoma. J Vasc Interv Radiol 2013;24:1218–1226.
115. Seidensticker R, Ricke J, Seidensticker M: Integration of chemoembolization and radioembolization into multimodal treatment of cholangiocarcinoma. Best Pract Research Clin Gastroenterol 2015;29:319–332.
116. Yang L, Shan J, Shan L, Saxena A, Bester L, Morris DL: Trans-arterial embolisation therapies for unresectable intrahepatic cholangiocarcinoma: a systematic review. J Gastrointest Oncol 2015;6:570–588.
117. Schiffman SC, Metzger T, Dubel G, et al. Precision hepatic arterial irinotecan therapy in the treatment of unresectable intrahepatic cholangiocellular carcinoma: optimal tolerance and prolonged overall survival. Ann Surg Oncol 2011; 18:431–438.
118. Burger, I., Hong, K., Schulick, R., Georgiades, C., Thuluvath, P., Choti, M., et. al, J. H. (2005). Transcatheter Arterial chemoembolization in unresectable cholangiocarcinoma: Initial experience in a single institution. *Journal of Vascular and Interventional Radiology, 16*(3), 353-361. doi:10.1097/01.rvi.0000143768.60751.78
119. Edeline J, Le Du F, Rayar M, et al. Glass microspheres 90y selective internal radiation therapy and chemotherapy as first-line treatment of intrahepatic cholangiocarcinoma. Clin Nucl Med 2015; 40: 851–855.
120. Konstantinidis IT, Groot Koerkamp B, Do RK, Gönen M, Fong Y, Allen PJ, D'Angelica MI, Kingham TP, DeMatteo RP, Klimstra DS, Kemeny NE, Jarnagin WR. Unresectable intrahepatic cholangiocarcinoma:

Systemic plus hepatic arterial infusion chemotherapy is associated with longer survival in comparison with systemic chemotherapy alone. Cancer. 2016 Mar 1;122(5):758-65. doi: 10.1002/cncr.29824. Epub 2015 Dec 22. PMID: 26695839; PMCID: PMC4764409

121. Chernyak V, Fowler KJ, Kamaya A, Kielar AZ, Elsayes KM, Bashir MR, et al. Liver imaging reporting and data system (li-rads) version 2018: imaging of hepatocellular carcinoma in at-risk patients. Radiology (2018) 289:816. doi: 10.1148/radiol.2018181494

CHAPTER 3

ABLATION IN PRIMARY HEPATIC LESIONS

BRANDON CUSTER MD

Introduction

Hepatocellular carcinoma (HCC), as discussed previously, is the sixth most common cancer in the world and fourth leading cause of cancer related death worldwide. Uniquely, liver cancer has also been steadily increasing in incidence of recent decades (1). The gold standard for management of liver masses is resection; however, because of anatomic limitations, the multifocal nature of the disease, insufficient functional liver reserve, or comorbidities, many patients are not surgical candidates. Due to the complex nature of hepatocellular carcinoma, leading hepatology societies around the world have developed treatment algorithms which include thermal ablation for curative intent, often as a first line treatment. For reasons described in the following chapter, microwave ablation has recently gained popularity over other thermal ablation techniques due to many reasons, including high temperature, fast ablation times, and less susceptibility to heat sink.

Common Ablation Techniques

Chemical – Percutaneous injection of sclerosant material to induce cell death. This was first described in 1983, with ethanol being the most well utilized and studied chemical ablation media. The injection of absolute ethanol into the tumor induces almost immediate coagulative necrosis at the cellular level due to dehydration and protein denaturation. Chemical ablation has been shown to be effective with small masses but commonly requires multiple treatments. Utilization is limited in larger tumors because of uneven diffusion of sclerosant throughout the tumor (2). Because of diffusion through the liver, it can be more difficult to control the treatment zone of chemical ablation compared to more contemporary techniques, which can lead to non-target ablation of healthy liver.

Thermal – Thermal ablation uses extreme temperature to induce cell death and has been growing in popularity over the years as a curative treatment option for early-stage hepatocellular carcinoma, not amenable to surgical resection. There are several types of thermal ablation which use differing mechanism of action to cause cell death. Radiofrequency ablation and Microwave ablation create extreme heat, with cell death occurring at 60 degrees Celsius. Cryoablation uses extreme cold, with cell death occurring at -20 degrees Celsius. Each ablative technique will be subsequently addressed.

Irreversible Electroporation (IRE) – IRE is a developing non-thermal ablative technique which offers some benefits compared to thermal ablation. With IRE, cell death is induced by applying a high-voltage current between antenna placed percutaneously around the target. This creates a strong external electric field that causes tiny pores to form in the cell membrane. The cell membrane loses its physiologic function and intracellular/extracellular solute transport becomes dysregulated, resulting in apoptosis. Thermal ablation techniques can be limited in efficacy because of heat sink effect and nontarget injury to adjacent structures, particularly bile ducts, blood vessels, the gallbladder, or bowel loops (3). In contrast, IRE induces cell death but does not affect the underlying extracellular matrix, allowing it to be more protective in treating sensitive areas.

Thermal Ablation

Radiofrequency Ablation- Radiofrequency ablation (RFA) is the most well established and researched of the available thermal ablation modalities. The effects of RFA on tissue was initially described as early as 1891, and its application was first applied to liver tumor in 1992. Radiofrequency is a portion of the electromagnetic spectrum between 3 Hz and 300 GHz (4). In its medical application, an RFA probe (Figure 1) acts as the cathode of an electrical circuit completed by pads placed on the patient's lower extremities. As an alternating current is applied, the dipolar water molecules in the tissue adjacent to the probe vibrate forcefully. This vibration leads to frictional heating between the molecules. Heat dispersion is then dependent upon thermal tissue conductivity and quickly tapers, which can limit the size of the ablation zone.

The greatest advantage of radiofrequency ablation is robust clinical research proving safe and effective treatment of liver masses, as it was adopted earliest of the thermal ablation techniques. This offers the provider and patients confidence in expected results, particularly in small liver masses measuring less than 3 cm in maximum dimension. Compared to other ablation techniques, RF is also relatively inexpensive, reducing cost to the hospital system and health care at large. Lastly, RF benefits from ubiquitous availability (5).

One major limitation of RF is that energy deposition is dependent on thermal conductivity. Conductive heating tapers quickly in tissue which limits RF ablation zone size at baseline. During treatment, other factors can further limit heat conduction. One factor is tissue charring and gas production due to extreme heat production during RF Ablation. Gas acts as an insulator and decreases thermal conduction and further reduces the size of effective treatment zone. RF is also susceptible to cooling effects of blood flow in adjacent vascular structures, of which there are many in the liver. This is commonly termed the "heat sink effect" and is a frequent cause of treatment failure using RF Ablation (6).

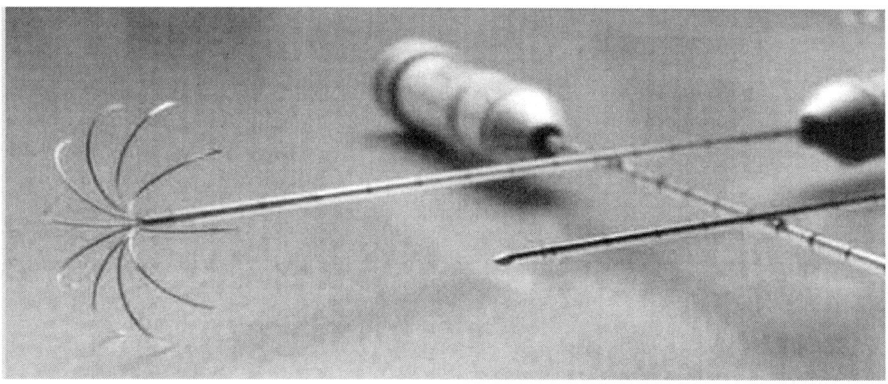

Figure 1: LeVeen (Boston Scientific, Nattick, MA) Radiofrequency antenna. The antenna introduced in the mass in the constrained position (Right) under imaging guidance. Once positioned, the tines can be extended to increase the size of the treatment zone.

Microwave Ablation – Microwave ablation (MWA) antenna (Figure 2) use a dielectric current to cause tissue heating and cell death. Like radiofrequency, microwaves are part of the electromagnetic energy spectrum. In contrast, the wavelengths are much shorter and therefore the frequency range is higher. Most microwaves are in the 900-2500 MHz range of the spectrum. The application of microwaves to tissue causes an oscillating electrical field that forces polar molecules, mostly water, to vibrate. This increases their kinetic energy and temperature. Unlike radiofrequency, which requires thermal conduction to disperse heat, microwaves are more adept at radiating through tissue. This means that microwaves are able to create a large treatment zone, better maintain the treatment zone size despite charring, and are better at heating a variety of tissue types regardless of specific impedance to conduction. Using multiple MWA antennas together can have synergistic effects and exponentially increase the effective treatment zone. Early MWA antenna' struggled with heat conduction along the shaft and resulted in skin burns. This has been greatly improved with modern systems that implement shaft cooling systems which utilize circulation of chilled saline or compressed gas (7).

The greatest advantage of MWA is decreased reliance on conductive heating, as microwaves are more effective at radiating through tissue. This means that MWA can create a larger effective treatment zone, with less tissue charring, and produce that treatment zone in much less time. It also means that microwaves are more effective in a larger range of tissues (lung, bone), independent of conductivity (8). The larger treatment zone equates to placement of less antenna and a decrease in associated complications. Reduced treatment times allows for more efficient use of procedure space, hospital personnel, and time under anesthesia (9). Ever increasing clinical data has also shown equal efficacy, safety, and survival compared RFA on small hepatic tumors (<3 cm). Due to the heating properties of MWA, there is also evidence of improved efficacy in larger tumors (8).

Clinically, MWA has many strengths over RFA. The largest limitations of MWA are cost and availability. Another limitation at our institution is the use of general anesthesia. The type of anesthesia (Moderate sedation vs Monitored anesthesia care vs General Anesthesia) used for microwave ablation is institution specific and dependent on multiple factors. While literature supports MWA may be performed using moderate sedation, many patients are unable to tolerate the associated pain/discomfort, leading to a trend of performing MWA under general anesthesia. The use of general anesthesia has its own risks which much be taken into account.

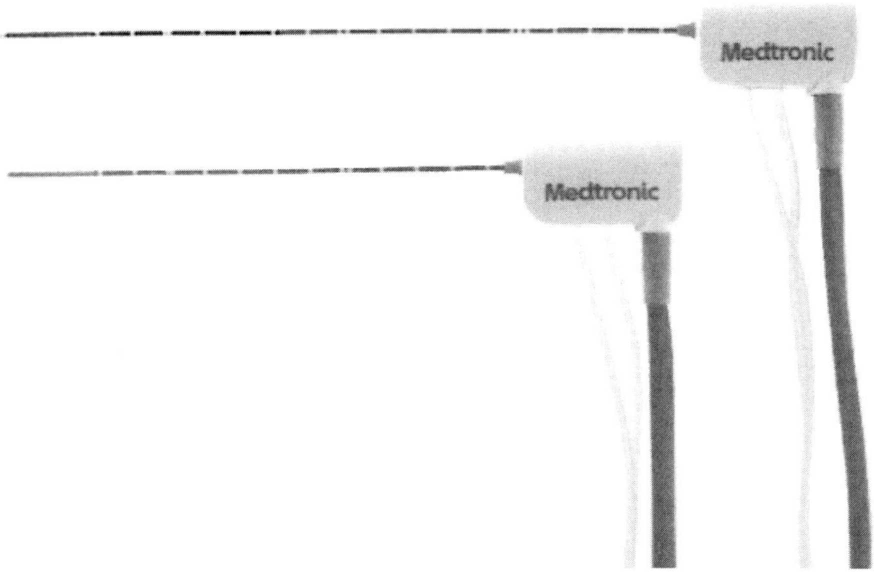

Figure 2: This is the Emprint Microwave ablation antenna (Medtronic). Because of the improved heat conduction through tissue, larger treatment zones can be obtained, even without tines.

Cryoablation – Cryoablation refers to induction of cell death through freezing. Once the cryoablation probe (Figure 3) or probes are positioned under imaging guidance, high pressure gas, most commonly argon, is forced though a small opening at the tip. The gas then rapidly expands to atmospheric pressure which induces rapid cooling by means of the Joule-Thompson effect, which states that rapid expansion of gas results in decrease in temperature. Cell death is caused through both direct cold-induced injury (protein denaturation) and indirect mechanisms (osmotic cellular dehydration from extracellular ice formation during freeze followed by fluid shifts during subsequent thaw which leads to cell rupture) from cold-induced changes in the surrounding structures. Almost all tissues exhibit cell death at temperatures below -20 degrees Celsius. Greater degrees of liquefactive necrosis have also been shown when using repeated freeze-thaw cycles (10). Treatment zones can be tailored by using antennae with different treatment shapes or using multiple antennae simultaneously with synergistic effects.

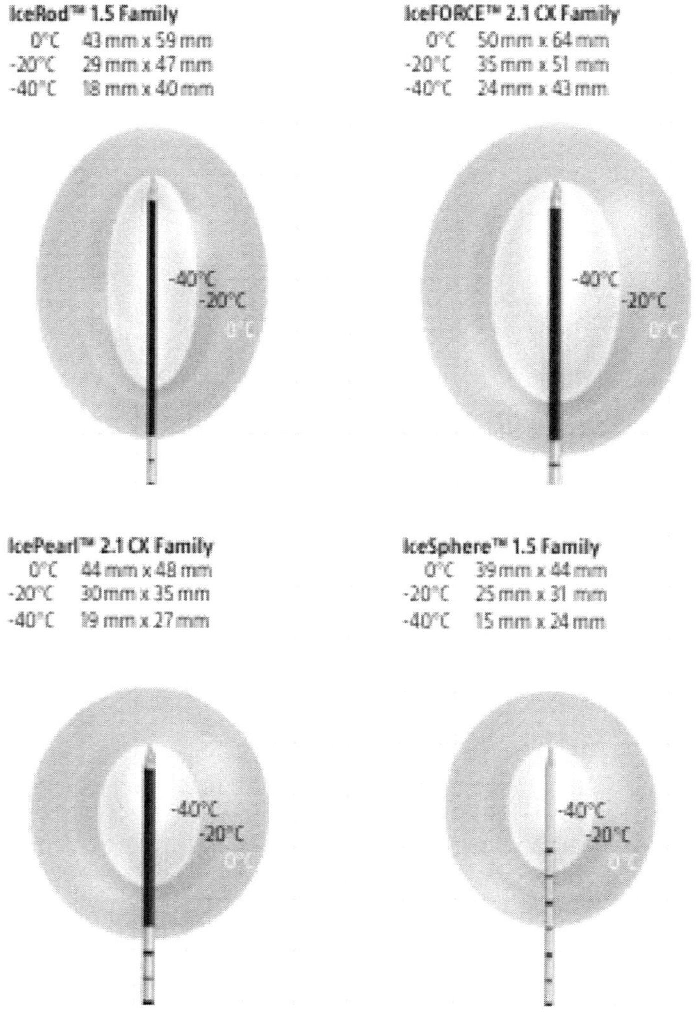

Cryoablation Product Catalogue (bostonscientific.com)

Figure 3: Example of different ablation zones created by cryoablation antenna (Boston Scientific, Nattick, MA). Unlike microwave ablation, where treatment zone is determined by power and duration of ablation, cryoablation zones are unique to the probe. The probe used is chosen to match the contour of the target lesion.

The most unique advantage of cryoablation compared to the other thermal techniques is the ability to visualize the ablation zone (11). The "ice ball" is visible under both CT and ultrasound, offering the provider confidence in the size of the treatment zone with a sufficient margin. Large ablation zones can also be obtained through the synergistic effects of multiple probes. Anecdotally, we find cryoablation to be better tolerated under moderate sedation. Some providers also feel as though cryoablation is less likely to cause non-target thermal injury to surrounding structures compared to RF or MWA.

Of thermal ablation techniques, cryoablation has the least robust clinical research verification proving safety, efficacy, or outcomes. Cryoablation treatment zones are also limited in size using a single antenna. Larger treatment zones can be obtained using several antennae synergistically, however this comes with increased procedural risks associated with the placement of multiple probes. Lastly, a major limitation is procedure time. Regardless of ablation zone size, all cryoablations require at least two freeze-thaw cycles to confidently cause cell death. Each cycle is a 10-minute freeze followed by 5-minutes of thawing.

Indications

The optimal treatment for any patient with liver malignancy is curative liver transplant or surgical resection. There are several different scoring criteria designed to help guide transplant centers in determining the appropriate utilization of transplant recipients. Each is institution specific, but common scoring criteria used are the Milan Criteria and the University of California San Francisco (UCSF) criteria. Minor differences in these criteria are listed in Table 1. Thermal ablation is indicated with curative intent as a stand-alone treatment in patients meeting transplant criteria, but who are not surgical candidates. It is also offered as a bridge therapy to transplant. Patients presenting outside of universal transplant criteria are more likely to be treated with endovascular therapies such as transarterial chemoembolization (TACE) or transarterial radioembolization (TARE).

Thermal Ablation is contraindicated in patients who can be treated with surgical resection. Other contraindications include vascular invasion by tumor, tumor location within 5 mm of a main bile duct, bile duct obstruction with dilation, widespread metastatic disease, and uncorrectable coagulopathy.

Milan Criteria	**UCSF Criteria**
• Single Tumor ≤ 5 cm, or • 2-3 tumors, none larger than 3 cm, and • No extrahepatic spread or vascular invasion	• Single Tumor ≤ 6.5 cm, or • 2-3 tumors, none larger than 4.5 cm, with total diameter ≤ 8 cm, and • No extrahepatic spread or vascular invasion

Table 1: The Milan Criteria and the UCSF criteria are the most commonly used criteria to determine liver transplant candidacy in patients with liver malignancy.

The American Association for the study of liver diseases (AASLD) further built off the Milan criteria and formulated a treatment algorithm to direct therapy for liver malignancy. A combination of tumor burden (Milan Criteria), liver function (Child-Pugh Classification, Table 2), and functional status (ECOG, Table 3) are used to determine treatment strategy in the Barcelona criteria liver cancer staging (BCLC, Table 4).

In general, thermal ablation is recommended for non-surgical patients within Milan Criteria, with generally good liver function (Child-Pugh A and B), with at least moderate functional status (ECOG < 3). This places thermal ablation in the curative intent section of the guidelines, with cure being achieved through ablation alone or by bridging to transplant. "Bridge to Transplant" is defined as a treatment designed to prevent intrahepatic disease progression and maintain the patient's curative transplant status within Milan criteria.

For more precise wording, the official AASLD guidelines state the following: (I) thermal ablation is the best modality for HCC smaller than 3 cm in diameter, with MWA now having the potential to show better tumoral control than RFA; (II) resection, local ablation, or transarterial chemoembolization (TACE) can be considered to minimize the risk of tumor progression as "bridge to transplant"; and (III) RFA or MWA may be considered as first-line treatment in very early-stage disease (BCLC 0) (13).

<table>
<tr><th>Clinical and Lab Criteria</th><th>1 point</th><th>2 points</th><th>3 points</th></tr>
<tr><td>Encephalopathy</td><td>None</td><td>Mild to Moderate</td><td>Severe</td></tr>
<tr><td>Ascites</td><td>None</td><td>Mild to Moderate (responsive to diuretics)</td><td>Severe (refractory to diuretics</td></tr>
<tr><td>Bilirubin (mg/dL)</td><td>< 2</td><td>2-3</td><td>>3</td></tr>
<tr><td>Albumin (g/dL)</td><td>>3.5</td><td>2.8-3.5</td><td><2.8</td></tr>
<tr><td>Prothrombin Time
INR</td><td><4
<1.7</td><td>4-6
1.7-2.3</td><td>>6
>2.3</td></tr>
<tr><td colspan="4">Child Pugh Classification calculated by adding total score
• Class A: 5-6 points, low operative mortality <5%
• Class B: 7-9 points, Moderate operative mortality 25%
• Class C: 10-15 points, High operative mortality > 50%</td></tr>
</table>

Table 2 – The Child Pugh classification system is designed to assess the prognosis of patients with chronic liver disease. It can be used to assess overall liver function and predict perioperative mortality associated with procedures.

Grade	Eastern Cooperative Oncology Group (ECOG)
0	Fully active, no restriction to function.
1	Restricted in physically strenuous activity, but ambulatory and able to carry out light work (i.e., house work and office work).
2	Ambulatory and up and about more than 50% of waking hours, capable of self care but incapable of any work activities.
3	Capable of only limited self care, confined to bed or chair >50% of waking hours.
4	Completely disabled, no ability to self care. Entirely bedbound.
5	Dead.

Table 3: The Eastern Cooperative Oncology Group (ECOG) created this scoring system in 1982 to evaluate a patient's level of function and ability to care for themselves. It has become the accepted gold standard for this task.

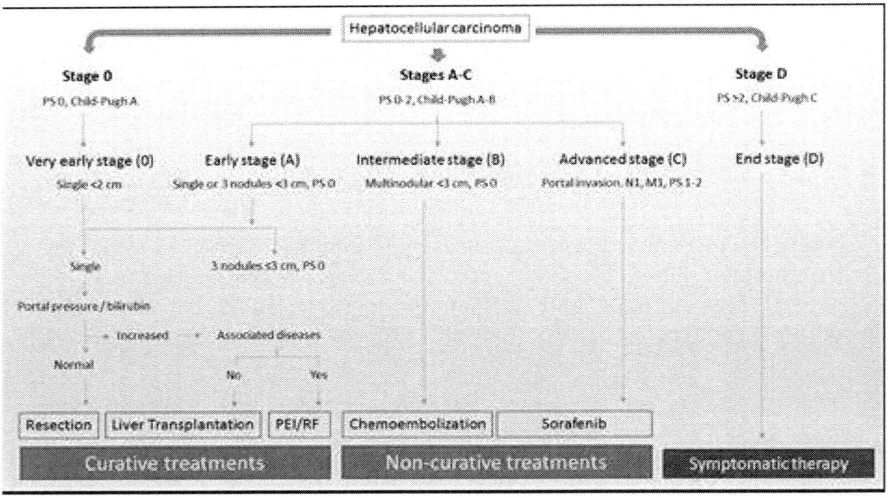

Table 4: This flow chart outlines the Barcelona criteria, a treatment algorithm for liver malignancy designed by the American Association for the study of Liver Diseases (AASLD)

Complications

Many studies have described safety and efficacy of thermal ablation in the liver. Major post procedure complications are rare (2.2%) including death (0.3%), peritoneal hemorrhage, tumor seeding, intrahepatic abscess requiring drainage, and intestinal perforation. The most common of these complications is abscess. Typically, if an abscess develops, the patient will represent at a range of 8 days to 5 months. The risk of abscess increases greatly in patients without a competent sphincter of Oddi. This will be further discussed later in the pre-procedure workup section of the chapter. Minor complications are also rare and occur in <5% of ablations. While not a true complication, it is important to discuss the development of Post-Ablation syndrome with your patients. Post ablation syndrome includes the development of low grade fever, nausea, vomiting, malaise, and myalgias which peaks about 5 days after the procedure and may last up to 2 weeks. Some studies report some level of post-ablation syndrome in up to 95% of ablations.

Outcomes

Several factors contribute to the efficacy of thermal ablation with tumor size and location having the strongest correlation with treatment outcome. In patients with solitary lesion less than 3 cm in size, overall survival is 50 months. With a solitary tumor greater than 3 cm, overall survival is reduced to 22 months (5).

Over the past decade, comparative studies have shown excellent outcomes and less adverse effects when comparing thermal ablation with surgical resection (14-22). Historically, metanalyses demonstrate no significant difference in survival rates between ablation and resection (23), but with ablation having inferior local tumor control. However, more recent studies have shown significant improvement in overall survival at five years with ablation (79.0% in masses < 2cm and 70.9 percent in masses > 2 cm), which is likely due to technological advancements in ablation and the development of post ablation antiviral therapies (24,25). A large study from 2019 comparing RFA with surgical resection for HCC including 18,296 subjects found ablation was superior to resection in terms of hospital stay duration, unplanned readmission, and 1-3 month mortality (25).

Most comparative studies between types of thermal ablation have contrasted MWA and RFA. Several retrospective comparative studies comparing MWA and RFA have shown no significant difference in survival between the two modalities, although some of the studies did show better local tumor control with MWA (26-29). There is no statistical difference in complication rates. The conclusion is that both MWA and RFA are suitable options for early stage HCC, but that MWA is more promising due to its higher thermal efficiency (30). Cryoablation and IRE are promising tools for safe ablation with studies showing similar efficacy, but more clinical data is needed to accurately compare them to RFA and MWA.

Adjuvant Locoregional Endovascular Treatment

Combining treatment modalities by concurrently treating with thermal ablation and an endovascular embolization (Bland Embolization, TACE, DEB-TACE) may have a synergistic effect. The ablation may sensitize tumor cells to chemotherapy and improve efficacy. As thermal ablation alone is highly effective on small tumors (<3 cm), this is most relevant for the treatment of larger masses. Studies have shown excellent tumor necrosis of 90% in masses treated with combination therapy. Most importantly, the rate of necrosis remains high on tumors greater than 3 cm. (31). The data suggests that combination therapy can be used effectively in tumors greater than 3 cm in size.

Our institution utilizes adjuvant DEB-TACE with Doxorubicin per provider preference, when treating masses that are variable in size, typically with 3-5 cm maximum dimension. These are performed in adjunct on the same day as an outpatient, but many studies consider combination therapy to be interventions performed within 2 weeks of each other (32). Ablation can be performed with either MWA or RFA, with some studies showing greater tumor necrosis when MWA is used in masses 3-5 cm in size, but no differences in overall survival, which is 27 months (32). Similar approaches performed on tumors up to 7 cm size have also showed significant improvements in overall survival when using combination embolization-ablation (33).

Procedure Planning

Any patient being considered for thermal ablation must undergo a full outpatient clinic visit for history and physical exam, discussion of the procedure risks, benefits, outcomes, and review of imaging. Functional status is evaluated at the clinic visit, also determining any limitations to patient positioning for the procedure through physical exam. This evaluation is vital in preparing a safe, successful, and uncomplicated procedure. During the clinic visit, relevant labs should also be reviewed including hematologic evaluation, coagulation panel, liver enzymes, bilirubin, albumin, creatinine. Laboratory analysis should be obtained within 30 days of the procedure.

The clinic visit should include a review of the patients past medical history with a particular interested in any prior biliary interventions. Patients without a competent sphincter of Oddi commonly have bacterial colonization of the biliary tree with enteric bacteria. These patients are high risk for biliary abscess after thermal ablation. Common causes for incompetent sphincter of Oddi include biliary stent placement, internal external biliary drain placement, prior sphincterotomy, or prior surgical hepaticojejunostomy. Patient with a high risk of biliary abscess formation should be treated with a prolonged course of outpatient antibiotics both before and after the procedure. There is no consensus antibiotic of choice in the Society of Interventional Radiology (SIR) literature; however, gram negative coverage is needed. At our institution, we use Levaquin 500 mg BID for 10 days before and 10 days after the procedure.

Up to date imaging is important in planning the procedure. At our institution we require liver mass protocol contrast enhanced MRI or CT within three months of the procedure date (Figure 4). Imaging is reviewed at the preprocedural clinic appointment to determine the size and number of masses, the location of the masses, the proximity of masses to vascular structures, and the proximity of masses to surrounding abdominal organs. Close proximity to vascular structures may reduce treatment efficacy due to heat sink, as detailed previously. Surrounding structures can be at risk of non-target thermal injury. The most worrisome some organ for non-target injury is the colon. It is more sensitive to thermal injury compared to the stomach or small bowel. A careful review of the imaging can help you determines treatment approach, the need for biopsy, and the possibility of needing advanced techniques to displace surrounding structures.

The clinic visit allows a complete review of all medications. Per SIR guidelines, deep intraprocedural biopsy or microwave ablation is considered a high bleeding risk procedure. This means target platelets of 50k, INR <1.7-2.0, and a hold of all anticoagulation until the patient is not therapeutic. The duration of hold varies based on the anticoagulant. Updated labs are necessary within 30 days of the procedure. Besides bleeding and infection, low risks for pneumothorax, bile duct injury, bile duct stenosis, and tumor seeding should be presented.

One major benefit to the safety profile of thermal ablation is the ability to be performed under conscious sedation or monitored anesthesia care. Literature has shown all types of thermal ablation to be tolerated at this level of sedation. We have anecdotal experience that patient's do not always tolerate MWA or RFA well using only conscious sedation, necessitating a multi-disciplinary approach with anesthesia. Cryoablation may be performed under conscious sedation. IRE requires general anesthesia. Ultimately the type of anesthesia used for ablation procedures will be institution specific.

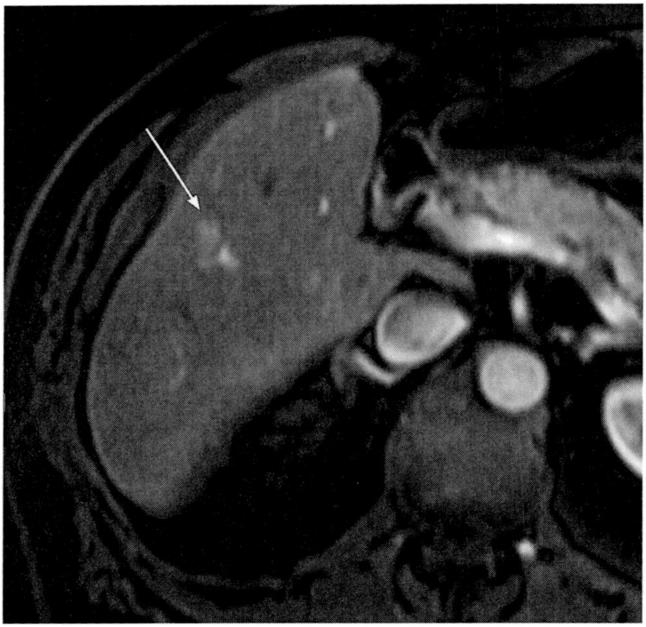

Figure 4: This is a good example of an ideal mass for treatment with Thermal Ablation. It is a small mass (< 3cm) located near the periphery of the liver, away from large bile ducts and vascular structures. The expectation is this lesion could be effectively treated with curative intent in a single ablation treatment.

Procedure

Thermal ablation is performed in the outpatient setting in most circumstances. The patient should arrive to the department at least one hour prior to the procedure start time. This allows time to review all relevant labs and ensure anesthesia adequate time to re-evaluate the patient prior to the procedure, as applicable. Per SIR consensus guidelines, periprocedural antibiotics should be provided within one hour of the procedure in all patients undergoing thermal ablation. The antibiotic can vary by institution or provider but gram-negative coverage is necessary. SIR provides a low-level recommendation of Cafazolin 1-2 g IV x 1 (34). As discussed above, a prolonged pre and post procedural antibiotic regimen is recommended for patients with increased risk of biliary abscess formation.

Once the patient has been sedated and positioned as desired, thermal ablation antenna placement can be guided by CT, Ultrasound, or MRI. At our institution we do almost all thermal ablation under CT Guidance (Figure 5). When choosing the optimal trajectory for antenna placement, there are several factors to consider. First is determining a safe percutaneous path to the target mass without traversing pleura, bowel, or major vascular structures. Next is determining the size and shape of the target lesion. Ideal positioning requires the antenna along the long axis of the mass. Most devices create the largest dimension of extreme temperature along the course of the antenna, extending back from the tip. If multiple overlapping treatment zones are required to obtain adequate margins of 5-10 mm, this can easily be performed simply by retracting the antenna. One must consider the size of the anticipated treatment zone and the risk for nontarget thermal injury to surrounding structures. The goal is to have no hollow viscera (stomach, small bowel, colon) within 1 cm of the anticipated ablation zone.

A)

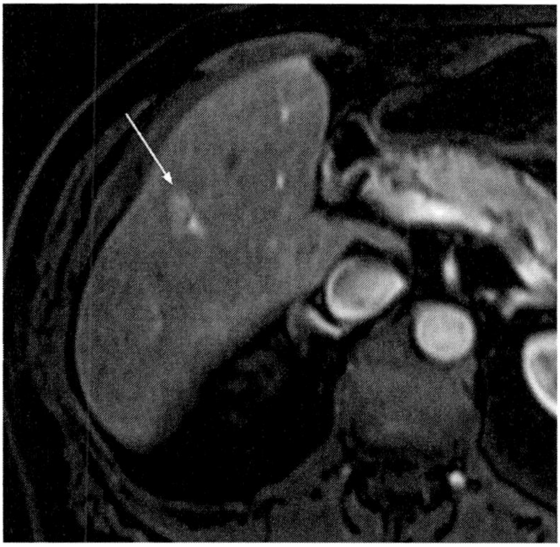

B)

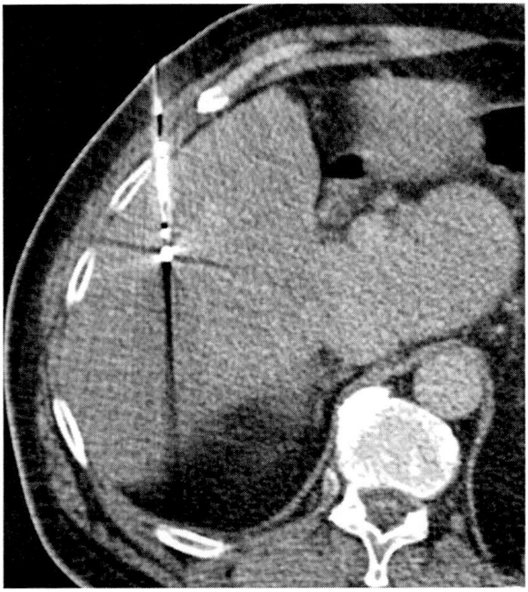

C)

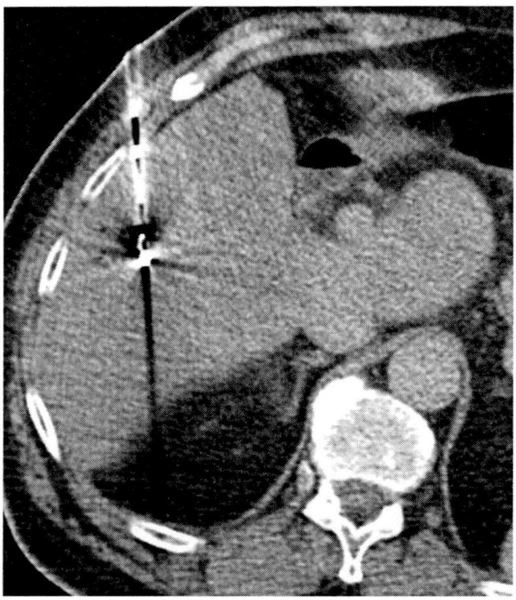

D)

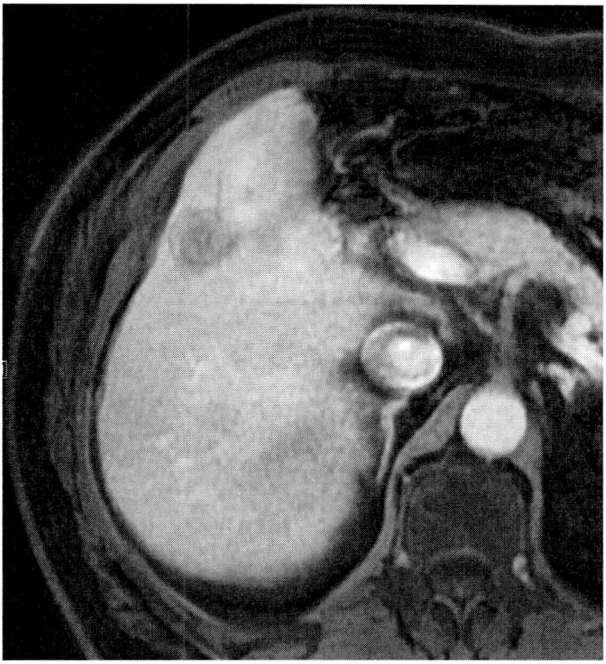

Figure 5: A) Preprocedure MRI showing a small solitary enhancing mass in the right hepatic lobe. B) CT guided positioning of the ablation antenna. The antenna is advanced to the distal aspect of the mass, as the ablation zone forms back from the tip. C) CT performed during ablation shows the formation of gas extending back from the tip. D) Post Procedural MRI showing a well-treated lesion. There is now a void of enhancement. The lesion appears larger because of a treatment zone and margin. This scan will serve as a new baseline for future surveillance.

There are several advanced techniques (Figure 6) that can be used to create a safe treatment margin when hollow abdominal viscera are within 1 cm of the ablation zone. The most well described is hydro-dissection. This involves placement of a needle into the space between the liver mass and bowel of concern. 5% Dextrose solution (D5) is then injected, commonly over 100 mL, to displace the bowel loops and create a safe margin. The use of D5 was historically important with RF Ablation, as the non-polar liquid is non-conductive. While this is less vital for modern Microwave Ablation, D5 is still used at our institution out of practice.

If hydro-dissection is unsuccessful, another option is the placement of high compliance balloon into the target space and inflating the balloon to displace the at-risk bowel. Through a hollowed needle, a microwire can be advanced. The needle is then exchanged for a transitional dilator, followed by a 0.035 working wire. The balloon is then advanced into position over the wire. The inflated balloon will displace the bowel and create a safe margin for ablation.

A)

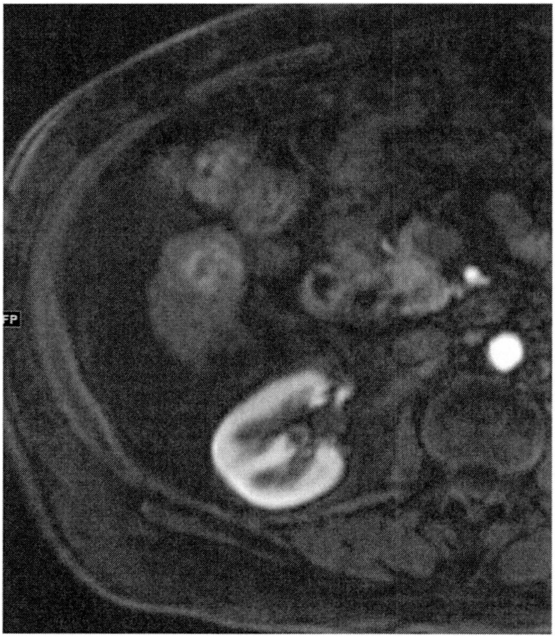

B)

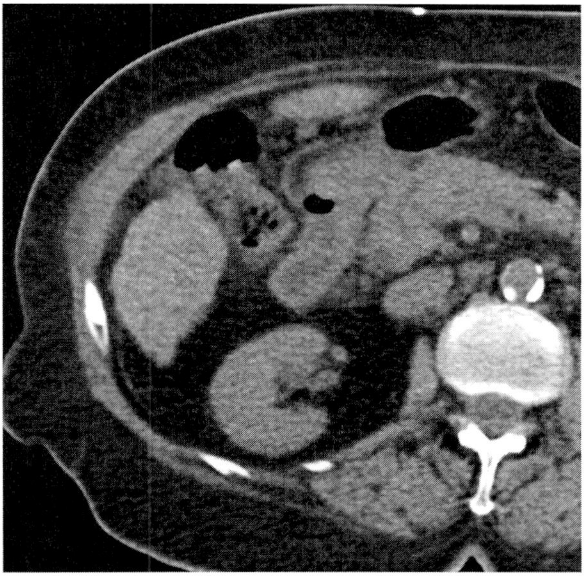

C)

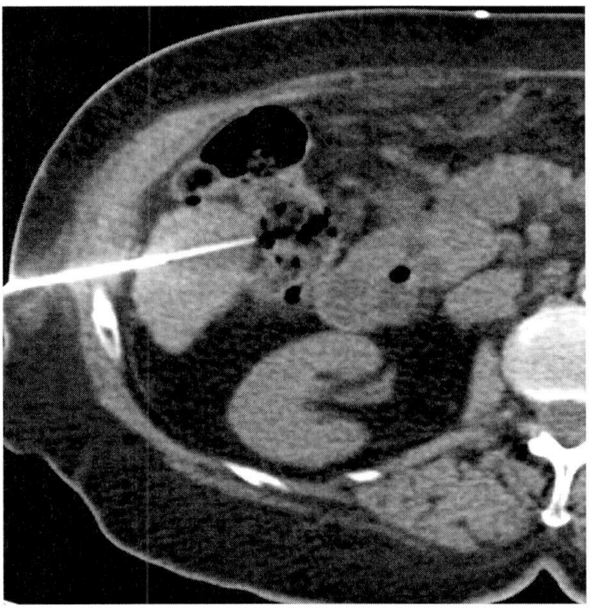

D)

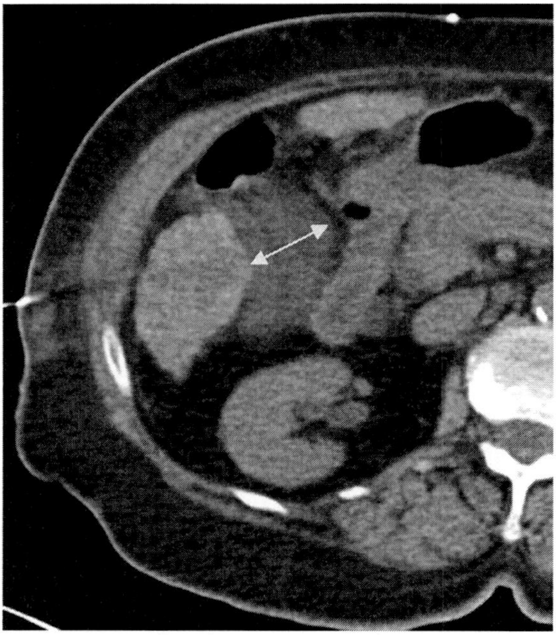

E)

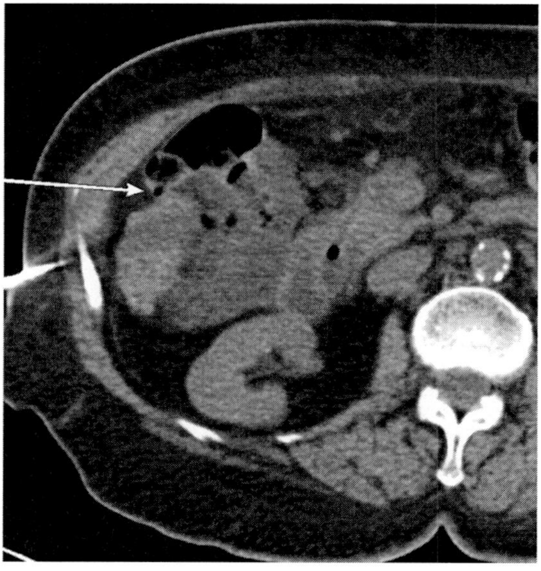

F)

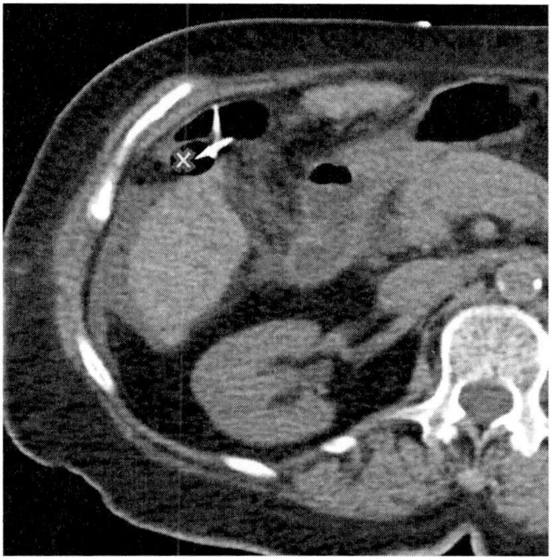

G)

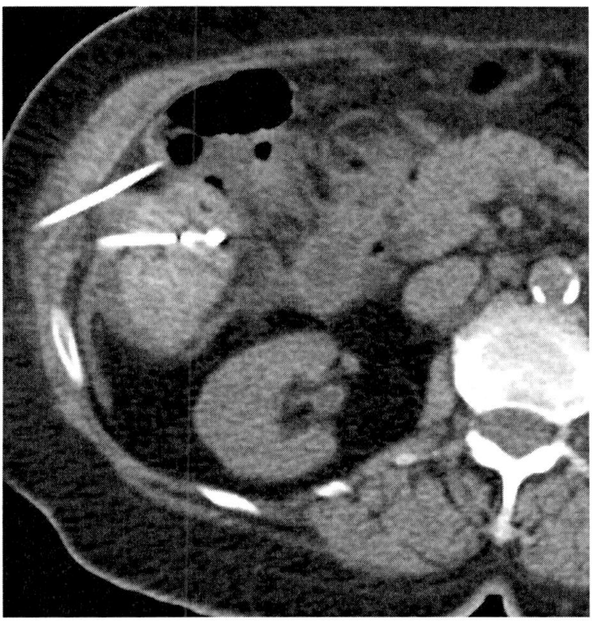

H)

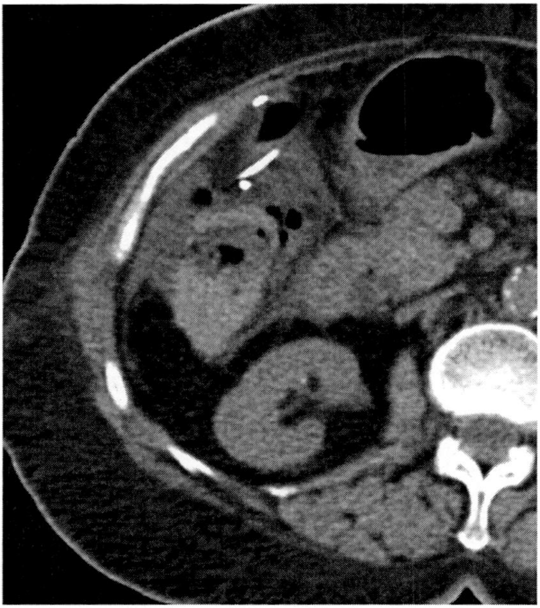

Figure 6: A) Preprocedural MRI showing a small arterially enhancing mass in the caudal tip of the right hepatic lobe. B) Procedural CT showing the mass with the adjacent hepatic flexure of colon within 1 cm of the anticipated treatment zone. C) A 22-gauge hollowed needle is advanced under CT guidance to the space between the mass and the colon. D) 5% Dextrose in water is injected to move colon a safe distance from the treatment zone. E) A small amount of colon (arrow) remains in close proximity to the treatment zone. F) After an 18-gauge hollowed needle is used to advance a 0.035 Amplatz wire between the colon and liver mass, the needle is exchanged for a balloon. The balloon is position under CT and inflated (x) to move the remaining colon a safe distance away and G) the ablation antenna is advanced through the central portion of the mass.H) Post ablation demonstrates gas and treatment zone that has replaced the mass.

Once you have optimally positioned the ablation antenna a safe treatment can be performed. Microwave ablation zones are determined by information provided by each specific vendor. Treatment times usually vary between 1-10 minutes with wattages between 60-100 W. Ablation zone size increases as power and duration increase and each power/time combination can create a different size ablation zone. Most modern microwave ablation antennas create ablation zones that are nearly spherical. With cryoablation, the shape of the ablation zone is determined by the type of antenna, with each manufacturer creating antennas of various shapes from spherical to elongated ovoid. The antenna you choose should be guided by the tumor shape and your desired treatment zone. For cryoablation, the antenna is what determines the ablation zone size/shape and all cryoablation requires two cycles of a 10-minute freeze followed by a 5-minute thaw, for a total ablation time of 30 minutes.

During ablation, an observatory CT can be performed at any interval of anticipated ablation time to confirm antenna position and potential adverse events. This is particularly important with patients who are deep breathers, as the motion can displace the antenna. This can also confirm the presence of gas when performing microwave ablation which confirms heat production. It is important to remember that gas formation is a poor correlate for overall ablation zone size. With cryoablation, you should be able to visualize the ice-ball being formed by the antenna and confirm coverage of the tumor with acceptable margins.

After satisfactory completion of the procedure, most modern microwave and cryoablation antenna have functionality to perform tract ablation. For MWA, heat is continually applied as the antenna is slowly retracted to the liver margin. Performing tract ablation has two purposes. One is the treatment of any potential track seeded tumor implants. The other is cauterization of blood vessels the antenna may have crossed, decreasing bleeding risk of the procedure. Cryoablation utilizes a de-thawing mechanism in a similar fashion.

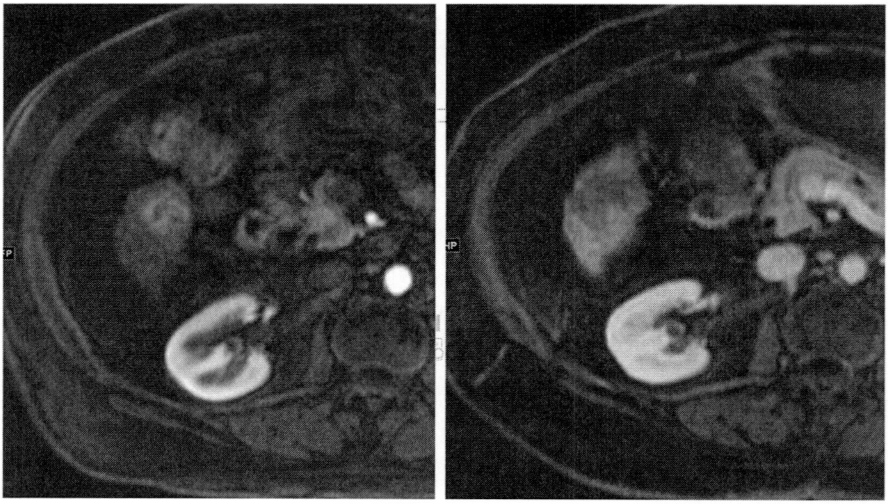

Figure 7: Pre (left) and Post (right) procedure MRI Images of the mass treated above. We see that the previously enhancing mass is now a void of enhancement with an appropriate treatment margin and no injuries to surrounding structures.

Post Procedure

Patients are observed in the post procedural area for 2-6 hours following the procedure depending on technical factors and provider preference. In the immediate post-procedural time, bleeding is the most significant complication for which to monitor. During this time, there should be continuous cardiac monitoring and frequent vitals (15-30 minutes). Prior to discharge, the patient should meet criteria which will be institution specific, but typically includes the patient being at baseline hemodynamics, tolerating oral intake, pain control, and passing urine. Once meeting the outlined criteria, the patient can be discharged home as an outpatient. Pain in the right upper quadrant and referred pain to the right shoulder should be anticipated. Patients can be re-assured that, while pain can rarely last up to two weeks. Immediate post procedure pain typically significantly improves within 48 hours and can be managed with oral pain medications.

Post ablation syndrome is common, occurring in up to one-third of patients. The patient can develop flu-like symptoms with low-grade fever, malaise, myalgia, nausea, and vomiting for 7-10 days after the procedure. Typically, we provide a short course of oxycodone and Zofran to manage post ablation symptoms. Worsening pain or new/worsening fevers after post-operative day 14 should raise concern for post-operative infection and may require further diagnostic workup for abscess formation.

Imaging surveillance for treatment response is frequent over the first two years. We perform post-operative cross-section imaging at 1, 3, 6, 9, 12, 18, and 24 months. There is no societal consensus for modality of post procedural imaging between CT or MRI. Imaging should be performed with contrast using a liver mass protocol including non-contrast, arterial phase, portal venous phase, and delayed phase series. It is not unexpected for the target lesion to appear larger in size on initial post treatment scan due to the treatment margin. Imaging features of a well-treated mass include smooth peripheral enhancement and high density internal necrotic material (Figure 7). The first post-treatment scan serves as a new baseline going forward. Tumor growth is not expected and should raise concern for recurrence. Any nodular enhancement (Figure 8) is also highly suspicious for residual/recurrent viable tumor and should be targeted with further therapy.

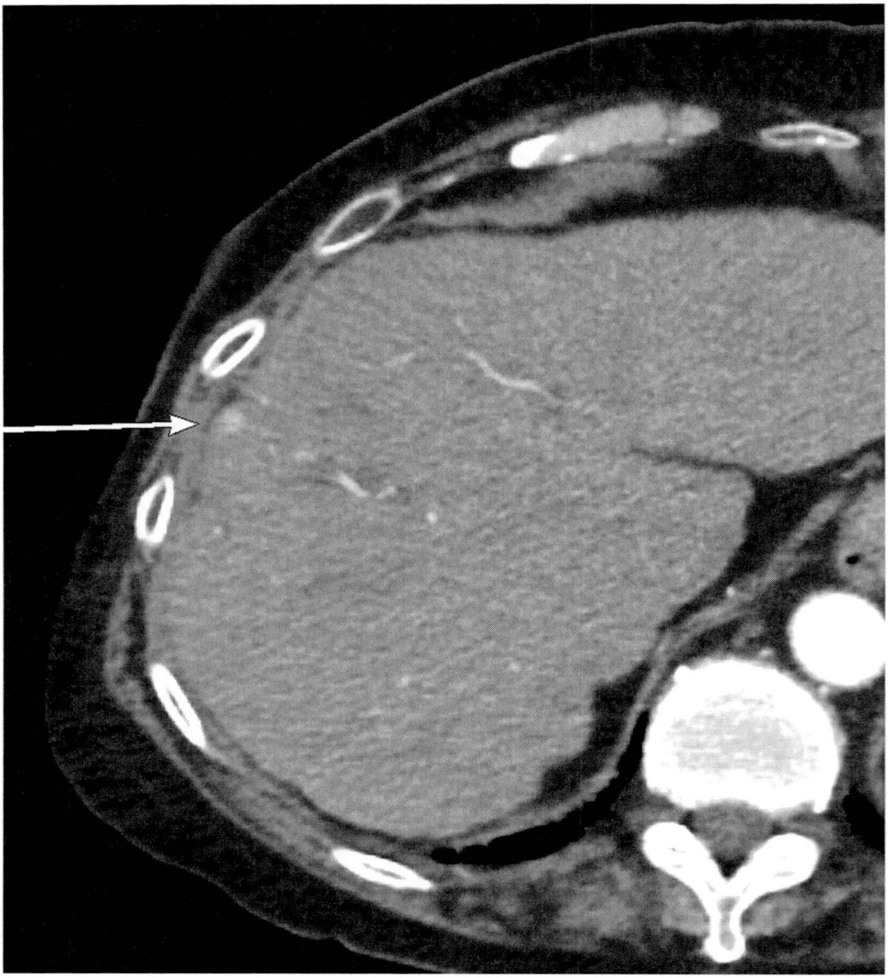

Figure 8: Surveillance imaging for a patient previously treated with thermal ablation to a right hepatic lobe mass shows a focus of nodular enhancement along the margin of the treatment cavity. This is highly concerning for recurrent disease and should be targeted for further treatment.

References

1. Parkin DM, Bray F, et al. Global Cancer statistics, 2002. CA Cancer J Clinic 2005; 55:74-108
2. Lee MJ, Mueller JR, et al. Percutaneous Ethanol Injection for the Treatment of Hepatic Tumors: Indications, Mechanism of Action, Technique, and Efficacy. 1995. American Journal of Roentgenol; 164: 215-220
3. Hsiao CY, Huang KW. Irreversible Electroporation: A Novel Ultrasound-Guided Modality for Non-thermal Tumor Ablation. 2017. Journal of Medical Ultrasound; 25: 195-200
4. Hong K, Georgiades CS. Radiofrequency Ablation: Mechanism of Action and Devices. 1 Radiofrequency Ablation: Mechanism of Action and Devices | Radiology Key
5. Izzo F, Granat V, et al. Radiofrequency Ablation and Microwave Ablation in Liver Tumors: An Update. 2019. The Oncologist; 24: 990-1005.
6. Pillai K, Akhter J, et al. Heat Sink Effect on Tumor Ablation Characteristics as Observed in Monopolar Radiofrequency, Bipolar Radiofrequency, and Microwave, Using Ex Vivo Calf Liver Model. 2015. Medicine; 94: 1-10
7. Lubner M, Brace C, et al. Microwave Tumor Ablation: Mechanism of Action, Clinical Results and Devices. 2010. J Vasc Interv Radiology; 21: 192-203
8. Brace CL. Radiofrequency and microwave ablation of the liver, lung, kidney, and bone: What are the differences? 2009. Curr Probl Diagn Rodiology; 38: 135-143
9. Awad M, Devgan L, et al. Microwave Ablation in a hepatic porcine model: correlation of CT and histopathologic findings. 2007. HPB; 9: 357-362
10. Erinjeri JP. Cryoablation: Mechanism of Action and Devices. 2010. J Vasc Interv Radiology; 21: 187-191.
11. Uppot RN, Silverman SG, et al. Imaging-guided percutaneous ablation of renal cell carcinoma: a primer of how we do it. 2009. Am J Roentgenol; 192:1558-1570
12. Omata M, Cheng AL, et al. Asia -acific clinical practice guidelines on the management of hepatocellular carcinoma: a 2017 update. 2017. Heatol Int; 11: 317-370
13. Zhu F, Rhim H. Thermal Ablation for hepatocellular carcinoma: What's new in 2019. 2019. Chin Clin Oncol; 8(6): 58

14. Huang J, Yan L, et al. A randomized trial comparing radiofrequency ablation and surgical resection for HCC conforming to the Milan Criteria. 2010. Ann Surg; 252:903-912
15. Shiina S, Rareishi R, et al. Radiofrequency ablation for hepatocellular carcinoma: 10-year outcome and prognostic factors. 2012. Am J Gastroenterol; 107:569-77
16. Kim YS, Lim HK, et al. Ten-year outcomes of percutaneous radiofrequency ablation as first-line therapy of early hepatocellular carcinoma: analysis of prognostic factors. 2013. J Hepatol; 58: 89-97
17. Cuchetti a, Piscaglia F, et al. Cost-Effectiveness of hepatic resection vs percutaneous radiofrequency ablation for early hepatocellular carcinoma. 2013. J Hepatol; 59: 300-307
18. Qi X, Zhao Y, et al. Management of hepatocellular carcinoma: an overview of major findings from meta-analyses. 2016. Oncotarget; 7: 34703-34751
19. Majumdar A, Roccarina D, et al. A randomized trial comparing radiofrequency ablation and surgical resection for HCC conforming to the Milan criteria. 2010. Ann Surg; 252: 903-912
20. Feng K, Yan J, et al. A randomized controlled trial of radiofrequency ablation and surgical resection in the treatment of small hepatocellular carcinoma. 2012. J Hepatol; 57: 794-802
21. Chen MS, Li JQ, et al. A prospective randomized trial comparing percutaneous local ablative therapy and partial hepatectomy for small hepatocellular carcinoma. 2006. Ann Surg; 243: 321-328
22. Wang Y, Luo Q, et al. Radiofrequency ablation versus hepatic resection for small hepatocellular carcinomas: a meta-analysis of randomized and nonrandomized controlled trials. 2014. PloS One; 9: e84484
23. Yu J, Liang P, et al. A comparison of microwave ablation and bipolar radiofrequency ablation both with an internally cooled probe: results in ex vivo and in vivo porcine livers. 2011. Eur J Radiol; 79: 124-130
24. Sohn W, Kang TW, et al. Effect of oral antiviral treatment on long-erm outcomes of radiofrequency ablation therapy for hepatitis B virus-related hepatocellular carcinoma. 2016. Oncotarget; 7: 47794-47807.
25. Uhlig J, Sellers CM, et al. Radiofrequency ablation versus surgical resection of hepatocellular carcinoma: contemporary treatment trends and outcomes from the United States National Cancer Database. 2019. Eur Radiol; 29: 2679-89
26. Potretzke TA, Ziemlewicz TJ, et al. Microwave versus radiofrequency ablation treatment for hepatocellular carcinoma: a comparison of efficacy at a single center. 2016. J Vasc Interv Radiol; 27: 631-638

27. Zhang L, Wang N, et al. Therapeutic efficacy of percutaneous radiofrequency ablation versus microwave ablation for hepatocellular carcinoma. 2013. PloS One; 8: e76119
28. Ding J, Jing X, et al. Comparison of two different thermal techniques for the treatment of hepatocellular carcinoma. 2013. Eur J Radiol; 82: 1379-1384
29. Qian GJ, Wang N, et al. Efficacy of microwave versus radiofrequency ablation for treatment of small hepatocellular carcinoma: experimental and clinical studies. 2012. Eur Radiol; 22: 1983-1990
30. Yu J, Yu XL, et al. Percutaneous colled-probe microwave versus radiofrequency ablation in early-stage hepatocellular carcinoma. A phase III randomized controlled trial. 2017. Gut; 66: 1172-1173
31. Vasnani R, Ginsburg M, et al. Radiofrequency and microwave ablation in combination with transarterial chemoembolization induce equivalent histopathologic coagulation necrosis in hepatocellular carcinoma patients bridged to liver transplantation. 2016. Hepatobiliary Surg Nutr; 5: 225-233
32. Abdelaziz AO, Abdelmaksoud AH, et al. Transarterial chemoembolization combined with either radiofrequency or microwave ablation in management of hepatocellular carcinoma. 2017. Pac J Cancer; 18: 189-194
33. YiY, Zhang Y, et al. Radiofrequency ablation or microwave ablation combined with transcatheter arterial chemoembolization in treatment of hepatocellular carcinoma by comparing with radiofrequency ablation alone. 2014. Chin J Cancer Res; 26: 112-118
34. Chehab m, Thakor A, et al. Adult and Pediatric Antibiotic Prophylaxis during Vascular and IR Procedures. A Society of Interventional Radiology Practice Parameter Update Endorsed by the Cardiovascular and Interventional Radiological Society of Europe and Canadian Association for Interventional Radiology. 2018. J Vasc Interv Radiol; 29: 1483-1501

CHAPTER 4

HEPATIC VASCULAR ANATOMY AND VARIANTS

ADAM ALLI MD, NICOLETTE DUMAS MD, VINCE GALATE MSIV

Celiac Artery

The celiac artery arises from the abdominal aorta, inferior to the diaphragmatic crura, at the level of T12-L1. The celiac artery supplies the stomach, duodenum, liver, spleen, and pancreas with important collateral vessels to the superior mesenteric artery (SMA). Traditional anatomy is seen approximately (63%) of the time. (1) Traditional celiac artery anatomy has been described as either a trifurcation of the left gastric, common hepatic, and splenic arteries and/or as bifurcation of left gastric and hepatosplenotrunk with further bifurcation into common hepatic and splenic arteries. Most authors consider traditional anatomy the latter; a bifurcation of the left gastric artery and hepatosplenotrunk with further bifurcation into splenic and common hepatic. (2, 3, 4) That is the definition that will be used in this text.

Celiac artery variations

Of the three main mesenteric arteries, the celiac artery is most likely to have variant anatomy as compared to either the superior mesenteric or inferior mesenteric arteries. In general, celiac artery variations can be broken down into three groups: complete celiac trunk, incomplete celiac trunk, and absence of the celiac trunk. (5) There are fifteen described variants of the celiac artery in the literature. Incomplete celiac trunk comprises six of the fifteen anatomic variations. Absence of the celiac trunk comprising eight of the fifteen variants. The last variant is ambiguous anatomy which includes all other variations that are very atypical and do not fit into the prior fourteen classifications. (3, 5, 6)

By far, the most common variation in the celiac trunk is with the hepatosplenic trunk arising from the aorta with the left gastric arising separately from the aorta. The next most common variation of the celiac trunk is to have a left gastric and splenic trunk arising from the aorta with the common hepatic arising separately from the aorta. The next most common variation is a common origin of the celiac trunk and the superior mesenteric arteries. The remainder of the variations are very rare and are listed in table below. (2, 3, 4, 5, 6, 7)

Anatomic Variations of Celiac Trunk (%)

Incomplete Celiac Trunk:	
Hepatosplenic trunk with left gastric replaced to the aorta	4.4%
Gastrosplenic trunk with common hepatic replaced to the aorta	2.6%
Gastrosplenic trunk with common hepatic replaced to the aorta, normal SMA	<1%
Hepatogastric trunk with the splenic artery replaced to the SMA	<<1%
Hepatogastric trunk with the splenic artery replaced to the aorta, normal SMA	<<1%
Hepatosplenic trunk with the left gastric artery replaced to the SMA	<<1%

Common origin of the celiac and superior mesenteric arteries	1.1%
Left gastric replaced to the aorta with common origin of superior mesenteric, common hepatic and splenic arteries	<1%
Left gastric and splenic arteries separately replaced to the aorta with common hepatic artery replaced to the superior mesenteric artery.	<1%
Common hepatic, splenic, and left gastric replaced separately to the aorta with a normal SMA	<1%
Common hepatic replaced to the aorta with the left gastric and splenic arteries replaced to the SMA	<1%
Common hepatic and left gastric replaced separately to the aorta with the splenic replaced to the SMA	<1%
Common origin of the common hepatic, gastric, and SMA with splenic artery replaced to the aorta	<<<1%
Common hepatic and splenic arteries separately replaced to the aorta with the left gastric replaced to the SMA	<<<1%

Anatomic Variations of the Hepatic Arteries

The common hepatic artery traditionally arises from the hepatosplenic trunk and conventionally branches into the gastroduodenal artery and the proper hepatic artery. The proper hepatic artery then bifurcates into the left and right hepatic arteries. (8) The cystic artery has the greatest variability in this vascular bed, but usually arises from the right hepatic artery. The normal branching pattern of the hepatic arteries, as described, is seen approximately 67% of the time. The most common variations of the hepatic arteries are described below. These anatomic variations can include replaced or accessory vessels to any of the mesenteric vessels. (2, 3, 4, 6, 9, 10)

Anatomic Variations of the Hepatic Arteries with Incidence (%)

Replaced right hepatic artery arising from the superior mesenteric artery	12%
Replaced left hepatic artery arising from the left gastric artery	11%
Accessory left hepatic artery arising from the left gastric artery	11%
Accessory right hepatic artery arising from the superior mesenteric artery	6%
Replaced right hepatic artery arising from the superior mesenteric artery and replaced left hepatic artery arising from the left gastric artery	2%
Replaced right hepatic artery arising from the celiac trunk	<1%

Superior Mesenteric Artery

The superior mesenteric artery arises from the anterior abdominal aorta, approximately 1-2 cm distal to the celiac artery, usually at the level of the L1-L2 intervertebral space. It passes posterior to the pancreas and over the left renal vein. The branches that originate from the SMA (in order) are the inferior pancreaticoduodenal, middle colic, right colic, ileocolic, jejunal and ileal branches. The previously described branches of the SMA may arise in a different order than described above but are only rarely replaced or duplicated to other vessels, such as celiac or inferior mesenteric artery, approximately 1% of the time. The ileocolic arteries are the most consistent vessels and rarely have aberrant anatomy. (12, 13) The right colic artery is the most variable branch arising from the SMA, arising from Ileocolic or middle colic approximately 40% of the time. As described previously, the most common celiac branch to arise from the SMA is the right hepatic artery. (3, 6, 14, 15)

Inferior Mesenteric Artery

The IMA comes off the anterolateral aspect of the left side of the aorta. The takeoff is usually at the level of L3, below the renal arteries, just above the bifurcation of the common iliac arteries. The first branch of the IMA is the left colic which supplies the descending colon. The sigmoid branches arise next and supply the sigmoid colon. The superior rectal artery is the terminal branch of the inferior mesenteric artery and supplies the upper rectum. (3, 16, 17)

Anatomic Variations

While there are variations in the branching pattern of the inferior mesenteric artery, the vessels are rarely replaced or accessory to the celiac or superior mesenteric arteries. A few case studies have shown a common trunk of the SMA and IMA. The common anatomic variations of the inferior mesenteric artery include a double IMA, absent left colic artery, Arc of Riolin, common left colic and sigmoid take off. (16, 17)

Extrahepatic Parasitized Vessels

Primary or metastatic tumors within the liver typically receive blood supply primarily from the hepatic arteries. These tumors can recruit extrahepatic vessels, leading to parasitized vessels feeding the tumor. Parasitized vessels are extremely important to identify as they can affect treatment outcomes and result in treatment failure. The most common tumor types to recruit extrahepatic parasitized vessels are typically hypervascular tumors, including hepatocellular carcinoma, breast, neuroendocrine, and renal cell carcinoma. Colorectal tumor metastases are common in the liver but rarely have parasitized vessels because it is a hypovascular tumor. The incidence of extrahepatic parasitized vessels varies depending on several variables, including size of tumor, location of the tumor within the liver, if tumor has extension beyond the capsule, exophytic tumor, and if prior treatments (surgical or endovascular) have been performed. (18, 19, 20)

The size of the tumor significantly influences whether the tumor will have extrahepatic arterial feeding vessels. Approximately, 3% of tumors 3.0 cm in size have parasitized vessels while approximately 93% of tumors 9cm in size have parasitized vessels. (18, 19, 20)

Previous treatment significantly impacts whether a tumor will develop extrahepatic vascular supply. Both endovascular and surgical treatments increase the likelihood of parasitized vessels. It has been found that approximately 98% of those undergoing a third transarterial chemoembolization (TACE) have extrahepatic parasitized vessels. Persistently elevated AFP, despite treatment, should spur the interventionist to seek out parasitized vessels. (18, 19, 20)

Tumors that are located near the periphery of the liver have a higher propensity to recruit parasitized vessels than are tumors located centrally within the liver itself. Tumors located near the bare area of the liver, where there is no protective capsule, have greater ability to recruit parasitized vessels. The location of the tumor within the liver usually dictates which vessels are most likely to be recruited given proximity. When the lesion is in direct contact with the right hemidiaphragm then the right inferior phrenic artery is usually recruited. If the lesion is near the left hemidiaphragm or in segments 2 and 3, then the left inferior phrenic artery should be suspected to be parasitized. Anteriorly located tumors may parasitize vessels from the omentum, particularly if the patient has had prior surgery and adhesions are present, adhering the omentum to the liver surface. If the lesion is in the anterior and superior aspect of the liver, abutting the diaphragm, then the internal mammary artery should be suspected. The right internal mammary artery can supply tumors in segments IV and VIII and the left internal mammary artery to segments II and III. If the tumor is located in segment VI, the right adrenal artery can parasite to that location. If the tumor is located in the inferior edge of the right liver, near the right kidney, then the right renal artery should be evaluated. A tumor along the posterior and lateral aspect of the right hepatic lobes (segments VI and VII) can recruit vessels from the intercostal arteries with the 9th, 10th, and 11th intercostal arteries being most common. A tumor that abuts the gallbladder can parasitize vessels from the cystic artery. Hepatic lesions that abut the lesser curvature of the stomach may recruit blood supply from the right or left gastric arteries. The left gastric can also supply tumors in hepatic segments II and III. Tumors along the posterior and inferior portion of the liver can recruit blood supply from the Lumbar arteries. Exophytic tumors from the inferior aspect of the liver, near the hepatic flexure, can parasitize vessels from the terminal branches of the colon, arising from the SMA. Hepatic tumors in segments V and VI which are in close proximity to the duodenum may have parasitized vessels from the gastroduodenal artery. (18, 19)

Prevalence of Commonly Extrahepatic Parasitized Arteries to Hepatic Masses

Parasitized Extrahepatic Artery	Prevalence
Right Inferior Phrenic a.	70-83%
Omental a.	13%
Left Inferior Phrenic a.	12%
Suprarenal a.	10%
Right Internal Mammary a.	8%
Right Renal a.	7%
Gastric a.	4%

Hepatic Vascular Shunts

Vascular shunts are an anomalous connection between vessels where there is a macroscopic opening between either the hepatic arteries, the portal veins, or the hepatic veins through physiological anastomoses, which become abnormally enlarged. The intervening capillary bed is bypassed. All intrahepatic vessels can be associated with the formation of shunts. These include arterioportal (AP), portosystemic and arteriosystemic venous shunts. Rarely, systemic venous (i.e., hepatic vein to hepatic vein) shunts and portal-to-portal communications are seen. (21, 22, 23)

Arterioportal shunts:

An arterioportal shunt is a communication between a hepatic arterial branch and a portal venous branch. This is the most common intrahepatic vascular shunt. This type of shunt may be acquired after biopsy, trauma, or drain placement. Masses, such as hepatocellular carcinoma and hemangioma can also result in arterioportal shunts. This type of shunt can also be seen in hereditary hemorrhagic telangiectasia. A segmental area of transient hepatic enhancement is seen during the arterial phase as a wedge-shaped geographic area of hyperenhancement, due to high-pressure arterial blood passing into a low-pressure portal vein branch. Given this abnormal flow, development of life threatening portal hypertension or high-output cardiac failure can rapidly occur. In this setting, treatment with imaging-guided intervention, such as embolization, is performed. If embolization fails, surgery is often necessary. (21, 22, 24, 25)

Arteriovenous Shunts:

Arteriovenous shunts are a connection between the hepatic arteries and the hepatic veins. These hepatic shunts are rare. AV shunts are seen in hypervascular tumors, such as hepatocellular carcinoma, hemangioma, focal nodular hyperplasia, and hemangioendotheliomas. They may also be seen in patients who have hereditary hemorrhagic telangiectasia. Early enhancement of a hepatic vein in the arterial phase is seen on CT or MRI imaging. The velocities in the IVC and hepatic veins on doppler ultrasound are increased as high-pressure arterial blood is entering the venous system. If the patients are asymptomatic then watchful waiting is employed. If patients become symptomatic and are refractory to medical treatments (specifically hemangioendothelioma), then embolization is performed. If endovascular treatment is not possible or fails then surgical intervention is necessary. (21, 24, 25)

A portosystemic shunt is a high-flow shunt between a portal vein and a systemic vein. These may be congenital or acquired and they may also be intrahepatic or extra hepatic. Acquired causes for portosystemic shunts include portal hypertension, iatrogenic (from transjugular intrahepatic portosystemic shunt TIPS), surgical portocaval shunt, trauma, rupture of a portal venous aneurysm, and mesentericocaval shunt. These types of shunts are most commonly seen in cirrhosis with portal hypertension. Increased portal pressure eventually leads to formation of collateral circulation that directly connects the portal blood vessels to systemic circulation, bypassing the liver parenchyma. The intrahepatic shunts can lead to high output cardiac failure and/or encephalopathy (potential side effects of TIPS). Extrahepatic portosystemic shunts are usually caused by congenital vascular malformations or portal hypertension (splenorenal shunt). CT demonstrates and aberrant connection between a systemic vein and portal vein and can help map the extent and size of the shunt. These are treated if they become symptomatic. Endovascular treatment includes occlusion of the shunt. If this is ultimately unsuccessful then surgery may be necessary. (21, 24, 25, 26)

A venovenous shunt (also known as systemic to systemic shunt) may develop when the normal venous drainage to the liver is obstructed, such as

Budd Chiari syndrome. This can also be caused by venous obstruction secondary to tumor compression or pregnancy. Imaging findings include decreased peripheral and increased central enhancement of the liver. Tortuous hepatic veins and collateral veins draining to the IVC or subcapsular veins may be seen. Therapeutic options can include thrombolytic therapy, angioplasty with or without stenting, TIPS, surgical shunting and liver transplantation. (21, 24, 25)

Portoportal Shunts:

Portoportal shunts are connections between the portal vein branches. They can be seen in patients with a normal liver, cirrhosis, or with portal vein thrombosis. In a normal liver, a portoportal shunt may be seen adjacent to the falciform ligament and is considered a normal variant. Heterogeneous patchy enhancement of the peripheral portions of the liver during the arterial phase is due to compensatory increased arterial blood flow. At Doppler US, hepatopetal flow without a typical respiratory wave is seen in the portal vein. Also, increased arterial blood flow results in a more prominent waveform. Embolization may be performed if treatment is required. (21, 24, 25)

References

1. Momeni, Mohammad, et al. "Anatomical Variation of Celiac Axis, Superior Mesenteric Artery, and Hepatic Artery: Evaluation with Multidetector Computed Tomography Angiography." *Journal of Research in Medical Sciences*, *21*(1), 26 Dec. 2016, p. 129. *PubMed*, https://doi.org/10.4103/1735-1995.196611. Accessed 2022.
2. Malviya, Kapil Kumar, et al. "Unraveling Variations in Celiac Trunk and Hepatic Artery by CT Angiography to Aid in Surgeries of Upper Abdominal Region." *Diagnostics*, *11*(12), 2021, p. 2262. *PubMed*, https://doi.org/10.3390/diagnostics11122262. Accessed 2022.
3. Kaufman, John A., and Michael J. Lee. "Chapter 11." *Vascular and Interventional Radiology the Requisites*, Elsevier Saunders, Philadelphia, Pa, 2014, pp. 229–264.
4. White, Richard D., et al. "The Celiac Axis Revisited: Anatomic Variants, Pathologic Features, and Implications for Modern Endovascular Management." *RadioGraphics*, *35*(3), 2015, pp. 879–898. *PubMed*, https://doi.org/10.1148/rg.2015140243. Accessed 2022.
5. Hemamalini. "Variations in the Branching Pattern of the Celiac Trunk and Its Clinical Significance." *Anatomy & Cell Biology*, *51*(3), Sept.

2018, p. 143. *PubMed*, https://doi.org/10.5115/acb.2018.51.3.143. Accessed 2022.
6. Song, Soon-Young, et al. "Celiac Axis and Common Hepatic Artery Variations in 5002 Patients: Systematic Analysis with Spiral CT and DSA." *Radiology*, *255*(1), July 2010, pp. 278–288. *PubMed*, https://doi.org/10.1148/radiol.09090389. Accessed 2022.
7. Mauro, Matthew A., et al. "Chapter 25." *Image-Guided Interventions*, Elsevier, Philadelphia, PA, 2021, pp. 229–264.
8. Hiatt, Jonathan R., et al. "Surgical Anatomy of the Hepatic Arteries in 1000 Cases." *Annals of Surgery*, *220*(1), July 1994, pp. 50–52. *PubMed*, https://doi.org/10.1097/00000658-199407000-00008. Accessed 2022.
9. Choi, Tae Won, et al. "Anatomic Variations of the Hepatic Artery in 5625 Patients." *Radiology: Cardiothoracic Imaging*, *3*(4), 19 Aug. 2021. *PubMed*, https://doi.org/10.1148/ryct.2021210007. Accessed 2022.
10. Covey, Anne M., et al. "Variant Hepatic Arterial Anatomy Revisited: Digital Subtraction Angiography Performed in 600 Patients." *Radiology*, *224*(2), 2002, pp. 542–547. *PubMed*, https://doi.org/10.1148/radiol.2242011283.
11. Abdullah, Siraj Saadaldin, et al. "Anatomical Variations of the Hepatic Artery: Study of 932 Cases in Liver Transplantation." *Surgical and Radiologic Anatomy*, *28*(5), 27 Oct. 2006, pp. 468–473. *PubMed*, https://doi.org/10.1007/s00276-006-0121-0. Accessed 2022.
12. Negoi, Ionut, et al. "Surgical Anatomy of the Superior Mesenteric Vessels Related to Colon and Pancreatic Surgery: A Systematic Review and Meta-Analysis." *Scientific Reports*, *8*(1), 8 Mar. 2018. *PubMed*, https://doi.org/10.1038/s41598-018-22641-x.
13. Xiao, Y, et al. "Clinical Anatomy Study of Superior Mesenteric Vessels and Its Branches." *Chinese Journal of Surgery*, *57*, 1 Sept. 2019, pp. 673–680. *PubMed*, Accessed 2022.
14. Silva, Natasha Gabriela, et al. "Anatomical Variations of the Superior Mesenteric Artery and Its Clinical and Surgical Implications in Humans." *ABCD. Arquivos Brasileiros De Cirurgia Digestiva (São Paulo)*, *33*(2), 24 Aug. 2020. *PubMed*, https://doi.org/10.1590/0102-672020190001e1508. Accessed 2022.
15. Alsabilah, J., et al. "Vascular Structures of the Right Colon: Incidence and Variations with Their Clinical Implications." *Scandinavian Journal of Surgery*, *106*(2), 2016, pp. 107–115. *PubMed*, https://doi.org/10.1177/1457496916650999. Accessed 2022.

16. Skinner, Dylan, et al. *Anatomy, Abdomen and Pelvis, Inferior Mesenteric Artery*. Stat Pearls Publishing, 2021. *PubMed*, Accessed 2022.
17. Ke, Jia, et al. "Anatomic Variations of Inferior Mesenteric Artery and Left Colic Artery Evaluated by 3-Dimensional CT Angiography: Insights into Rectal Cancer Surgery – A Retrospective Observational Study." *International Journal of Surgery*, *41*, 18 Mar. 2017, pp. 106–111. *PubMed*, Accessed 2022.
18. Moustafa, Amr Soliman, et al. "Chemoembolization of Hepatocellular Carcinoma with Extrahepatic Collateral Blood Supply: Anatomic and Technical Considerations." *RadioGraphics*, *37*(3), 2017, pp. 963–977. *PubMed*, https://doi.org/10.1148/rg.2017160122. Accessed 2022.
19. Kim, Hyo-Cheol, et al. "Recognizing Extrahepatic Collateral Vessels That Supply Hepatocellular Carcinoma to Avoid Complications of Transcatheter Arterial Chemoembolization." *RadioGraphics*, *25* suppl_1, Oct. 2005. *PubMed*, https://doi.org/10.1148/rg.25si055508. Accessed 2022.
20. Zhao, Yilin et al. "Evaluation of Extrahepatic Collateral Arteries in Hepatocellular Carcinoma in Three Independent Groups in a Single Center." *Experimental and Therapeutic Medicine*, *10*(6), 2015, pp. 2366–2374. *PubMed*, https://doi.org/10.3892/etm.2015.2822. Accessed 2022.
21. Bhargava, P, et al. "Hepatic Vascular Shunts: Embryology and Imaging Appearances." *The British Journal of Radiology*, *84*(1008), Dec. 2011, pp. 1142–1152. *PubMed*, https://doi.org/10.1259/bjr/82649468. Accessed 2022.
22. Choi BI, Lee KH, Han JK, Lee JM. Hepatic arterioportal shunts: dynamic CT and MR features. Korean J Radiol. 2002 Jan-Mar;3(1):1-15. doi: 10.3348/kjr.2002.3.1.1. PMID: 11919473; PMCID: PMC2713981.
23. Dessouky, B. A., El Abd, O. L., & Abdel Aal, E. S. (2011). Intrahepatic vascular shunts: Strategy for early diagnosis, Evaluation and Management. *The Egyptian Journal of Radiology and Nuclear Medicine*, *42*(1), 19–34. https://doi.org/10.1016/j.ejrnm.2011.02.005
24. Elsayes, Khaled M., et al. "A Comprehensive Approach to Hepatic Vascular Disease." *RadioGraphics*, vol. *37*(3), 2017, pp. 813–836. *PubMed*, https://doi.org/10.1148/rg.2017160161. Accessed 2022.
25. Bodner, G., Peer, S., Karner, M., Perkmann, R., Neuhauser, B., Vogel, W., & Jaschke, W. (2002). Nontumorous vascular malformations in the liver. *Journal of Ultrasound in Medicine*, *21*(2), 187–197. https://doi.org/10.7863/jum.2002.21.2.187

26. Remer, E. M., Motta-Ramirez, G. A., & Henderson, J. M. (2007). Imaging findings in incidental intrahepatic portal venous shunts. *American Journal of Roentgenology*, *188*(2). https://doi.org/10.2214/ajr.05.1115

CHAPTER 5

TRANSARTERIAL CHEMOEMBOLIZATION (TACE) FOR PRIMARY HEPATIC TUMORS

STEVE LEMONS MD, BRENT SMITH MD, CAROLINE MUSSATTO MD

Introduction

Transarterial chemoembolization (TACE) is a procedure performed by interventional radiologists which delivers chemotherapeutic and embolic agents simultaneously to a tumor via intraarterial blood supply.[1] First trialed in the late 1970s and early 1980s,[2] this minimally invasive procedure offers the advantage of delivering chemotherapeutic drugs directly to the tissue of interest and thereby minimizing systemic toxicity. The addition of an embolic agent aims to prolong the chemotherapeutic drug effect on the involved tissue by decreased blood flow.[1] TACE is performed under fluoroscopic image guidance with addition of a contrast agent to visualize the arterial supply in real time.

The primary application of TACE is management of hepatocellular carcinoma (HCC) and other liver neoplasms.[3] The dual blood supply of the liver via the hepatic artery and portal vein creates a unique advantage when it comes to treatment of liver neoplasms. Healthy hepatic tissue receives approximately 75% of its blood supply from the portal vein with the hepatic artery supplying the remaining 25%. By contrast, liver neoplasms generally rely on the hepatic artery for the vast majority of their blood supply by means of neovascularization.[4] Due to this natural propensity for liver tumors to derive their blood supply from the hepatic artery, transarterial delivery of embolic chemotherapy is well suited to target neoplastic tissue while sparing native hepatic parenchyma.[3-5]

Historical review of TACE

Common limitations to treating any tumor with systemic chemotherapy include drug toxicity and difficulty in delivering the chemotherapeutic to the tissue of interest in sufficient quantities and concentrations for cytotoxic effects. TACE offers a solution to both concerns by delivering chemotherapeutic agents directly to the tumor via its rich arterial blood supply.[2] Early descriptions of TACE in scientific literature date back to Japan during the late 1970s and early 1980s, where TACE was first applied to renal cell carcinoma.[6] Early TACE utilized ethylcellulose microcapsules of mitomycin mc.[2, 6] Instillation of the microcapsules led to temporary embolic occlusion of the feeding tumor vessels, with subsequent gradual and steady delivery of a chemotherapeutic drug over time. Not only does this delivery mechanism minimize systemic toxicity of the chemotherapeutic drug, but it increases the duration of cytotoxic effect toward the tumor tissue.[2, 4] TACE demonstrated efficacy in a variety of tumor types at providing palliative symptom relief, pain relief and reducing tumor burden, which in some cases facilitates bridging to surgical resection.[2, 7]

Over the following decades, a variety of chemotherapeutic agents and combinations of chemotherapeutic agents were pioneered in TACE including cisplatin, 5-fluorouracil, doxorubicin (Adriamycin), and others.[8-10] The most frequently utilized chemotherapeutic agents today are combinations of mitomycin C, doxorubicin, and cisplatin. These agents may be administered emulsified in lipiodol, a radiopaque iodized oil which carries the chemotherapy or drug eluting beads (DEB).[3-5] The embolic component of TACE may consist of Gelfoam, lipiodol or other microparticles such as DEB and degradable starch microspheres (DSM).[3, 5]

Procedural Description

The primary application of TACE is treatment of hepatic tumors, whether metastatic lesions or primary hepatic malignancy. For each patient, a multidisciplinary team of specialists are typically involved to determine treatment options prior to TACE administration.[3, 4] Obtaining preprocedural cross-sectional imaging is necessary to characterize the tumor, evaluate tumor blood supply, identify any contraindications, and facilitate interventional planning.[3] For liver masses, contrast-enhanced CT abdomen or MRI abdomen are the imaging studies most frequently utilized for preprocedural planning (Fig. 1).[3, 11] Patients should remain NPO for 8 hours prior to anesthesia administration, or per institutional protocol.

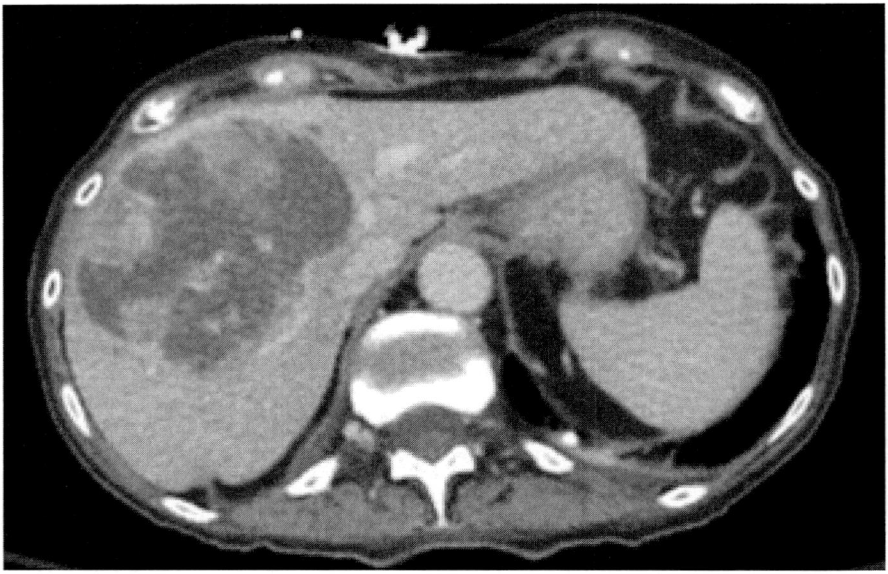

Fig. 1: Computed tomography (CT) image of a large biopsy proven right hepatic lobe hepatocellular carcinoma.

Periprocedural intravenous hydration in the form of isotonic fluids should be utilized for protection against acute kidney injury, dehydration, contrast nephrotoxicity, and nephrotoxic chemotherapy agents.[11]

Anesthesia requirements may vary but moderate conscious sedation is sufficient for most patients undergoing TACE procedure.[3, 11] Following adequate anesthesia, the bilateral groin is sterilized and prepared. The right common femoral artery is the typical arterial access point. Diagnostic arteriograms may first be performed in the abdominal aorta and superior mesenteric artery to elicit any collateral tumor blood supply and exclude accessory hepatic arteries.[3] The arterial supply of the liver is classically derived from the celiac artery which gives rise to the common hepatic artery, though variant anatomy is not uncommon. The most common hepatic arterial variant anatomy is a replaced right hepatic artery arising from the superior mesenteric artery and given the prevalence of variable vasculature a preoperative angiography is necessary.[11] Once the configuration of arterial supply to the tumor is known, optimal placement of the catheter for chemoembolization is determined using selective angiography (Fig. 2A).[4] This placement will be dependent upon individual vascular anatomy, tumor size and tumor location. Catheter placement should be proximal enough in the vessel such that the entire mass will receive chemoembolization, yet distal enough to minimize the cytotoxic effect on surrounding nontarget tissue.[3, 4] Optimizing this balance will aid in decreasing side effects while maximizing therapeutic treatment. Once catheter placement is adequate, the chemotherapy mixture is administered under continuous fluoroscopic guidance.[3] Angiography is repeated after administration to demonstrate and confirm change in blood flow (Fig. 2B). All catheters are removed and hemostasis of the arteriotomy site is achieved prior to departure from the interventional radiology suite.[4]

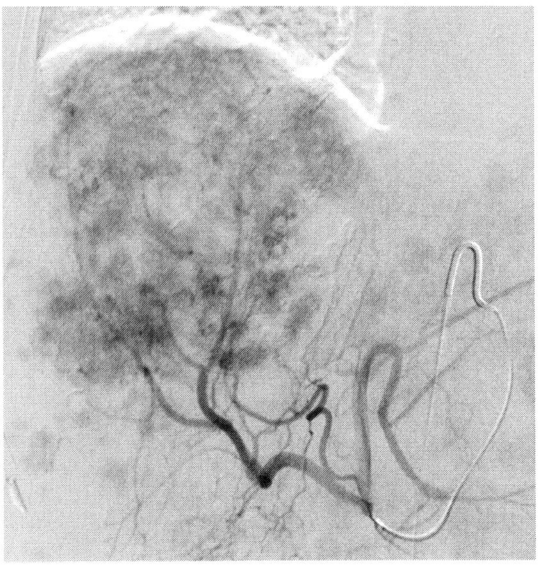

Fig. 2A: AP projection digital subtraction angiography of the common hepatic artery demonstrating extensive tumoral blush within the right hepatic lobe.

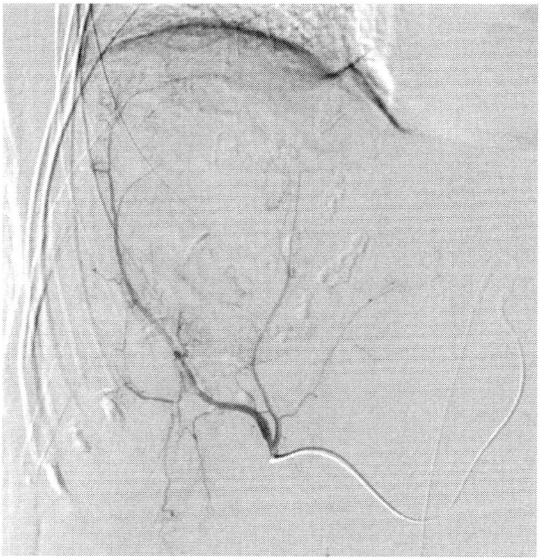

Fig. 2B: Postembolization selective digital subtraction angiography of the right hepatic artery demonstrates substantially diminished tumoral vascularity following delivery of doxorubicin coated embolization beads.

Post-Procedural Management

Abdominal pain, nausea/vomiting and fever are very common following TACE and thought to be directly related to hepatic tissue embolization. This triad together is known as postembolization syndrome and occurs in up to 80% of patients or more.[3, 4] Postembolization syndrome should be thought of as an expected potential side effect of TACE rather than a complication. General post-procedural management following TACE includes analgesia and antiemetics in anticipation of postembolization syndrome. Vigorous hydration is recommended to protect from acute kidney injury. Prophylactic corticosteroids such as dexamethasone have been utilized for postembolization syndrome with some efficacy.[5]

Utility of antibiotic prophylaxis following TACE is debated. Existing research shows evidence for efficacy of antibiotics in reducing rates of liver abscess, while other studies show no correlation between prophylactic antibiotics and decreased infection risk.[12, 13] Unified guidelines for antibiotic use in TACE have not been developed. However, use of antibiotic prophylaxis is generally applied in all patients who have preexisting sphincter of Oddi dysfunction, biliary stent placement, and/or evidence of bilio-enteric colonization.[1, 3] TACE aims to induce tissue necrosis, and theoretically will create a necrotic bed of tissue in which an abscess may form. A majority of institutions currently prescribe antibiotic prophylaxis during TACE due to the high morbidity and mortality associated with development of liver abscess.[11]

Patients should be instructed to remain supine for a period of time while femoral arterial access site hemostasis is achieved (or to remain seated for a period of time while radial arterial access site hemostasis is achieved). Most patients tolerate TACE well and return to PO diet, ambulate and produce urine appropriately for discharge within 24 hours.[3, 4] Pain control may be managed with scheduled dosages of pain medication or patient-controlled anesthesia. Temporary as-needed pain medication is often prescribed for the outpatient setting.

Subtypes of TACE

Conventional TACE (c-TACE) as described above utilizes cytotoxic agent(s) emulsified in radiopaque lipiodol, followed by an embolic agent. Variations of c-TACE exist in the form of drug-eluting bead transarterial chemoembolization (DEB-TACE), balloon-occluded transarterial chemoembolization (B-TACE), selective occlusion of feeding arteries in transarterial chemoembolization (SOFA-TACE) and more.

DEB-TACE utilizes non-resorbable embolic microspheres that are coated with cytotoxic chemotherapy agents and delivered via arterial supply as one unit.[3, 5, 11] DEB are typically 100 – 300 μm in size, but beads as small as 30 μm have been studied (Fig. 3).[14] The coated embolic beads then lead to sustained release of chemotherapy to the tumor over time as compared to c-TACE. Effectiveness of DEB-TACE in comparison to c-TACE has been found to be comparable for most outcomes, though some research appears to demonstrate that DEB-TACE has lower rates of side effects such as postembolization syndrome.[3, 5, 14] Further research is needed to clarify whether significant differences in outcomes and complications exist between c-TACE and DEB-TACE.

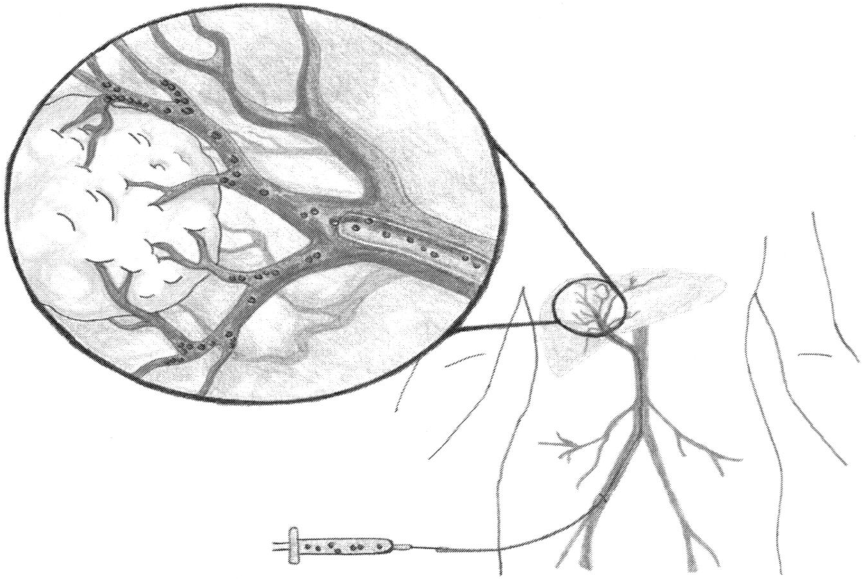

Fig. 3: Illustration demonstrating components of a transarterial chemoembolization (TACE) procedure. The delivery catheter is seen accessing the right common femoral artery with the catheter tip in a right hepatic artery branch. Tumoral neovascularity is seen with drug eluting beads preferentially accumulating within the tumoral vasculature.

B-TACE is an additional variation in development over the past decade.[15, 16] This method involves the use of a micro balloon catheter for occlusion of the vessel proximally during delivery of chemoembolization with the goal of preventing proximal migration, increasing accumulation of cytotoxic drug in the target tissue, and increasing overall selectivity of TACE. B-TACE decreases balloon-occluded arterial stump pressure (BOASP), allowing for more forceful delivery of chemoembolic mixture to the tumor.[15, 16] Studies have shown potential for greater therapeutic effect from B-TACE compared to c-TACE in the form of increased complete response of the tumor and lower re-treatment rates.[15-17]

Selective occlusion of feeding arteries in TACE (SOFA-TACE) is another procedural variant which seeks to deliver chemoembolic agents with higher precision. During SOFA-TACE, arterial inflow from feeding arteries is selectively occluded with a balloon catheter. This has been observed to result in complete filling of the tumor vasculature with chemoembolic agents.[18] The SOFA-TACE method is proposed to facilitate TACE treatment in anatomically challenging cases.[18]

Complications

While TACE is generally well tolerated, serious complications can and do occur. Liver failure and liver abscess are two potential complications of TACE which carry high morbidity and mortality.[1, 11] Risk of liver failure is unsurprisingly increased in the presence of underlying liver disease and impaired liver function. This risk may be mitigated by selecting TACE candidates with care, and using extreme caution when considering TACE in patients who are Child-Pugh C, total bilirubin level $\geq$ 4 mg/dL, serum albumin $\leq$ 2 mg/dL, encephalopathy or poor performance status.[1, 3] Liver abscess following TACE tends to affect patients with preexisting sphincter of Oddi dysfunction, occurring in 25–80% of patients with prior sphincterotomy, biliary-enteric anastomosis or biliary stent.[1, 3] In such individuals with presumed enteric colonization of the biliary tree, biliary ischemia induced by TACE may create ideal conditions for abscess to form and this complication is difficult to avoid. Broad-spectrum antibiotic coverage is generally always given for prophylaxis of liver abscess in these individuals.[1, 3] Luckily, liver abscess is a very rare outcome for patients with functional sphincter of Oddi.[1, 3]

Additional complications after TACE include tumor rupture, cholecystitis, pancreatitis, biloma, biliary stricture, gastrointestinal hemorrhage, and others.[5, 11] Chemoembolization of nontarget tissue may lead to such complications, and should be avoided through careful selection of arterial supply and meticulous catheter placement.[11] Coil embolization of arteries near the target tissue may also be performed to reduce nontarget tissue chemoembolization and subsequent complications.[11] Death following TACE is rare and occurs in less than 1% of patients.[5, 11]

Applications of TACE

Hepatocellular Carcinoma

The primary application of TACE is treatment of hepatocellular carcinoma (HCC). As previously described, the dual blood supply of the liver and the predilection of liver tumors for hepatic arterial supply creates an ideal setup for TACE which naturally targets tumors and spares native liver tissue.[1, 3] HCC is the most common primary liver malignancy and is a major cause of cancer mortality, representing the third leading cause of cancer death worldwide.[19] Key risk factors include chronic liver disease, cirrhosis, chronic hepatitis B/C and aflatoxin B1 exposure.[4, 19] HCC develops in roughly one third of patients with cirrhosis, making it crucial to screen and detect cancer early to preserve treatment options and maximize prognosis.[5]

When considering treatment options for HCC, TACE is less effective than surgical resection or liver transplantation yet more effective and bearing less morbidity than systemic chemotherapy or palliative treatments.[11] The ideal candidates for TACE are patients with disease that is advanced enough to preclude surgery or minimally invasive ablative therapies, yet contained such that liver function and overall ECOG (Eastern Cooperative Oncology Group) performance status is mostly preserved.[11, 19] The Barcelona Clinic Liver Cancer (BCLC) staging system recommends TACE as first-line treatment for patients with intermediate-stage (B) hepatocellular carcinoma.[4, 19] Tumors in the intermediate-stage (B) category are those which are confined to the liver with relatively preserved liver function, are not amenable to resection, without vascular invasion, and ECOG performance status 0.[5, 11, 19] HCC which is very early stage (0) or early stage (A) may be candidates for curative therapies such as liver transplantation or surgical resection, or benefit from local ablation with radiofrequency or microwave ablation; HCC which are advanced stage (C) or terminal stage (D) are managed with systemic chemotherapy or supportive care.[19]

Greater than 50% of HCC patients treated with TACE demonstrate a positive response via extensive tumor necrosis, translating to improved survival.[11, 19] Some studies report improved survival rate and fewer side effects following DEB-TACE compared to c-TACE in patients with HCC, yet conclusive evidence for one therapy over the other is yet to come.[5] TACE may result in downstaging of a patient such that they become a candidate for liver transplantation or surgical resection. It may also aid in successfully maintaining a patient as a candidate awaiting liver transplantation ("bridging" therapy).[11] TACE has been utilized and studied as neoadjuvant therapy prior to surgical resection of HCC. While neoadjuvant TACE prior to surgical resection may theoretically shrink tumors for easier resection, systematic reviews have not shown demonstrable benefit to disease-free survival or overall survival from this application of TACE.[20]

Combination therapies involving TACE are being actively investigated as HCC treatment options.[5] TACE + microwave ablation and TACE + radiofrequency ablation have been applied to medium- to large-sized HCC (3–10 cm) which are ineligible for ablation monotherapy. Randomized controlled trials demonstrate safety and efficacy of these combination therapies without significant difference in survival rates between TACE + radiofrequency ablation or TACE + microwave ablation, though TACE + microwave ablation may offer improved efficacy for tumors greater than 5 cm.[5]

In cases which demonstrate significant tumor progression after TACE (development of extrahepatic metastasis, extensive liver involvement, significantly impaired ECOG performance status), retreatment with TACE should not be attempted.[19] Tumors which do not demonstrate any substantial necrosis after two rounds of TACE should be managed with alternative therapy rather than reattempting TACE.[19] TACE may be utilized as an investigative treatment option for patients which have failed initial chemotherapy or other treatment options, patients with recurrence, and/or patients who may receive palliative symptomatic benefit from reduced tumor burden.[11] In such cases, it is important to emphasize the investigative nature of the treatment and involve the patient in discussions of the relative benefits, risks and alternatives.

Intrahepatic cholangiocarcinoma

TACE has served as a viable treatment option for intrahepatic cholangiocarcinoma.[21-23] Intrahepatic cholangiocarcinoma is a rare primary liver tumor arising from biliary epithelium with poor prognosis, in large part due to the advanced unresectable disease often present at diagnosis. Approximately 80–85% of intrahepatic cholangiocarcinoma cases are unresectable at diagnosis.[22, 24] Five-year survival for unresectable intrahepatic cholangiocarcinoma is dismal at less than 5%.[22] TACE has demonstrated benefit in extending overall survival in patients with unresectable disease as compared to palliative therapy and is an established treatment option.[21, 23] TACE has also been used with success as adjuvant treatment for previously resected intrahepatic cholangiocarcinoma, with efficacy in improving overall survival and recurrence-free survival in such patients.[21, 24]

Summary and Conclusions

The current and future applications of TACE are ever expanding. TACE is a minimally invasive procedure which simultaneously delivers chemotherapy and embolic agent(s) via arterial blood supply, thereby minimizing systemic toxicity and maximizing selective therapeutic effect.

TACE remains a well-established therapeutic treatment for intermediate-stage hepatocellular carcinoma (HCC) as well as forms of early-stage HCC and advanced-stage HCC which are unresectable or recurrent. It is increasingly being utilized as a tool for treatment of advanced intrahepatic cholangiocarcinoma, colorectal liver metastases, and various other liver metastases. Tolerability of TACE continues to improve over time as technology improves the ability of radiologists to target chemoembolization to the tissue of interest. Refinement in the selectivity of TACE will continue to reduce incidence of postembolization syndrome, thus improving tolerability. It will also reduce nontarget embolization and subsequently reduce risk of related complications such as cholecystitis, biliary stricture, biloma, pancreatitis and hemorrhage. Overall rates of complications following TACE are low, and risks of TACE can be mitigated through appropriate patient selection. Prognostic grading scores to identify which patients will derive benefit from TACE have been developed for select scenarios, and will aid in guiding individual patient management.[5] Additional research will be needed to elucidate any advantages of existing TACE variants (c-TACE, DEB-TACE, B-TACE, and so on) for specific treatment populations.

The heterogeneity in research study populations is a limiting factor for establishing conclusive benefit of TACE as compared to various alternative therapies. However, TACE has demonstrable survival benefit in a variety of tumors at various stages and its applications are likely to continue expanding as research evidence identifies appropriate candidates for whom TACE may provide benefit. The contraindications and risks of TACE are known and can be weighed against the risks of alternative treatment options or supportive therapy. The balance of benefits and risks to the individual patient case should naturally guide the discussion of TACE as a treatment option for any neoplastic tumor in the absence of established treatment guidelines.

References

1 Lee MJ. Vascular and interventional radiology : the requisites. St. Louis, Mo. ; [London]: Mosby; 2004.

2 Kato T, Nemoto R, Mori H, et al. Arterial chemoembolization with microencapsulated anticancer drug. An approach to selective cancer chemotherapy with sustained effects. JAMA 1981;245(11):1123-7.

3 Kandarpa K, Machan L. Handbook of interventional radiologic procedures. 4th ed. [Place of publication not identified]: LWW; 2012.

4 Angle JF, Haskal ZJ, Keefe NA, et al. IR Playbook : A Comprehensive Introduction to Interventional Radiology. Cham: Springer International Publishing : Imprint: Springer,; 2018.
5 Kotsifa E, Vergadis C, Vailas M, et al. Transarterial Chemoembolization for Hepatocellular Carcinoma: Why, When, How? J Pers Med 2022;12(3).
6 Kato T, Nemoto R, Mori H, et al. Transcatheter arterial chemoembolization of renal cell carcinoma with microencapsulated mitomycin C. J Urol 1981;125(1):19-24.
7 Kato T. [Selective arterial chemo-embolization with microencapsulated anticancer drugs]. Gan To Kagaku Ryoho 1983;10(2 Pt 2):333-9.
8 Nakamura H, Hashimoto T, Taguchi T, et al. [Oily chemoembolization of hepatoma]. Gan To Kagaku Ryoho 1987;14(2):381-7.
9 Courtheoux P, Berthelin JL, Segol P, et al. [Chemoembolization of hepatic metastases. Preliminary study]. J Radiol 1987;68(4):247-53.
10 Sasaki Y, Imaoka S, Kasugai H, et al. A new approach to chemoembolization therapy for hepatoma using ethiodized oil, cisplatin, and gelatin sponge. Cancer 1987;60(6):1194-203.
11 Young M, John S. Hepatic Chemoembolization. StatPearls. Treasure Island (FL)2022.
12 Li B. Prophylactic Use of Antibiotics for Postsurgical Infection in c-TACE and DEB-TACE High-Risk Patients: A Case-Control Study. J Healthc Eng 2022;2022:6203817.
13 Yoshihara S, Yamana H, Akahane M, et al. Association between prophylactic antibiotic use for transarterial chemoembolization and occurrence of liver abscess: a retrospective cohort study. Clin Microbiol Infect 2021;27(10):1514 e5- e10.
14 Chang Y, Jeong SW, Young Jang J, et al. Recent Updates of Transarterial Chemoembolilzation in Hepatocellular Carcinoma. Int J Mol Sci 2020;21(21).
15 Irie T, Kuramochi M, Takahashi N. Dense accumulation of lipiodol emulsion in hepatocellular carcinoma nodule during selective balloon-occluded transarterial chemoembolization: measurement of balloon-occluded arterial stump pressure. Cardiovasc Intervent Radiol 2013;36(3):706-13.
16 Golfieri R, Bezzi M, Verset G, et al. Balloon-Occluded Transarterial Chemoembolization: In Which Size Range Does It Perform Best? A Comparison of Its Efficacy versus Conventional Transarterial Chemoembolization, Using Propensity Score Matching. Liver Cancer 2021;10(5):522-34.

17 Golfieri R, Bezzi M, Verset G, et al. Retrospective European Multicentric Evaluation of Selective Transarterial Chemoembolisation with and without Balloon-Occlusion in Patients with Hepatocellular Carcinoma: A Propensity Score Matched Analysis. Cardiovasc Intervent Radiol 2021;44(7):1048-59.
18 Yu SCH. Blood Flow Diversion Within Hepatocellular Carcinoma (HCC) after Selective Occlusion of Feeding Arteries (SOFA) and Feasibility of Utilizing the SOFA Technique in Transarterial Chemoembolization (SOFA-TACE). Cardiovasc Intervent Radiol 2022;45(1):121-6.
19 Forner A, Reig M, Bruix J. Hepatocellular carcinoma. Lancet 2018;391(10127):1301-14.
20 Chua TC, Liauw W, Saxena A, et al. Systematic review of neoadjuvant transarterial chemoembolization for resectable hepatocellular carcinoma. Liver Int 2010;30(2):166-74.
21 Lv TR, Hu HJ, Liu F, et al. The effect of trans arterial chemoembolization in the management of intrahepatic cholangiocarcinoma. A systematic review and meta-analysis. Eur J Surg Oncol 2022.
22 Krenzien F, Nevermann N, Krombholz A, et al. Treatment of Intrahepatic Cholangiocarcinoma-A Multidisciplinary Approach. Cancers (Basel) 2022;14(2).
23 Mosconi C, Calandri M, Javle M, et al. Interventional radiology approaches for intra-hepatic cholangiocarcinoma. Chin Clin Oncol 2020;9(1):8.
24 Ke Q, Lin N, Deng M, et al. The effect of adjuvant therapy for patients with intrahepatic cholangiocarcinoma after surgical resection: A systematic review and meta-analysis. PLoS One 2020;15(2):e0229292.

CHAPTER 6

YTTRIUM-90 IN REVIEW

ZACHARY COLLINS MD, IAN KOZLOWSKI MD, MAXIMILIAN MAYR MS IV, AARON BRAKE MS IV

History of Y90

The mineral Yttrium was found by Swedish lieutenant and part time chemist, Carl Axel Arrhenius, in 1787 [1]. While there are conflicting notes on when the actual date the mineral was discovered, it is well documented that it was discovered in the late 18th century. The newly discovered mineral was originally named Ytterbite, after it was shipped to Arrhenius's friend, Johan Gadolin, a Flemish chemistry professor. After numerous name changes over the next several years, the number 39 element on the periodic table was finally named Yttrium, after the Swedish town for which it was found nearby, Ytterby, Sweden [1].

Yttrium comes in an abundance of isotopes. To be exact, there are currently 44 recognized isotopes of yttrium, the most common isotope found is Y88.9, which is the natural isotope 100% of the time [2]. This natural isotope of yttrium also happens to be the most stable form of the element [3]. All yttrium isotopes other than Y88 and Y89 are artificially produced and radioactive.

The earliest clinical use of Y90 can be traced back to the 1950s when investigators discovered that hepatocellular carcinoma (HCC) derived 80% of its blood supply from the arterial system compared to normal hepatic parenchyma which derived mainly from the portal venous system [4]. In 1965, Irving Ariel was the first to describe using Y90 in 4 patients with inoperable primary pancreatic and liver cancer [5]. His technique utilized

Y90 attached to ceramic microspheres and administered intra-arterially through the celiac axis [5].

Over the next 30 years, several studies and clinical trials began utilizing Y90 to determine its clinical usefulness and safety profile. In the late 1980s and early 1990s, both TheraSphere and SIR-Spheres data emerged from phase 1 and 2 clinical trials showing early stability and efficacy of Y90 [6-8]. Significantly greater interest was sought into the treatment of both hepatocellular carcinoma (HCC) and metastatic colorectal cancer (mCRC) to the liver over the next 10 years into the early 2000s. In 1999, the Food and Drug Administration (FDA) approved the use of TheraSpheres under the Humanitarian Device Exemption Guidelines for unresectable HCC [9]. Three years later, in 2002, SIR-Spheres also received premarket approval (PMA) from the FDA for usage in combination with floxuridine for mCRC [10]. The subsequent two decades continue to show improved data from both SIR-Spheres and TheraSpheres with increased mortality benefits. As of latest, TheraSpheres Y90 was recently granted full FDA approval for the treatment of HCC. This approval was mainly granted due to the results of The LEGACY Study, by Salem et al., which was a multicenter retrospective study evaluating outcomes of patients with solitary, unresectable HCC [11].

The Why, How, and Why Not

Y90 is part of a group of therapies called locoregional therapy. Additional therapies include microwave (MWA), radiofrequency (RFA), cryoablation, and irreversible electroporation (IRE) also known as Nanoknife (Angiodynamics. Latham, NY). There is also chemoembolization also known as transarterial chemoembolization (TACE) and transarterial radioembolization (TARE) which incorporates Y90. It is also known as selective internal radiation therapy (SIRT). The goal of Y90 is to selectively target a high-dose radioactive isotope to a neoplasm using a catheter directed through a vascular supply as a channel.

Y90 serves as a palliative treatment and/or bridge to hepatic transplantation or resection. Hepatic transplantation, as previously described, is one of the treatment options for patients with HCC and mCRC. Y90 can be utilized to downstage patients in order to be eligible for hepatic transplantation. Downstaging for transplantation utilizes the administration of locoregional therapies in order to reduce tumor burden enough to make a patient eligible for transplantation. Bridging therapies are a similar process that are used to slow or lessen the progression of tumor burden for those already on the waitlist for liver transplantation. This kind of management helps lower the dropout rate from the transplant list.

The Milan transplant criteria was introduced by Vincenzo Mazzaferro in 1996 strictly for HCC as a portion of the exclusion criteria. The original study included several criteria: (1) a single mass with a diameter less than 5 cm; (2) no more than three tumor foci with each not exceeding 3 cm; (3) no angioinvasion (including portal venous tumor thrombus); (4) no extrahepatic metastasis or involvement [12]. These exclusion criteria have since been the benchmark for hepatic transplantation, along with several other biochemical tests. However, there have been several studies since the Milan criteria's inauguration that have shown it can be expanded. Yao et al. argues that the criteria should be expanded to include a greater breadth of tumor burden [13]. The now termed University of California San Francisco (UCSF) criteria allows for greater individual nodule size and total tumor size as follows: (1) a single lesion less than 8 cm, or (2) two to three lesions each equal to or less than 5 cm, with the sum of maximum tumor diameters equal to or less than 8 cm, or (3) four or five lesions each equal to or less than 3 cm, with the sum of the maximum tumor diameters equal to or less than 8 cm, and (4) the absence of vascular invasion on imaging [13]. Ultimately a systematic review and meta-analysis performed by de Sousa et al. demonstrated that there was no variation in survival rates between the Milan and UCSF criteria [14].

These criteria were ultimately implemented to maximize the overall post-transplant survival in transplant recipients. Y90 has also been shown to be useful in the treatment of unresectable metastatic neuroendocrine tumors (NET). Kennedy et al. showed that Y90 in NET produced high response rates even with extensive tumor burden and replacement of normal liver parenchyma [15]. One systematic review by Jia and Wang showed that Y90 can also be utilized for patients who have undergone unsuccessful TACE or transarterial bland embolization (TABE) treatment [16]. However, additional studies may still be required to fully delineate the full potential of Y90 in the treatment of NET. Y90 is also indicated for patients who are not transplant candidates, such that it can be used as a palliative therapy. Salem et al. demonstrated that when Y90 is compared to cTACE in the treatment of HCC, patients receiving Y90 radioembolization had significantly prolonged median time to progression (TTP) greater than 26 months, compared to 6.8 months for patients receiving cTACE [17]. The same study also proved that Y90 can significantly prolong survival time when compared to conventional transarterial chemoembolization (cTACE) and censored by liver transplantation, 18.6 months versus 17.7 months, respectively [17]. TACE microsphere particles are also significantly larger than Y90 microspheres. TACE particles are between 200 and 500 microns compared to the 20 to 30 microns of Y90. This creates a greater embolic phenomenon in TACE. The treatments for advanced liver cancer are increasing with new targeted systemic therapies and combinations with chemotherapy. This includes both primary disease such as hepatocellular carcinoma and metastatic disease, such as colorectal carcinoma.

There are several contraindications to Y90 that must be considered prior to treatment. Absolute contraindications include: exaggerated hepatopulmonary shunting calculated as greater than 20% during by Technetium MAA scan, uncorrectable gastrointestinal reflux, pregnancy, and those who have been treated with cabecitabine in the previous two months or anytime thereafter, especially while breastfeeding (SIR-Spheres only) [10] [18] [19]. Radiation pneumonitis and gastro-duodenal ulcers are two of the more serious, but rarely seen due to standards in proper administration, complications associated with Y90 treatment. Reflux of Y90 through the gastroduodenal artery during treatment is usually prevented with placement of the catheter tip distal to the feeding vessel or prophylactic coil embolization of the vessel during mapping or prior to microsphere administration. For TheraSphere, the upper limit of injected activity to the lungs for safety is 30 Gy for a single treatment and 50 Gy for all treatments combined in a single lifetime. These numbers are relative contraindications include prior hepatic radiotherapy, portal vein compromise, fulminant liver failure (including hepatic encephalopathy and greater than a Child-Pugh Score A for cirrhosis), renal failure, right to left cardiopulmonary shunting, biliary obstruction, patients who cannot undergo hepatic artery catheterization (such as patients with vascular abnormalities or abnormal bleeding diatheses), pulmonary insufficiency, portal venous thrombosis (PVT), greater than 70% replacement of liver parenchyma with tumor, and those comorbidities or overall health that make a patient a poor procedural candidate [18] [19].

As previously stated, Y90 therapy is not a curable alternative. Curable therapies include hepatic transplantation, resection, and ablation, both microwave and radiofrequency. A study by Lewandowski et al. in 2018 demonstrated that radiation segmentectomy utilizing TheraSphere Y90 produced outcomes that are consistent with treatments considered curative in patients with solitary tumors less than 5 cm in diameter [20]. Similarly, Cardarelli-Leite et al. demonstrated similar outcomes in a more diverse population utilizing both glass and resin Y90 in radiation segmentectomy or lobectomy [21]. This study concluded that there were no significant differences at 1-year survival and overall survival [21]. However, there are benefits associated with Y90. These includes disease stabilization until transplant becomes available, palliative treatment, or resection. Y90 treatment requires a mutli-specialty approach including a combination of providers from transplant hepatology, diagnostic radiology, medical oncology, surgical oncology, and interventional radiology/oncology. Other benefits of Y90 include a minimally invasive procedure that can be performed on an outpatient basis. Y90 is a two-step process. The initial encounter includes a hepatic arteriogram, also known as a mapping, where a provider visualizes the feeding arteries and branches that supply the tumor. A radiotracer composed of technetium-99m (Tc99m) with macroaggregated albumin (MAA) is delivered to the target site. This Tc99m MAA contains the gamma-emitting Tc99m, which houses the metastable nuclear isomer of technetium-99 (Tc99). The gamma radiation is able to be visualized with subsequent single photon emission computed tomography (SPECT). The main purpose of this process is to confirm that there are no collateral vessels that would allow the distribution of Y90 to surrounding tissues, mainly the lungs, stomach, and duodenum. Nearby feeding branches can also be prophylactically coil-embolized to prevent any reflux. The main arteries embolized are usually the right gastric or gastroduodenal arteries. It also gives a prediction of where the target Y90 will distribute to. This step is usually performed between 1 to 7 days prior to the Y90 treatment; however, some centers have shown that same day mapping and treatment area also possible.

The mapping itself can be thought of in two steps. The first step includes angiography with any desired preparatory interventions (e.g., embolization). The angiography should provide a comprehensive understanding of liver and tumor vascular supply. In addition, angiography should provide a good understanding of the vessels at risk for potential non-target embolization. The second step is a trial run with the infusion of technetium-99m-macroagregated albumin (MAA) into the target vessel and subsequent scintigraphy. The goal of Tc-MAA is to provide details regarding a real time calculation of the pulmonary radiation exposure secondary to shunting as well as dosimetric calculations of tumor radiation dosage.

After acquiring pre-procedural abdominal MRI and/or CT scans, the use of angiographic mapping is important for delineating segmental vascular anatomy and blood-flow patterns that can only be detailed by angiographic observation. This allows for a more comprehensive understanding of the appropriate target vessels for Y90 embolization. Angiography also allows for identification and preventative embolization of vessels at risk for off-target embolization. When performing the initial angiography, it is important to be thorough in the evaluation of the celiac trunk paying special attention to the hepatic arterial supply. Some notable arteries that should be identified include the gastroduodenal, right gastric, falciform, supra-duodenal, and cystic. Attention should be paid to any notable variants including accessory or replaced left gastric arteries and variant right gastric artery origins. First vessel reflux should be noted because reflux and undesired filling of off target vessels can lead to inaccurate mapping and be a risk for non-target embolization during Y90 treatment. Contrast injection should be at a manageable flow rate to avoid reflux while providing sufficient opacification of target vasculature. Certain anatomy with high reflux or high shunting may benefit from embolization pre-operatively, a topic described earlier. In addition to celiac arteriogram, angiographic interrogation of the superior mesenteric artery (SMA) is commonplace. In some instances, evaluation of the inferior mesenteric artery (IMA), intercostals and phrenic arteries can facilitate planning and may identify any important variant anatomy or arterial supply to tumor. However, the decision to pursue SMA or IMA angiography should be determined based on patient anatomy from initial imaging (CT/MRI) and should be weighed against the risk of potential kidney damage from contrast agents.

Shunting patterns such as arteriovenous or arterioportal shunting can also be identified based on angiographic findings even before Tc-MAA infusion studies. High grade shunting can be managed by various embolic approaches, modified dosing, and hepatic venous outflow occlusion.

Prophylactic embolization used to be a standard practice for all Y90 cases. However, a more selective approach to prophylactic embolization is becoming the standard of practice. It is generally preferable to pursue prophylactic embolization only of the high-risk vessels likely to be source of off-target embolization based on angiographic/CBCT findings and avoid unnecessary embolization. Prophylactic embolization can be done with coils, plugs, or glue, although coils are the most common approach. The most common arterial sources of off target embolization include the gastroduodenal, right gastric, and falciform arteries [22]. The indications for prophylactic coil embolization are individual based on each case but some general patterns tend to be true and should be taken into consideration [22]. The most common situation requiring gastroduodenal artery embolization includes lobar Y90 treatment, particularly if there is a short proper-hepatic artery which would be a higher risk for infusion reflux to the gastroduodenal artery. In the case of variant anatomy embolization should be considered based on the flow patterns on angiography. Identification of a falciform artery should be noted and this artery may be coil embolized to prevent the potential complication of abdominal wall radiation dermatitis, however this practice varies and it is not an absolute indication. Alternatively, an ice pack could be placed over the abdomen at the site of arterial supply to the cutaneous surface prior to and during treatment. This will vasoconstrict vessels in this location decreasing distal embolization. Variant anatomy can present challenges when it comes to radioembolization as flow patterns can be unpredictable and the tumor vasculature may be more difficult to delineate. Therefore, it is important to have prior knowledge of the baseline CT and MRI imaging before beginning angiography. Some common variants include a right hepatic artery from the SMA and left hepatic artery from the left gastric artery. These replaced hepatic artery variants pose a potential risk by their branching from enteric vessels and as such they are a source of potential reflux into enteric vasculature. It is possible to coil embolize these variant arteries in attempt to force collateralization from the contralateral hepatic artery lobe, but this will preclude selective lobar treatment and prevents re-access to the vessel in question. Alternatively, Y90 embolization can be delivered safely from the variant vessel themselves so long as there is sufficient distance between the catheter tip and the nearest proximal enteric side branch to prevent reflux embolization.

After angiographic planning and preoperative embolization, the second step of mapping is the infusion of Tc-MAA. MAA particles range in diameter between 0 to 150um with 90% falling between 10 and 90um. Being comparable in size to Y-90 particles allows a simulation embolization pattern of the resin or glass beads while also being biodegradable. Because Technetium-99m radioisotope possesses a short half-life (6 hours) and emits gamma rays making it an ideal radioisotope label. The Tc-MAA can be used to effectively simulate Y90 treatment without risk of harm. Following Tc-MAA infusion at the target vessel the patient is immediately sent for scintigraphy. A planar view has historically been used, but the use of more advanced tomographic imaging such as single photon emission CT (SPECT) allows for more accurate detection of Tc99 distribution, particularly in extra-hepatic tissues. With more accurate imaging, dosimetrists can simulate the expected deposition of Y90, and advanced dosimetry calculations based on these findings allows for the calculation of the hepato-pulmonary shunt fraction which is the proportion of radiation dose delivered to the lung parenchyma given as a percentage. The hepato-pulmonary shunt fraction, also called the lung-shunt fraction (LSF), should be minimized.

In terms of total doses, it is recommended that the lung total exposure be less than 30 Gy in one given treatment, and that the lifetime exposure be less than 50 Gy for TheraSphere. A LSF higher than this puts the patient at high risk for developing radiation pneumonitis. MAA scintigraphy can give an estimate for the dose delivery to the tumor and liver parenchyma. Extrahepatic deposition of Tc-MAA should also be investigated to determine if it is true off target embolization or simply free technetium-99 released from degraded MAA particles. There are a few key arteries listed above that are potential sources for off-target embolization, particularly the GDA, supra duodenal, high gastric, cystic, and falciform arteries. This distinction can be made by observing whether the pattern of deposition is focal or diffuse. True off target embolization will present with focal Tc-MAA deposition, often in the gastric or duodenal mucosa. Free Tc-MAA will appear diffusely through gastric mucosa, thyroid, and kidneys [23].

Alternative Brachytherapy

There are three types of brachytherapy utilized for the treatment of cancer. There are low-dose rate (LDR) implants which keeps a radiation source in place for a short amount of time, typically 1 to 7 days, which usually requires hospitalization during that time. The source of radiation is subsequently removed after the treatment period. High-dose rate (HDR) implants where the radiation source is left in place for 10 to 20 minutes at a time. There may be multiple treatments: a patient may receive two treatments per day for a duration of 2 to 5 days. However, because the radiation source is removed after a short period of time, the advantage over LDR implants is that this can be performed on an outpatient basis. Scheduling is variable depending on the cancer type and location of the neoplasm. Once treatment has been completed, the source can also be removed. The earliest published reports on seed brachytherapy came from Memorial Hospital, New York, USA, in which Barringer experimented with radon-222 (Rn-222) seeds for prostate carcinoma [24]. The earliest radioisotopes included Radon-222 (222Rn), Aurium-198 (198Au), and Iodine-125 (125I) [24]. After several years of experimentation, the most commonly used sources of radioisotopes include Iodine-125 (125I), Palladium-103 (103Pd), Cesium-131 (131Cs), and Iridium-192 (192-Ir) [24] [25]. The third category of brachy therapy includes permanent implants. Y90 is a type of manual permanent brachytherapy implant as it is user-operated for select targeting and super-selection of neoplasms.

Microbrachytherapy is a type of brachytherapy utilizing lower doses of radiation to radioablate tumors. Y90 has been known to be a microtherapy and is usually catheter-directed. However, some earlier studies have shown to be effective by reducing tumor size with direct intra-tumoral injection of Y90 microspheres [26] [27]. Other studies have also utilized holmium-166 (166Ho) as a type of brachytherapy. Holmium is an interesting isotope because it mainly emits beta particles, just like Y90, but also emits a small fraction of gamma radiation [28]. Therefore, it has the potential to emit dual electromagnetic radiation to help selectively target and ablate tumor cells. The gamma rays can then be accurately measured for precise location using gamma scintigraphy. Studies continue to evaluate the effectiveness of holmium and its stability as a microsphere. One study on rabbits however, showed that when holmium is attached to acetylacetonate microspheres, it remains attached to particles after 30 days without any leakage into bodily fluids and tissues including femur, blood, feces, or urine [28]. One pilot study investigated the administration of holmium-166 in felines with unresectable liver cancer [29]. Results were promising and showed no adverse effects, although there were limitations to the study including 3 total participants [29].

Y90 in Practical Detail

Yttrium-90 has the electron configuration [Kr] 4d15s2 which decays into Zirconium-90 (^{90}Zr) after the emission of a beta particle. Beta decay can be either beta plus (β+) where a high energy positron is emitted or beta minus (β-) where a high speed electron is emitted. Y90 undergoes beta minus decay, therefore emitting an electron and also an antineutrino along with it. In this process, a neutron is also converted to a proton therefore increasing the atomic number of the element by 1. This transforms it into the next highest element on the periodic table. Y90 is a pure beta-emitter with an average decay energy of .94MeV [30] and maximum energy of 2.27 MeV [31].

The half-life of Yttrium-90 is 64.2 hours, or roughly 2.68 days. As with any radiation source, there can be a given radioactive period. Following Y90 administration, patients are said to be "hot" or radioactive for several days where 95% of the material will have decayed within 12 days.

The penetration of Y90 is an average of 2.5 mm through human tissue and air with a maximal distance of 11 mm [32]. This makes Y90 a relatively safe isotope compared to other radioactive elements.

The microspheres to which Y90 is attached to (SIR-Sphere) or integrated with (TheraSphere) have a similar density to that of a red blood cell. The resin is isodense but the glass matrix of TheraSpheres have 3 times the density and are thus hyperdense to red blood cells. For this reason, resin microspheres may have a higher propensity to more uniformly distribute within the tumor [33].

There are two main producers of Y90. TheraSphere is produced by Boston scientific. It is composed of a 15-35 μm glass sphere and approximately 1.2-8 million spheres are injected per dose. Theraspheres are created utilizing yttrium-89 (89Y) that is mixed with ultrapure aluminum oxide and silicone dioxide. This mixture is then heated and smelted at 1500 degrees Celsius, subsequent cooled, crushed, and passed through a flame sprayer causing the mixture to spheridize [34]. These spheres are subsequently sifted to select the proper size. The 89Y is then bombarded with neutrons to convert 89Y into 90Y. With this production, several impurities can be created including 88Y and Europium-154 (154Eu), which both have significantly longer half-lives than Y90.

The calculated dose is 2500 becquerel (Bq) per sphere at the time of calibration [34]. TheraSpheres come in sizes between 3 to 20 gigabecquerel (GBq) in 0.5 GBq increments for vial sizes. This allows for the delivery of between 1.2 and 8 million microspheres per vial depending on the radioactivity and subsequently the administration per treatment [34]. The high specific activity of the product enables a high radiation dose to be delivered to the perfused volume without concerns for embolization. Due to its calibration, insitutions have the option to perform radioembolization up to 12 days after delivery creating an extended shelf life. What this translates to is that a given radioactivity can be achieved and administered with varying number of beads based off how many half-lives have passed. Similar outcomes were reported in patients who received an increased number of beads compared to less beads [35].

Current indications for use include local tumor control of solitary tumors with a diameter of 1 to 8 cm, patients with unresectable hepatocellular carcinoma (HCC) who have well-compensated liver function, no macrovascular invasion, and good performance status.

SIR-Spheres are microspheres which are composed of a sulfonated divinyl benzene-styrene copolymer. The production process creates resin spheres ranging from 20 to 30 μm. Contrary to TheraSpheres, which incorporate Y90 into the sphere, SIR-Spheres are coated in Y90. A series of reactions take place which convert the Y90 into a phosphate salt. The salt is subsequently immobilized through a partially cross-linked exchange resin

[36]. SIR-Spheres production creates no impurities as pure Y90 is attached to the resin bead.

Each SIR-Spheres also has a significantly lower radioactivity at 75 Bq per sphere at the time of calibration. SIR-Spheres are calibrated at 6pm EST every day of the week. However, prior to the time of calibration the specific radioactivity can be significantly higher per microsphere as they can be delivered up to 5 days pre-calribration increasing the per sphere Bq considerably. For this reason, significantly greater number of SIR-Spheres are required to be injected in order to reach the same radioactive dose as TheraSphere. The production was standardized so that each batch created contains the same amount of microspheres per vial, which is approximately 44 ±2.6 million [37]. Contrary to how TheraSpheres are designed, SIR-Spheres can be administered up to 5 days pre-calibration time and up to 1 day post-calibration. They are calibrated so that the dose is equivalent to 3 GBq at 18:00 hours the next day, with a variation of ± 10%. Therefore, a 1 GBq aliquot of SIR-Spheres will deliver approximately 13 million microspheres at the time of calibration, which is to be expected due to the radioactive decay [34].

SIR-Spheres Y-90 resin microspheres received pre-market approval by the FDA in 2002 for for the treatment of unresectable metastatic liver tumors from primary colorectal cancer with adjuvant intrahepatic artery chemotherapy (IHAC) of FUDR (Floxuridine). It is awaiting full FDA approval, which will most likely come in the coming years or months.

Initial SIRTex studies on mCRC showed a time to progressive disease of 18.6 months when combined with first-line chemotherapy fluorouracil/leucovorin versus fluorouracil/leucovorin alone [38]. Median survival was also increased in the Y90 + chemotherapy group with a median of 29.4 months compared to 12.8 months in the chemotherapy alone group [38]. The first multi-centre phase II clinical trial by Cosimelli et al. in patients with mCRC who failed previous systemic chemotherapy demonstrated a median overall survival of 12.6 months and 1- and 2-year survival rates of 50.4% and 19.6%, respectively [39]. An early phase III clinical trial by Hendlisz et al. evaluated for time to progression (TTP) and time to liver progression (TTLP) in patients with mCRC receiving fluorouracil alone and resin Y90 radioembolization in combination with fluorouracil [40]. This study demonstrated longer TTLP at 2.1 and 5.5 months and TTP of 2.1 and 4.5 months when comparing fluorouracil alone with combination fluorouracil and Y90, respectively [40]. A more recent prospective study of 1027 patients performed by the Cardiovascular and Interventional Radiological

Society of Europe (CIRSE) addressed the outcomes of Y90 resin microspheres for primary or metastatic liver tumors and their overall survival [41]. For primary tumors, median overall survival was: 16.5 months for hepatocellular carcinoma and 14.6 months for intrahepatic cholangiocarcinoma. For primary liver metastasis, medial overall survival was: 9.8 months for mCRC, 5.6 months for pancreatic cancer, 10.6 months for breast cancer, 14.6 months for melanoma, and 33.1 months for neuroendocrine cancer [41].

Initial practices utilized pure water as the diluent. However, it has since been switched to D5W as data showed lower rates of stasis and higher rates of prescribed activity when compared to sterile water [42]. This ultimately resulted in a more complete dose delivery [42].

Why not external radiation?

Stereotactic body radiotherapy (SBRT) or stereotactic ablative radiotherapy (SABR) are a type of external beam radiation therapy (EBRT) where external sources or radiation are positioned to specifically target lesions in the body to induce cell death. This is a type of non-invasive procedure in comparison to selective internal radiation therapy. It also serves as a bridge to transplant just as TARE does. However, some studies have demonstrated that it is underutilized in today's clinical practice for the treatment of HCC, even though it's overall utilization has increased in the last 10 years [43]. EBRT has similar use indications to SIRT including curative treatment as well as palliation for patients with intractable disease and vessel invasion [44]. The National Comprehensive Cancer Network (NCCN) has even increased the treatment categorization of EBRT to the same level as intra-arterial radioembolization (from 2B to 2A) [44]. Reasons for underutilization are currently unclear but could be related to additional damage to surrounding tissues caused by the external radiation leading to tissue necrosis and/or fibrosis.

There are currently no studies that have directly compared SBRT with SIRT. Two retrospective studies were able to demonstrate similar outcomes with regards to overall and disease-specific survival benefits [45] [46]. Further prospective comparison studies are required to truly determine the overall benefits and determine a superior treatment. At this time, both have equal recommendations when it comes to the treatment of HCC.

Mechanism of cell death in Y90 treatment

Radiation induced cell death from Y90 is the same kind of process as would be expected from other radiation sources. The primary mechanism by which cells die after a significant amount of radiation is due to a deficiency in DNA repair mechanisms that ultimately leads to double stranded DNA breaks [47]. The exact process that these DNA breaks occur is through the high energy electrons that are released. These particles are able to break covalent bonds between atoms which then weaken the structure causing it to denature.

Secondary effects of ionizing radiation cause the production of reactive oxygen species (ROS). ROS are nucleophilic molecules that can lead to the oxidation of several molecules including lipids, proteins, and lead to changes within the DNA structure. Changes in the DNA structure include the production of single stranded DNA breaks and the production of apurinic or apyrimidinic (abasic) sites. Cells are able to repair DNA damage to a given extent. Once a specific threshold is met and the cell is unable to repair a significant portion of the damage, it undergoes programmed cell death or apoptosis [48, 49]. The two pathways double stranded breaks are repaired include non-homologous end joining (which is error prone) and homologous recombination (which requires an undamaged sister chromatid as the template strand).

Y90 radioembolization induces cell death in two ways: through oxygen starvation and through electromagnetic radiation. The microspheres have an embolic effect limiting blood flow to the tumor causing infarction and ischemia. One study was able to demonstrate the immunohistochemical and genetic changes that take place with Y90 [50]. This study showed that Caspase 8 had more pronounced activation in Y90 treated tumor cells which suggests a stronger activation of the apoptotic pathway [50]. In addition to apoptosis, the autophagy pathway was also significantly more active when compared to controls by demonstrating increased Atg12-Atg5 complexes [50]. Other studies demonstrated local immune activation with increased populations of CD4 and CD8 T cells, antigen presenting cells, and NK cells suggesting, an inflammatory component to cell death [51]. These studies have laid the groundwork to determine pre-treatment response in specific patient populations. Further studies are required to investigate additional molecular pathways.

References

1. Diner, P., *Yttrium from Ytterby.* Nat Chem, 2016. **8**(2): p. 192.
2. Lide, D.R., *CRC Handbook of Chemistry and Physics, 86th Edition.* 2005: Taylor & Francis.
3. Baum, E.M., Knolls Atomic Power Laboratory., and Bechtel Marine Propulsion Corporation., *Nuclides and isotopes : chart of the nuclides.* 17th / ed. 2010, Schenectady, N.Y.: KAPL : Bechtel. vi, 94 pages.
4. Bierman, H.R., et al., *Studies on the blood supply of tumors in man. III. Vascular patterns of the liver by hepatic arteriography in vivo.* J Natl Cancer Inst, 1951. **12**(1): p. 107-31.
5. Ariel, I.M., *Treatment of Inoperable Primary Pancreatic and Liver Cancer by the Intra-Arterial Administration of Radioactive Isotopes (Y90 Radiating Microspheres).* Ann Surg, 1965. **162**: p. 267-78.
6. Wollner, I., et al., *Effects of hepatic arterial yttrium 90 glass microspheres in dogs.* Cancer, 1988. **61**(7): p. 1336-44.
7. Gray, B.N., et al., *Regression of liver metastases following treatment with yttrium-90 microspheres.* Aust N Z J Surg, 1992. **62**(2): p. 105-10.
8. Gray, B.N., et al., *Selective internal radiation (SIR) therapy for treatment of liver metastases: measurement of response rate.* J Surg Oncol, 1989. **42**(3): p. 192-6.
9. Services, U.D.o.H.a.H., *TheraSphere: Summary of safety and probable benefit 1999*, P.H.S.F.a.D. Administration, Editor. 1999.
10. Services, U.D.o.H.a.H., *SIR-Spheres: Summary of safety and effectiveness data 2002*, P.H.S.F.a.D. Administration, Editor. 2002.
11. Salem, R., et al., *Yttrium-90 Radioembolization for the Treatment of Solitary, Unresectable HCC: The LEGACY Study.* Hepatology, 2021. **74**(5): p. 2342-2352.
12. Mazzaferro, V., et al., *Liver transplantation for the treatment of small hepatocellular carcinomas in patients with cirrhosis.* N Engl J Med, 1996. **334**(11): p. 693-9.
13. Yao, F.Y., et al., *Downstaging of hepatocellular cancer before liver transplant: Long-term outcome compared to tumors within Milan criteria.* Hepatology, 2015. **61**(6): p. 1968-1977.
14. Bento de Sousa, J.H., et al., *Comparison between Milan and UCSF criteria for liver transplantation in patients with hepatocellular carcinoma: a systematic review and meta-analysis.* Transl Gastroenterol Hepatol, 2021. **6**: p. 11.
15. Kennedy, A.S., et al., *Radioembolization for Unresectable Neuroendocrine Hepatic Metastases Using Resin 90Y-Microspheres:*

Early Results in 148 Patients. American Journal of Clinical Oncology, 2008. **31**(3): p. 271-279.

16. Jia, Z. and W. Wang, *Yttrium-90 radioembolization for unresectable metastatic neuroendocrine liver tumor: A systematic review.* Eur J Radiol, 2018. **100**: p. 23-29.
17. Salem, R., et al., *Y90 radioembolization significantly prolongs time to progression compared with chemoembolization in patients with hepatocellular carcinoma.* Gastroenterology, 2016. **151**(6): p. 1155-1163. e2.
18. Murthy, R., et al., *Radioembolization of yttrium-90 microspheres for hepatic malignancy.* Semin Intervent Radiol, 2008. **25**(1): p. 48-57.
19. Scientific, B. *Instructions for Use TheraSphere ™ Yttrium-90 Glass Microspheres*. 2021 March 2021 [cited 2022; Available from: https://www.bostonscientific.com/content/dam/elabeling/pi/OTT-00221_Rev1_TheraSphere_en_s.pdf.
20. Lewandowski, R.J., et al., *Radiation Segmentectomy: Potential Curative Therapy for Early Hepatocellular Carcinoma.* Radiology, 2018. **287**(3): p. 1050-1058.
21. Cardarelli-Leite, L., et al., *Ablative Transarterial Radioembolization Improves Survival in Patients with HCC and Portal Vein Tumor Thrombus.* Cardiovasc Intervent Radiol, 2020. **43**(3): p. 411-422.
22. Borggreve, A.S., et al., *Radioembolization: Is Prophylactic Embolization of Hepaticoenteric Arteries Necessary? A Systematic Review.* Cardiovasc Intervent Radiol, 2016. **39**(5): p. 696-704.
23. Bailey, J.J., et al., *Biodistribution of 99mTc-MAA on SPECT/CT performed for 90Y radioembolization therapy planning: a pictorial review.* Clin Transl Imaging, 2017. **5**(5): p. 473-485.
24. BARRINGER, B.S., *RADIUM IN THE TREATMENT OF CARCINOMA OF THE BLADDER AND PROSTATE: REVIEW OF ONE YEAR'S WORK.* Journal of the American Medical Association, 1917. **LXVIII**(17): p. 1227-1230.
25. Stish, B.J., et al., *Low dose rate prostate brachytherapy.* Transl Androl Urol, 2018. **7**(3): p. 341-356.
26. Jia-He, T., et al., *Ultrasound-guided internal radiotherapy using yttrium-90-glass microspheres for liver malignancies.* The Journal of Nuclear Medicine, 1996. **37**(6): p. 958.
27. Ho, S., et al., *Ultrasound guided internal radiotherapy using yttrium-90 glass microspheres for liver malignancies.* The Journal of Nuclear Medicine, 1997. **38**(7): p. 1169.

28. Bult, W., et al., *Radioactive holmium acetylacetonate microspheres for interstitial microbrachytherapy: an in vitro and in vivo stability study.* Pharm Res, 2012. **29**(3): p. 827-36.
29. Bult, W., et al., *Interstitial microbrachytherapy using holmium-166 acetylacetonate microspheres: a feasibility study in feline liver cancer patients.* Holmium microparticles for intratumoral radioablation, 2010: p. 75.
30. Tong, M., *Radiation safety post liver Y90 therapy - Is the hospital ward safe?* Journal of Nuclear Medicine, 2018. **59**(supplement 1): p. 1806-1806.
31. Kim, S.P., et al., *A guide to (90)Y radioembolization and its dosimetry.* Phys Med, 2019. **68**: p. 132-145.
32. Kim, Y.-C., et al., *Radiation safety issues in Y-90 microsphere selective hepatic radioembolization therapy: possible radiation exposure from the patients.* Nuclear medicine and molecular imaging, 2010. **44**(4): p. 252-260.
33. Burrill, J., U. Hafeli, and D. Liu, *Advances in radioembolization-Embolics and isotopes.* J Nucl Med Radiat Ther, 2011. **2**(1): p. 107.
34. Westcott, M.A., et al., *The development, commercialization, and clinical context of yttrium-90 radiolabeled resin and glass microspheres.* Adv Radiat Oncol, 2016. **1**(4): p. 351-364.
35. Lewandowski, R.J., et al., *Sustained safety and efficacy of extended-shelf-life (90)Y glass microspheres: long-term follow-up in a 134-patient cohort.* Eur J Nucl Med Mol Imaging, 2014. **41**(3): p. 486-93.
36. Gray, B.N., *Polymer based radionuclide containing particulate material*, S.M. Limited, Editor. 2002.
37. Incorporated, S.M. *About SIR-Spheres* [cited 2022 09-12-2022]; Available from: https://www.sirtex.com/us/products/sir-spheres-y-90-resin-microspheres/about-sir-spheres/.
38. Van Hazel, G., et al., *Randomised phase 2 trial of SIR-Spheres® plus fluorouracil/leucovorin chemotherapy versus fluorouracil/leucovorin chemotherapy alone in advanced colorectal cancer.* Journal of Surgical Oncology, 2004. **88**(2): p. 78-85.
39. Cosimelli, M., et al., *Multi-centre phase II clinical trial of yttrium-90 resin microspheres alone in unresectable, chemotherapy refractory colorectal liver metastases.* Br J Cancer, 2010. **103**(3): p. 324-31.
40. Hendlisz, A., et al., *Phase III trial comparing protracted intravenous fluorouracil infusion alone or with yttrium-90 resin microspheres radioembolization for liver-limited metastatic colorectal cancer refractory to standard chemotherapy.* J Clin Oncol, 2010. **28**(23): p. 3687-94.

41. Helmberger, T., et al., *Clinical Application of Trans-Arterial Radioembolization in Hepatic Malignancies in Europe: First Results from the Prospective Multicentre Observational Study CIRSE Registry for SIR-Spheres Therapy (CIRT).* Cardiovasc Intervent Radiol, 2021. **44**(1): p. 21-35.
42. Koran, M.E., et al., *Five percent dextrose maximizes dose delivery of Yttrium-90 resin microspheres and reduces rates of premature stasis compared to sterile water.* Biomed Rep, 2016. **5**(6): p. 745-748.
43. Herman, T., et al., *Bridge-to-transplant external-beam radiation therapy in patients with hepatocellular carcinoma: A utilization analysis of the United Network for Organ Sharing (UNOS) database.* International Journal of Radiation Oncology, Biology, Physics, 2021. **111**(3): p. e62-e63.
44. Park, S., W.S. Yoon, and C.H. Rim, *Indications of external radiotherapy for hepatocellular carcinoma from updated clinical guidelines: Diverse global viewpoints.* World journal of gastroenterology, 2020. **26**(4): p. 393.
45. Oladeru, O.T., et al., *Conformal external beam radiation or selective internal radiation therapy—a comparison of treatment outcomes for hepatocellular carcinoma.* Journal of Gastrointestinal Oncology, 2016. **7**(3): p. 433.
46. Oladeru, O., et al., *External Beam Radiation Therapy or Selective Internal Radiation Therapy? A Comparison of Treatment Outcomes for Hepatocellular Carcinoma.* International Journal of Radiation Oncology, Biology, Physics, 2015. **93**(3): p. E123.
47. Borrego-Soto, G., R. Ortiz-López, and A. Rojas-Martínez, *Ionizing radiation-induced DNA injury and damage detection in patients with breast cancer.* Genet Mol Biol, 2015. **38**(4): p. 420-32.
48. Deckbar, D., P.A. Jeggo, and M. Löbrich, *Understanding the limitations of radiation-induced cell cycle checkpoints.* Crit Rev Biochem Mol Biol, 2011. **46**(4): p. 271-83.
49. Guo, G.S., et al., *DNA repair and synthetic lethality.* Int J Oral Sci, 2011. **3**(4): p. 176-9.
50. Meller, R., et al., *Programmed cell death in a patient with hepatocellular carcinoma treated with yttrium-90 and doxorubicin-loaded beads.* Journal of Vascular and Interventional Radiology, 2013. **24**(10): p. 1537-1542. e2.
51. Chew, V., et al., *Immune activation underlies a sustained clinical response to Yttrium-90 radioembolisation in hepatocellular carcinoma.* Gut, 2019. **68**(2): p. 335-346.

CHAPTER 7

^{90}YTTRIUM FOR PRIMARY HEPATIC TUMORS

ZACHARY S. COLLINS MD, FSIR,
PATRICIA TOWNSEND MD, DEVON O'GUINN MD,
STEPHEN MARKHAM DO

Prevalence/Incidence/At Risk Population

As discussed earlier, though in short review, hepatocellular carcinoma (HCC) is the principal liver cancer accounting for approximately 75% of liver cancers worldwide. It is the seventh most frequently occurring cancer in the world and the third leading cause of cancer-related deaths [1, 2]. Annually, 700,000 new cases and 600,000 deaths attributable to HCC worldwide [2]. In 2021, the incidence of liver and intrahepatic bile duct cancers was approximated to be 42,230 with 30,230 deaths [3]. Incidence rates among men are 2-3 times higher than women [1, 3]. The incidence rate correlates directly with age until 75 years of age. In the United States (US), the median age of diagnosis is between 60-64 years [1]. In the US, per 100,000 people, the prevalence of HCC was greatest in Native Americans/Native Alaskans (11.4), followed by Hispanics (9.8), Asians/Pacific Islanders (9/1), Non-Hispanic Black people (8.1) and Non-Hispanic White people (4.6) [1]. The age at diagnosis of HCC is generally lower in areas where HBV is more prevalent, while the prevalence of obesity, metabolic syndrome and non-alcoholic fatty liver disease (NAFLD) are directly related to incidence of HCC [4]. Hepatitis B Virus (HBV) Hepatitis C Virus (HCV) carriers have risk of developing HCC is 10-25% and 10-20% respectively while NAFLD and non-alcoholic Steatohepatitis are also major factors in the onset of HCC [1].

General treatment options

Up until the 1980's, surgical resection was the only intervention for HCC until the acceptance of liver transplantation as a curative solution [4]. Overall survival for HCC within the United States is <20% [5]. The Barcelona Clinic Liver Cancer guidelines denote patients with very early or early-stage disease are eligible for curative therapies including surgical resection or liver transplantation [6]. However, 80% of patients first present with advanced stage HCC making alternative treatment modalities essential [5]. Liver transplantation for non-resectable tumors is limited by availability of transplant livers and patient eligibility. These factors are defined by patient preserved liver function and associated Milan criteria [6]. Non-curative ablation therapies have been developed out of necessity including transarterial chemoembolization (TACE) and transarterial radioembolization (TARE, also referred to as Y90). Surgical resection remains the gold standard primary treatment option for well-defined tumors and can be associated with excellent results.

Yttrium

As discussed thoroughly in the prior chapter, Y90 is a decay product of strontium and is a pure beta-particle emitter [7]. It has a half-life of 64.1 hours [7]. Y90 is produced in a resin and glass form. Sirtex (SIR-Spheres®, Sirtex Medical Inc., Woburn, MA, USA) a resin microsphere, received FDA approval for unresectable HCC in in 2002 [8] while Thera-Sphere®, (BTG Inc. West Conshohocken, PA, USA) which produces glass microspheres and received the same approval in 2021 [9].

Phase 1 trials began in the 1980s and 1990s that lead to an FDA Humanitarian Device exemption in 1999. Premarket approval for colorectal cancer liver metastases followed in 2002 [6]. In 2004, the safety of Y90 glass microspheres was first evaluated in 15 patients with unresectable HCC patients with Portal Vein Thrombosis (PVT) demonstrating minimal non-serious adverse events. Y90 treatment was found to not preclude additional therapy with TACE or hepatic artery infusion chemotherapy, opening the opportunity for TARE utilization as an adjuvant therapy [6]. In 2008, Y90 therapy was evaluated to include HCC patients without PVT and demonstrated a similarly acceptable safety profile [10]. The establishment of Y90 as a therapy for patients without PVT prompted an investigation into the efficacy of Y90 for patient's ineligible for systemic treatment. This population was evaluated in 2013, demonstrating that the application of Y90 for patients in Child Pugh B or C as an adjuvant therapy demonstrated comparable results in the patient population to current therapies [6].

Y90's first HCC usage was in the setting of PVT in 2004. TACE has been contraindicated in the setting of PVT due to iatrogenic induced acute liver failure, unless super selective or segmental embolization could be achieved, leading to the investigation of Y90 as a potential therapy. A cohort of 15 patients underwent treatment with Y90 glass microspheres in unresectable HCC with PVT. No patients in the cohort experienced acute liver failure and it was determined that Y90 treatment did not preclude future treatments such as TACE or hepatic artery infusion chemotherapy [6, 11]. A similar study conducted in 2008 evaluated 108 patients with unresectable HCC with and without PVT demonstrating similar outcomes: no cases of radiation induced gastritis, pneumonitis. However, an increased incidence of elevated bilirubin and development of ascites was observed in the group with main PVT, though no treatment related complications or treatment related deaths [10]. The establishment of the Y90 safety profile encouraged research into long term outcomes associated with Y90 therapy. In 2010, Salem et al evaluated 291 patients treated for HCC using Y90 glass microspheres. This single center prospective longitudinal cohort study measured objective response rates (ORRs) of 42% and 57% based on WHO and EASL criteria respectively. The total time to progression (TTP) was noted at 7.9 months with survival and TTP correlating to severity of Child-Pugh Classification. [12]. The demonstration of Y90s effectiveness led to the development of trials investigating a direct comparison of Y90 against existing therapies or in combination with other therapies. In 2021, the conclusion of the LEGACY trial led to the FDA approval of a second Y90 device, Therasphere glass microspheres. The grant indication is for treatment of local tumor control of unresectable solitary HCC <8cm in patient with Child-Pugh Grade A cirrhosis and ECOG performance status 0 and 1. The glass microspheres were previously utilized under humanitarian device exemption [13].

Comparison to Existing Therapies

Y90 has been compared to the current standard of care treatments as a bridge to therapy, in measuring overall effectiveness, and as a combination therapy. In 2009, a comparative analysis evaluated the efficacy of TARE-Y90 vs TACE in downstaging HCC patient from the United Network for Organ (UNO) sharing. A total of 86 patients with comparable tumor sizes who underwent TACE or TARE were followed. In downstaging from T3 to

T2, partial response rates favored TARE over TACE (61% vs 37% respectively). Time to progression also favored TARE (18.2 months TACE; 33.3 months TARE-Y90). Ultimately, downstaging was achieved in 58% of TARE-Y90 and 31% of cases for TACE, supporting the conclusion that TARE-Y90 outperforms TACE in downstaging HCC from UNOs T3 to T2 [14]. The PRIMIERE study, a randomized Phase 2 study comparing effects of cTACE and Y90 in patients with HCC demonstrated a longer median TTP ($\geq$ 26 months) in the Y90 randomized group compared to the TACE (6.8 months). Results indicated significantly increased local tumor control. Furthermore, 87% of Y90 showed complete and partial responses compared to 73.7% resulting from cTACE. However, this study noted increased time to progression did not correlate with an overall increase in survival [15].

Overall effectiveness was evaluated in the Salem 2016 retrospective analysis of 60 patients comparing stereotactic body radiation therapy (SBRT), Y90, radiofrequency ablation, and transarterial chemoembolization as bridge to liver transplant. In this review, Y90 and SBRT demonstrated no Grade 3 toxicities post treatment while Grade 3 or 4 toxicities were seen in TACE (n=4) and RFA (n=3). Rates of pathological complete response were highest in Y90 among all the locoregional therapies [15]. The European Association for the Study of the Liver (EASL) Clinical Practice Guidelines note patients undergoing TARE versus TACE demonstrated increased median survival of 16.9 months to 17.2 months for patients at intermediate stages and 10 months to 12 months for patients at advanced stages with portal vein invasion, decreased toxicity, and a longer TTP. TARE demonstrated better tumor control while maintaining higher quality of life. Notably, there was no difference in survival is noted between the two therapies [16]. Liver hypertrophy post treatment for TARE recipients was also noted for the non-target lobes. In doing so, this could better prepare a candidate for curative surgical resection [16].

As of 2022, a Phase 2 study, "Transarterial RAdioembolization versus ChemoEmbolization for the treatment of hepatocellular carcinoma (TRACE)," comparing 66 patients who underwent either TARE or DEB-TACE for intermediate and early-stage unresectable HCC completed their interim analysis. Interim analysis revealed a median TTP was 17.1 months vs 9.5 months in TARE vs DEB-TACE respectively. A subgroup analysis revealed of those patients with BCLC stage B, there was a median TTP of 12.8 months vs 9.6 months in TARE vs DEB-TACE respectively (p= .009). TARE demonstrated a lower incidence of serious adverse events of Grade 3 or higher compared to DEB-TACE however these results were not statistically significant. [17]. The interim results of this trial support previous conclusions of similar trials but the study is still ongoing.

Two meta-analyses of 5 and 10 studies respectively reviewed the outcomes of TARE versus TACE. Both meta-analyses concluded there were no significant differences in survival at 1 year. However, there was increased overall survival at 2 and 3 years in the TARE cohorts compared to TACE [18, 19]. Progression free survival was greater in TARE at 1 year [18]. Grade 3 and 4 adverse events were found to be reduced in TARE compared to TACE. This relationship was statistically significant in the Lobo meta-analysis [18]. While TARE demonstrated decreased adverse events in the Facciorusso meta-analysis, it was not found to be statistically significant [19]. The Facciorusso meta-analysis included all five studies included in the Lobo analysis plus an additional five. No significant difference was demonstrated in partial or complete response between treatments [19].

Combination therapies

Combination therapies in 2017 and 2018 including Nexavar (Sorafenib, Bayer USA, Whippany NJ) in locally advanced and inoperable hepatocellular carcinoma (SARAH) and SIRT versus Sorafenib (SIRveNIB) trials were evaluated to determine survival outcomes between Y90 and systemic chemotherapy for advanced HCC. In the SARAH Phase 3 randomized control trial of 459 patients, there was no significant different to overall survival or progression free survival between the groups. This study demonstrated a higher rate of adverse events in the sorafenib group when compared to Y90 [20]. Similarly, the results of SIRvsNIB, also a Phase 3 randomized control trial of 360 patients, demonstrated no significant differences in overall survival, even with increased tumor response found in SIRT. Adverse events were less frequently reported in SIRT versus Sorafenib [21]. In 2019, the SORAMIC study, a Phase 2 randomized control trial, evaluated the impact of Sorafenib versus Sorafenib plus Y90 treatment in 529 patients with unresectable locally advanced HCC. No difference in overall survival or adverse events was found between. However, a sub-group analysis demonstrated a possible survival benefit for: patients less than 65 years old, those with non-alcoholic cirrhosis, and those without cirrhosis [22]. A randomized Phase 3 clinical trial of intra-arterial TheraSphere in treatment of patients with unresectable hepatocellular carcinoma plus sorafenib versus sorafenib standard of care (STOP-HCC) is underway. Results are not available as of 2022.

Patient selection

The selection of patients is based on tumor staging criteria as well as determinations by tumor board influenced by current standards for treatment (Example, Fig. 1). Treatment based on tumor classification, extension, and liver disease status can influence the choice of locoregional and systemic approaches for unresectable tumors [4]. There is no consensus as to the optimal use of this therapy, particularly when and if it should be chosen over TACE for treatment of unresectable HCC. TARE is superior to TACE in in the setting of HCC complicated by malignant main or lobar branch portal vein thrombosis [23]. TARE is not recommended for metastatic disease due to the localized nature of the therapy. Systemic therapy for patients of Child-Pugh Class A with extrahepatic metastasis is recommended. Individualized and supportive care are recommended for patients staged Child-Pugh Class B or C respectively [23].

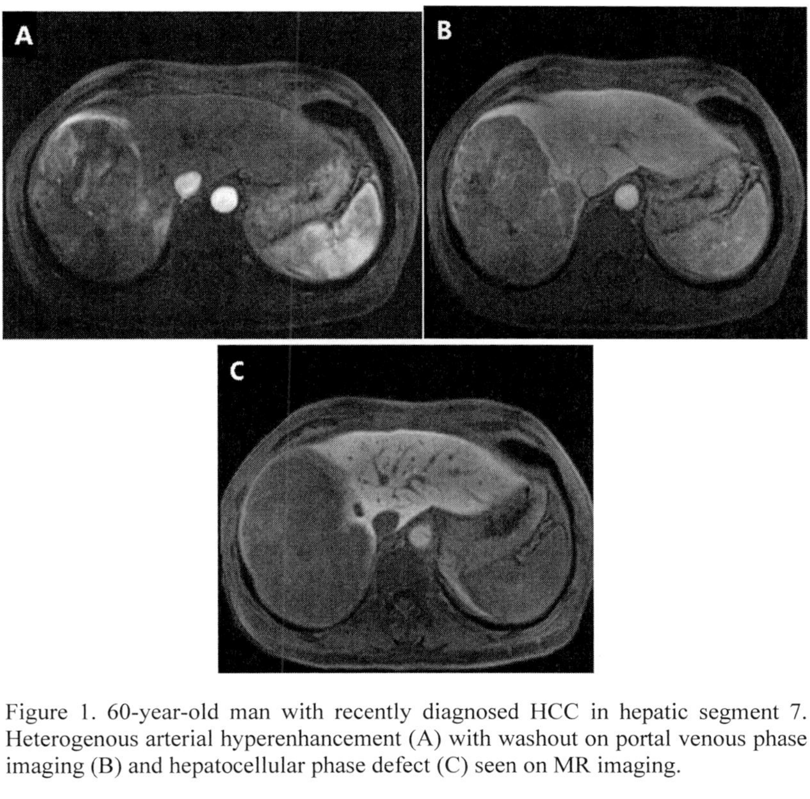

Figure 1. 60-year-old man with recently diagnosed HCC in hepatic segment 7. Heterogenous arterial hyperenhancement (A) with washout on portal venous phase imaging (B) and hepatocellular phase defect (C) seen on MR imaging.

Guidelines

Evidence based guidelines from the EASL and American Association for the Study of Liver Disease (AASLD) agree on the utilization of BCLC as the most evidence based practice for tumor staging [16, 24]. The BCLC 2022 model incorporates Child-Pugh Staging, α-fetoprotein, albumin-bilirubin, and Eastern Cooperative Oncology group performance status into the staging model. EASL notes current TARE data in BCLC stages B and C have not demonstrated survival benefit compared to TACE or sorafenib, yet it is noted that TARE does have a good safety profile and could reduce patient drop-out from the transplant waiting list due to increased tumor control, longer time to progression, higher quality of life, and contralateral liver lobe hypertrophy. When bridging patients to transplant in BCLC criteria, TARE has not demonstrated increased overall survival benefit compared to sorafenib [16]. AASLD notes TARE has been utilized by some centers in BCLC B patients who are poor candidates for TACE, progressive disease post TACE, and patients with >2 nodules with portal vein invasion. In BCLC stage C patients, sorafenib is still recommended as the first line therapy. TARE studies have demonstrated moderate levels of benefit but have not demonstrated benefit over sorafenib [25]. Asia-Pacific Clinical Practice Guidelines note that TARE can be a good option for patients who are not good candidates for TACE due to bulky tumor and/or portal vein invasion and may be used as an alternative locoregional treatment for unresectable HCC.

Y-90 mapping - Mapping via angiography

Understanding variable anatomies within hepatic arterial blood supply and collaterals is essential to effective embolization and Y-90 delivery, decreasing the incidence of non-target deliveries. Pretreatment planning utilizing angiography enables increased vascular mapping for identification of variable arterial and vascular anatomies of the liver, assessment of specific Y90 delivery to the target tumor, and prevention of Y90 shunting via collateral circulation to the lungs, biliary tract, and gastrointestinal tract (Fig. 2) [26].

Cone beam radiation during ^{90m}Tc-MAA shunt examination allows for detection and exclusion of extra-hepatic enhancement more precisely than conventional angiography. This may also be performed during the procedure to track flow of contrast. Technetium TC 99m macroaggregated

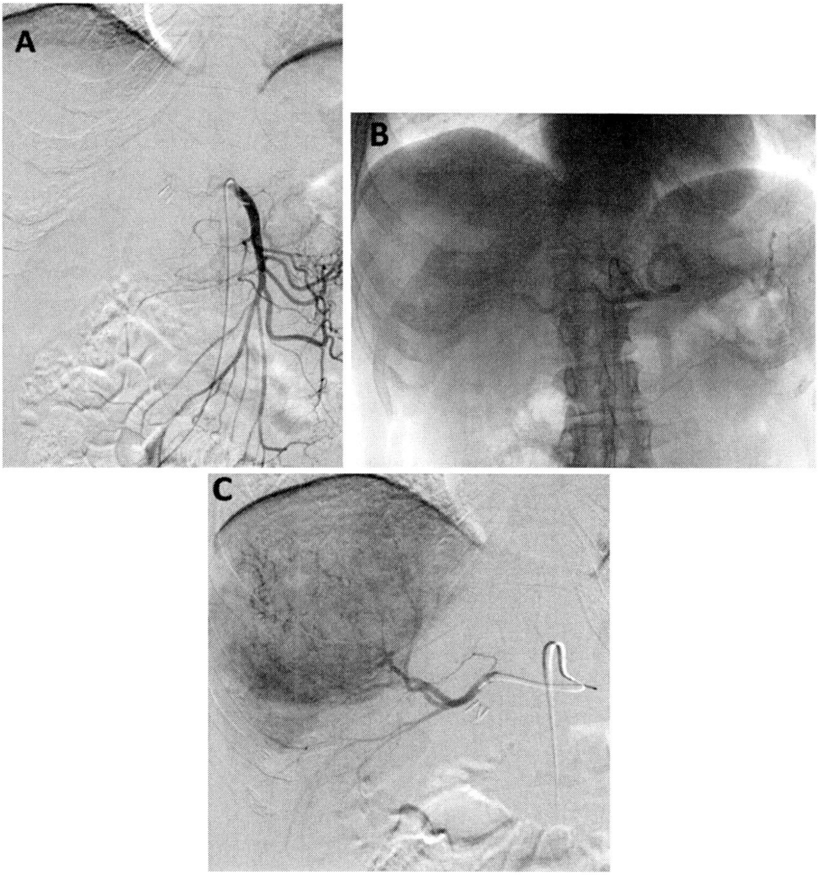

Figure 2. Diagnostic angiogram performed to evaluate extrahepatic vascular supply, extent of disease, and anatomy. Diagnostic subtraction angiogram (DSA) of the SMA (A) and celiac axis (B) demonstrates conventional anatomy. Microcatheter positioned into the right hepatic artery with large tumor blush and neovascularity related to known mass (C).

albumin (MAA) is the most common radiotracer used for mapping radioactive material up into the lungs. [26]. Single-photon emission computed tomography (SPECT/CT) provides the most sensitivity and specificity in imaging technetium Tc99m [7]. Calculation of the dose to the tumor, healthy liver tissue, hepato-pulmonary shunt fraction, and tracer distribution are evaluated.

$$Lung\ Shunt\ Fraction\ (\%) = 100\ x\ \frac{\%\ ID\ Lung}{\%\ ID\ lung + \%\ ID\ Liver}$$

ID = Injected Dose

Patients with >20% shunt fraction are not ideal candidates due to increased risk of radiation pneumonitis. The lung shunt fraction is then applied to calculate the potential activity that might reach the lungs.

$$A_{lung}(GBq) = A_{total}x\ \frac{L}{100}$$

A = activity

L = Lung Shunt Fraction (%)

Treatment may still be delivered provided total activity delivered to the lungs is <30 Gy per treatment session and 50 Gy for the cumulative dose [7]. If Tc 99m MAA microsphere distribution is complete and homogenous without non-target shunting, the procedure may proceed (Example Fig 3) [26].

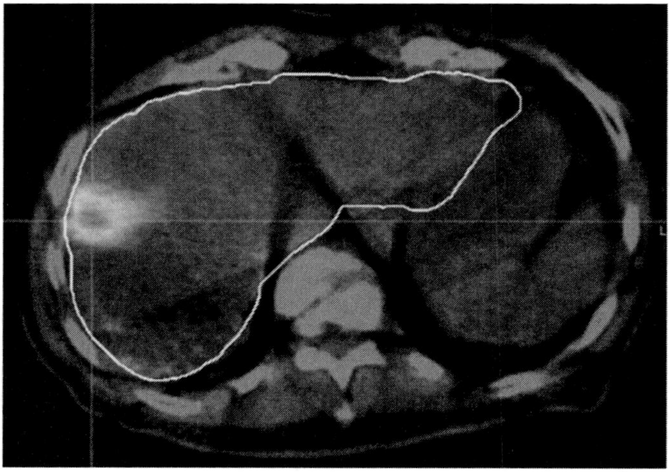

Figure 3. Image-guided dosimetry for Y-90 therapy using converted dose nuclear medicine imaging software by RapidSphere Dosimetry Reporting (Varian Medical Systems, Atlanta, GA).

Dosing

Dosing Guidelines are determined by the selected vehicle for administration and the device instructions for use. The most current version of the product instructions for use should be consulted on a product specific basis. The TheraSphere and Sirtex devices include an interactive dose ordering calculator that are available online. These calculators are based on desired absorbed dosage, timing of administration, lung shunt fraction, anticipated residual waste, and previous dose to the lungs [27, 28].

Side effects/complications (AEs and Toxicities)

Mapping angiograms in pretreatment can decrease incidences of radiation induced stomach ulcers, cholecystitis, hepatocirrhosis, pancreatitis, and pneumonitis [26]. Absolute contraindications to TARE include Tc 99m MAA microsphere $\geq$ 30 Gy shunted to liver, gastrointestinal collaterals that cannot be corrected with embolization, clinically overt hepatic encephalopathy, biliary obstruction, or Child-Pugh Class C Cirrhosis. Relative contraindications include: Bilirubin > 2mg/dL and ascites [23]. Unlike TACE, extensive vein thrombosis or obstruction is not a contraindication to TARE [6].

Hepatocellular Carcinoma Treatment

As discussed previously, Y-90 can be used as a bridge to transplant liver by downstaging tumors (Fig. 4). Qualification is decided using the Milan Criteria (MC) to categorize patients. Milan Criteria: 1 lesion greater than or equal to 2 cm and less than or equal to 5 cm, OR up to 3 lesions, each greater than or equal to 1 cm and less than or equal to 3 cm (Fig. 1) [29]. Since the passage of the MC approximately 20 years ago, additional expanded criteria have been published, citing concerns that the MC is too rigorous [30, 31]. The Milan Criteria remains most known and well adopted [32].

When tumor size and/or number is outside the MC, Y-90 can be used as local-regional therapy for downstaging [14]. In 2017, a standardized UNOS/Region 5 down-staging protocol was adopted [33]. clinical and imaging prognosticators associated with successful bridging or downstaging to transplant have been proposed, including lower albumin-bilirubin score, lower AFP, lower Child-Pugh class and lower Barcelona Clinic Liver Cancer Stage, as well as absence of fatigue and abdominal pain [34, 35].

Other indications for Y-90 include local-regional therapy of HCC for tumor control if the expected wait time for OLT is greater than 6 months [36].

The use of radiation therapy is the cornerstone of primary liver neoplasm treatment. The traditional radiation options for local control of liver disease include whole liver treatments with external beam radiation or targeted therapy with the radioactive isotope Y90 [37-41]. Selective internal radiation therapy (SIRT) uses resin or glass microspheres to carry the Y90 directly into the hepatic arterial system for treatment of primary liver cancer. The primary advantage of radioembolization with Y90, when compared to external beam radiation therapy, is the ability to deliver local tumoricidal effects while causing minimal effects to surrounding normal hepatic tissue [42]. SIRT has replaced external beam radiation by interventional radiologists for liver-directed therapy.

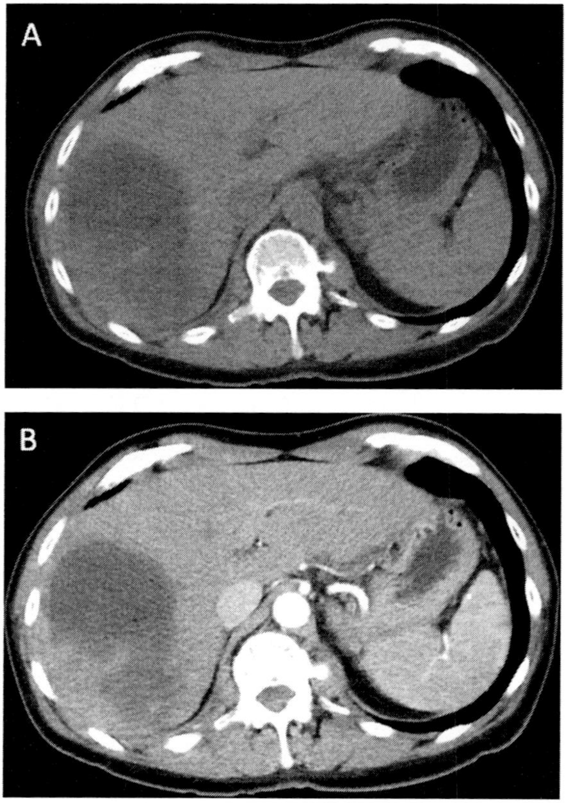

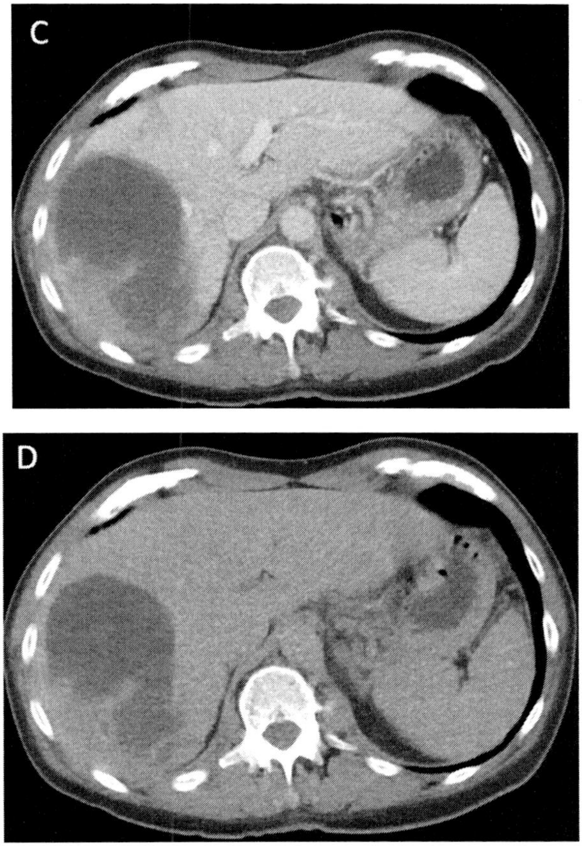

Figure 4. Status post-Y-90 embolization of segment 7 HCC approximately 2 months post-treatment. Precontrast (A), arterial phase (B), portal venous (C), and delayed phase (D) imaging demonstrates slight decreased size of the heterogeneous right hepatic lobe mass with expected post-procedural edema and blood.

Y-90 Combination Therapy

For patients with more advanced HCC, a combined systemic and liver-directed radioembolization approach is often used, based on the discretion of the referring provider/tumor board. These recommendations stem from SIRFLOX, a landmark randomized control trial on patients with liver metastases from colorectal cancer demonstrating the efficacy of adding

SIRT in combination to Y90 versus standard FOLFOX-based chemotherapy treatment alone [43].

Since the SIRFLOX trial, numerous parallel studies (FOXFIRE, FOXFIRE Global for primary HCC, FOL- FOXIRI, FOLFIRI) have emerged studying different combinations of chemotherapy, SIRT, and the timing of each [44]. While trials are ongoing, results demonstrate importance of SIRT in treatment of HCC, with continued evolution and advancement [45-46]. Most recently, the multicenter, retrospective LEGACY study evaluated patients who underwent radioembolization using Y-90 and demonstrated meaningful clinical response rates and prolonged duration of response in patients with unresectable HCC [13]. Detailed discussion of systemic therapies is outside the scope of view for this chapter.

Role of Y-90 in HCC recurrence after OLT

Recurrence rate of HCC after OLT is approximately 15% and is the most common cause of death in this population. Several risk-stratification models have been proposed (including MORAL and RETREAT scores) which attempt to predict risk of recurrence, and include size, number/differentiation of tumors within the explanted liver, AFP levels, and microvascular invasion [36, 47, 48]. Treatment options for post-transplant HCC recurrence remain similar to those in the native liver [49]. There is currently no standardized treatment protocol for disease recurrence, again relying on a multi-disciplinary approach. Recurrence with a solitary lesion is often managed with locoregional therapy such as Y-90 [50-52]. Attempts at prophylactic therapies to reduce HCC post-liver transplant, such as SiLVER trial, have failed to demonstrate long term recurrence-free survival [53]. Further research in this field is needed.

Y-90 for Unresectable HCC

HCC is an aggressive malignancy which often presents late in the disease course. Many patients are not candidates for curative treatment due to advanced disease stage, social factors, comorbidities, and limited availability of liver transplant donors. For these patients, several treatment options exist, including TACE, TARE, or systemic chemotherapy [54]. Y-90 plays an important role in disease control/delaying progression due to low side effect profile and good treatment response. The SORAMIC trial was a randomized control trial evaluating tumor response to sorafenib or sorafenib plus SIRT with Y-90 resin microspheres. The study showed no significant difference in overall survival between the treatment groups, however there was a survival benefit found in patients without cirrhosis, cirrhosis of non-alcoholic etiology, or patients < 65 y/o [22]. Significant protocol deviations occurred in this study, most importantly, delays in Y-90 treatment initiation.

Other trials evaluated benefits of TARE vs TACE in patients with unresectable HCC. Findings showed similar survival outcomes, but when considering the heterogeneity between treatment groups, there was longer time to progression and decreased toxicity compared to TACE, urging towards sub staging HCC even further [55-58]. The consensus recommendations recently published by Salem et al. should be consulted [59].

Cholangiocarcinoma

Cholangiocarcinoma is the second most common primary liver cancer in the US and Europe, with limited treatment options, and poor prognosis. Like HCC, complex surgical resection is considered the only curative treatment, though is often not feasible for patients with this disease [60]. Systemic chemotherapy using gemcitabine and cisplatin is often used [61]. Recent implementation of TARE has shown promising results [62]. A study comparing surgical resection with intra-arterial therapy (defined as either TACE, TARE, or HAI) demonstrated no survival benefit in surgical resection vs IAT [63-64]. Additional retrospective studies show significant overall survival in patients treated with TACE; however no randomized control trials have been performed to date [65].

Hepatocholangiocarcinoma

Hepatocholangiocarcinoma is a rare form of primary liver malignancy featuring histopathologic features of both cholangiocarcinoma and hepatocellular carcinoma (cICC-HCC). This form of liver malignancy has a poor overall prognosis and survival, with only a minority of patients being surgical candidates. As seen with many other forms of primary liver cancer, Y-90 radioembolization is a well-tolerated and effective form of treatment, with some studies citing up to 65% of patients achieving disease control [66-68]. Like cholangiocarcinoma, no randomized control trials for cICC-HCC have been performed, likely due to the rarity of this disease [69].

Hepatoblastoma

Hepatoblastoma (HB) is the most common primary liver cancer in pediatric population. In keeping with primary liver neoplasms, primary treatment is transplant or resection. For those who don't qualify for surgery, systemic chemotherapy is attempted, however HB is often resistant to standard chemotherapy regimens. Treatment with TARE is a novel approach, with increased survival rates and decreased OLT in patients with HB [70]. In a case study, two toddlers with HB proceeded to TARE after suboptimal response to oral chemotherapy. Both patient's tumors responded to TARE without complications, developed hypertrophy of the future liver remnant, received hepatectomies, and went into complete remission [70]. In a separate case study of three toddlers with chemotherapy-resistant HB, TARE allowed for curative treatment in two out of the three toddlers. Unfortunately, one patient developed AML secondary to prior chemotherapy and died [71]. Again, there is limited data and no randomized control trials using TARE on HB given the rarity of this disease and the population affected.

Voxel based dosimetry

As discussed above, determination of the correct Y90 dose is a delicate balance, as under-dosing patients leads to residual/recurrent tumor, and over-dosing can lead to radiation pneumonitis or hepatonecrosis [26]. Currently, there are two well-known methods to calculate liver dose: the body-surface-area (BSA) and partition models, both of which generally under-dose patients with the radioactive substance. The voxel-based dosimetry model considers tumor to normal liver ratio (T/N), liver volume, and dose distribution heterogeneity (tumor necrosis) [72-73]. This is evaluated using average dose and dose-volume histogram of the anatomically defined tumors leading to more accurate evaluation of tumor dose and absorption [74-75].

Retrospective studies using the voxel-based dosimetry model confirm that patients are frequently underdosed with Y90. Dosage delivered during each treatment can be evaluated and may be used to evaluate response after radioembolization [76].

Unfortunately, there are limited studies using the voxel-based dosimetry method to calculate Y90 dosing. Current research is promising, and further investigation is needed to validate the use of this model.

Glass vs resin beads

Continued debates regarding resin and glass microspheres continues in medical literature and in clinical practice. Both resin and glass microspheres act as delivery vehicles for Y-90 radioactive material and are both used in clinical practice for Y-90 treatment. There has been significant research exploring the differences between glass and resin treatments.

Due to the size of glass particles (20–30 µm), glass beads deliver much larger activity per bead (2500 Bq vs 50 Bq, for resin) [78-81]. Resin beads, however, due to their larger size (20–60 µm), produces an embolization effect in addition to the radiation effect [82]. This phenomenon is further compounded by the sheer number of microspheres needed to achieve treatment doses, due to the lower density of Y90 per sphere in the resin than glass [83]. Complete dose delivery for glass microspheres is accomplished without detectable angiographic evidence of embolization, whereas full delivery of resin microspheres is not always possible, as the target artery can develop stasis prior to completion of infusion [82].

Ultimately, it is postulated that these differences may result in increased tumor ischemia by resin microspheres rather than increased radiation dose, however no formal studies have been performed to prove this theory.

A meta-analysis comparing glass versus resin Y90 microspheres reported a significant benefit in HCC patients when treated with resin compared to glass [84]. In a retrospective review, patients who received Y90 with resin beads had statistically significantly longer survival times compared to those treated with glass, with resin patients experiencing a 44% reduction in the likelihood of death within 1 year after initiation of Y90 treatment. However, when examined by liver disease pathology and presence of portal vein invasion (PVI), no statistically significant differences could be determined for patients with HCC, mCRC, or other pathologies. This inability to detect statistically significant differences in these subgroups may be attributable to their relatively small sample sizes, though this remains somewhat perplexing [81, 85].

Further research is needed to establish a true statistically significant difference of survival rates between glass and resin beads.

Sir-Sphere recently began a prospective, multi-center, open-label FDA approved study, DOORwaY90, to evaluate the safety and efficacy of SIRT using SIR-Spheres as a first line treatment for HCC patients [86].

Radiomics

Radiomics is a promising new field in diagnostic and interventional radiology, using algorithms to find associations between qualitative and quantitative information from patient's imaging [87-89]. These imaging features, including tumor texture, shape, and spatial relationships are evaluated via reconstruction algorithms and are converted to mineable data [88]. Radiographic patterns may reveal tumor signatures and further quantify tumor response and outcomes. Currently, the RECIST 1.1 criteria is used to evaluate treatment response, however, as previously discussed, this criterion only accounts for tumoral size, which may be variable depending on the type of treatment administered [90].

Radiomic research on liver neoplasms have been conducted on patients with metastatic colorectal cancer [91]. Using morphologic criteria such as homogeneity, density, and border lines, a radiomic signature was created and validated for each patient. Results showed that 'radiomic signature' was better able to identify "good responders" from Y-90 treatment on follow-up imaging when compared the RECIST1.1 criteria [92].

While not studying HCC, these studies demonstrate the importance of using pretreatment imaging features when assigning therapies. Patients stratified as "poor responders" may begin with a more aggressive treatment therapy to improve disease free survival, whereas "good responders" may take a less toxic treatment course to avoid side effects.

Future research should evaluate the use of radiomic signatures for HCC.

EYE-90 Microspheres

EYe^{90} microspheres (ABK Biomedical, Inc., Halifax, NS, Canada) is a novel, investigational device for TARE of primary liver cancers, acting as the delivery vehicle for Y-90 material (similar to TheraSpheres and SIR-Spheres). Unlike its current counterparts, eYe^{90} microspheres contain radiopaque elements within the glass matrix, allowing for peri and post-procedure tumor target confirmation and distribution. In comparison to existing technologies, eYe^{90} demonstrates a similar microsphere size but increased radioactivity and specify to targeting tumor cells. Additionally, eYe^{90} cites advantages include physician injection control and unique patient specific dosages [93].

The proprietary Dual-syringe System delivers the physician-controlled infusion in two different methods; a continuous delivery (administers a 2cc infusion at the rate of 0.3cc/s) and intermittent delivery (administers two doses of 1cc infusions at the rate of 0.33cc/s with a 180 second pause between dosages). The entire system contains 100 mg of microspheres total or 50g/mL. In comparison, the Therasphere Bolus Delivery system delivers a single bolus: a 3cc infusion at the rate of 0.6cc/s, totaling 100mg of microspheres. When visualized in-vivo using a rabbit liver model, the Dual syringe system demonstrated increased particle counts in microvascular trees downstream when compared to Bolus Delivery [94].

First in man studies using eYe^{90} began late 2022 for treatment of unresectable hepatocellular carcinoma and metastatic colorectal cancer. Key safety evaluations will include the incidence of Grade 3 toxicities at 90- and 180-days post treatment as well as incidence of serious adverse events related treatment (CTCAE Ver. 5). The primary endpoints include response rate using RECIST 1.1 criteria for tumor size and enhancement reduction.

ROUTE90 is planned as a prospective 20-25 site Phase 2 study intended to enroll up to 140 patients. The primary endpoint will evaluate the odds ratio using local mRECIST criteria and Duration of Response (DoR) greater than 6 months.

Holmium-166 Microspheres

Another current field of active research is in the use of holmium-166 as the source of radioactive particle, instead of yttrium-90. The holmium-166 radioisotope is similar in size and activity to Y-90 but has a much shorter half-life. Due to the shorter half-life, HO-166 could replace the traditional MAA used in diagnostic workup and dose prediction. Advantages include paramagnetic activity of HO-166, making it easily visualized by MRI, as well as more accurate dose prediction. Currently, this product, QuiremSpheres microspheres (Terumo Medical Corporation, Somerset, NJ, USA), is available in Europe

Since 2009, several clinical trials have taken place using HO-166 both in patients with primary HCC and liver metastases [95]. Studies using HO-166 in HCC demonstrate promising results, with outcomes and side effect profiles similar to Y-90 [96, 97].

HistoSonics

HistoSonics (HistoSonics, Inc., Ann Arbor, MI, USA) is a new noninvasive, non-radioactive form of therapy using ultrasound waves to create a discrete zone of tissue destruction. Using pulsed sound waves to induce 'bubble clouds' histotripsy mechanically destroys tissue through cavitation [98, 99]. A clinical trial is currently underway using histosonics for treatment of HCC, with promising results [100].

References

1. McGlynn KA, Petrick JL, El-Serag HB. Epidemiology of Hepatocellular Carcinoma. Hepatology. 2021;73 Suppl 1(Suppl 1):4-13.
2. Sung H, Ferlay J, Siegel RL, Laversanne M, Soerjomataram I, Jemal A, et al. Global Cancer Statistics 2020: GLOBOCAN Estimates of Incidence and Mortality Worldwide for 36 Cancers in 185 Countries. CA Cancer J Clin. 2021;71(3):209-49.
3. Siegel RL, Miller KD, Fuchs HE, Jemal A. Cancer Statistics, 2021. CA Cancer J Clin. 2021;71(1):7-33.
4. Konyn P, Ahmed A, Kim D. Current epidemiology in hepatocellular carcinoma. Expert Rev Gastroenterol Hepatol. 2021;15(11):1295-307.
5. Akateh C, Black SM, Conteh L, Miller ED, Noonan A, Elliott E, et al. Neoadjuvant and adjuvant treatment strategies for hepatocellular carcinoma. World J Gastroenterol. 2019;25(28):3704-21.
6. Saini A, Wallace A, Alzubaidi S, Knuttinen MG, Naidu S, Sheth R, et al. History and Evolution of Yttrium-90 Radioembolization for Hepatocellular Carcinoma. J Clin Med. 2019;8(1).
7. Camacho JC, Moncayo V, Kokabi N, Reavey HE, Galt JR, Yamada K, et al. (90)Y Radioembolization: Multimodality Imaging Pattern Approach with Angiographic Correlation for Optimized Target Therapy Delivery. Radiographics. 2015;35(5):1602-18.
8. Premarket Approval SIR-Spheres: FDA; 2002 [Available from: https://www.accessdata.fda.gov/scripts/cdrh/cfdocs/cfpma/pma.cfm?id=P990065.
9. Premarket Approval Therasphere: FDA; 2021 [updated 12/12/2022. Available from: https://www.accessdata.fda.gov/scripts/cdrh/cfdocs/cfpma/pma.cfm?id=P200029.
10. Kulik LM, Carr BI, Mulcahy MF, Lewandowski RJ, Atassi B, Ryu RK, et al. Safety and efficacy of 90Y radiotherapy for hepatocellular

carcinoma with and without portal vein thrombosis. Hepatology. 2008;47(1):71-81.
11. Salem R, Lewandowski R, Roberts C, Goin J, Thurston K, Abouljoud M, et al. Use of Yttrium-90 glass microspheres (TheraSphere) for the treatment of unresectable hepatocellular carcinoma in patients with portal vein thrombosis. J Vasc Interv Radiol. 2004;15(4):335-45.
12. Salem R, Lewandowski RJ, Mulcahy MF, Riaz A, Ryu RK, Ibrahim S, et al. Radioembolization for hepatocellular carcinoma using Yttrium-90 microspheres: a comprehensive report of long-term outcomes. Gastroenterology. 2010;138(1):52-64.
13. Salem R, Johnson GE, Kim E, Riaz A, Bishay V, Boucher E, et al. Yttrium-90 Radioembolization for the Treatment of Solitary, Unresectable HCC: The LEGACY Study. Hepatology. 2021;74(5): 2342-52.
14. Lewandowski RJ, Kulik LM, Riaz A, Senthilnathan S, Mulcahy MF, Ryu RK, et al. A comparative analysis of transarterial downstaging for hepatocellular carcinoma: chemoembolization versus radioembolization. Am J Transplant. 2009;9(8):1920-8.
15. Salem R, Gordon AC, Mouli S, Hickey R, Kallini J, Gabr A, et al. Y90 Radioembolization Significantly Prolongs Time to Progression Compared With Chemoembolization in Patients With Hepatocellular Carcinoma. Gastroenterology. 2016;151(6):1155-63.e2.
16. EASL Clinical Practice Guidelines: Management of hepatocellular carcinoma. J Hepatol. 2018;69(1):182-236.
17. Dhondt E, Lambert B, Hermie L, Huyck L, Vanlangenhove P, Geerts A, et al. (90)Y Radioembolization versus Drug-eluting Bead Chemoembolization for Unresectable Hepatocellular Carcinoma: Results from the TRACE Phase II Randomized Controlled Trial. Radiology. 2022;303(3):699-710.
18. Facciorusso A, Serviddio G, Muscatiello N. Transarterial radioembolization vs chemoembolization for hepatocarcinoma patients: A systematic review and meta-analysis. World J Hepatol. 2016;8(18):770-8.
19. Lobo L, Yakoub D, Picado O, Ripat C, Pendola F, Sharma R, et al. Unresectable Hepatocellular Carcinoma: Radioembolization Versus Chemoembolization: A Systematic Review and Meta-analysis. Cardiovasc Intervent Radiol. 2016;39(11):1580-8.
20. Vilgrain V, Pereira H, Assenat E, Guiu B, Ilonca AD, Pageaux GP, et al. Efficacy and safety of selective internal radiotherapy with yttrium-90 resin microspheres compared with sorafenib in locally advanced and inoperable hepatocellular carcinoma (SARAH): an open-label randomised controlled phase 3 trial. Lancet Oncol. 2017;18(12):1624-36.

21. Chow PKH, Gandhi M, Tan SB, Khin MW, Khasbazar A, Ong J, et al. SIRveNIB: Selective Internal Radiation Therapy Versus Sorafenib in Asia-Pacific Patients With Hepatocellular Carcinoma. J Clin Oncol. 2018;36(19):1913-21.
22. Ricke J, Klümpen HJ, Amthauer H, Bargellini I, Bartenstein P, de Toni EN, et al. Impact of combined selective internal radiation therapy and sorafenib on survival in advanced hepatocellular carcinoma. J Hepatol. 2019;71(6):1164-74.
23. Eddie K Abdalla M, FACSKeith E Stuart; MD, Amit G Singal, MD. Overview of treatment approaches for hepatocellular carcinoma. In: Kenneth K Tanabe MRMG, MD Diane MF Savarese, MD, editor. UpToDate2022.
24. Heimbach JK, Kulik LM, Finn RS, Sirlin CB, Abecassis MM, Roberts LR, et al. AASLD guidelines for the treatment of hepatocellular carcinoma. Hepatology. 2018;67(1):358-80.
25. Reig M, Forner A, Rimola J, Ferrer-Fàbrega J, Burrel M, Garcia-Criado Á, et al. BCLC strategy for prognosis prediction and treatment recommendation: The 2022 update. J Hepatol. 2022;76(3):681-93.
26. Omata M, Cheng AL, Kokudo N, Kudo M, Lee JM, Jia J, et al. Asia-Pacific clinical practice guidelines on the management of hepatocellular carcinoma: a 2017 update. Hepatol Int. 2017;11(4):317-70.
27. Howerton L. Yttrium 90 Radioembolization for Hepatocellular Carcinoma. Radiol Technol. 2021;93(2):197-215.
28. TheraSphere iDOC™ interactive Dose Ordering Calculator: Boston Scientific; 2022 [Available from: https://www.bostonscientific.com/en-US/products/cancer-therapies/therasphere-y90-glass-microspheres/ordering-information/therasphere-idoc.html.
29. SIR-Spheres® Microspheres Activity Calculator (SMAC) 2022 [Available from: https://smac.sirtex.com/.
30. Mazzaferro V. Liver Transplantation Criteria for Hepatocellular Carcinoma, Including Posttransplant Management. The New England Journal of Medicine1996.
31. Lingiah VA, Niazi M, Olivo R, Paterno F, Guarrera JV, Pyrsopoulos NT. Liver Transplantation Beyond Milan Criteria. J Clin Transl Hepatol. 2020;8(1):69-75.
32. Pavel MC, Fuster J. Expansion of the hepatocellular carcinoma Milan criteria in liver transplantation: Future directions. World J Gastroenterol. 2018;24(32):3626-36.
33. Mazzaferro V, Bhoori S, Sposito C, Bongini M, Langer M, Miceli R, et al. Milan criteria in liver transplantation for hepatocellular

carcinoma: an evidence-based analysis of 15 years of experience. Liver Transpl. 2011;17 Suppl 2:S44-57.

34. Organ Procurement and Transplantation Network (OPTN) Policies Online2022 [Available from: https://optn.transplant.hrsa.gov/media/eavh5bf3/optn_policies.pdf.
35. Villalobos A, Wagstaff W, Guo M, Zhang J, Bercu Z, Whitmore MJ, et al. Predictors of Successful Yttrium-90 Radioembolization Bridging or Downstaging in Patients with Hepatocellular Carcinoma. Can J Gastroenterol Hepatol. 2021;2021:9926704.
36. Mehta N, Guy J, Frenette CT, Dodge JL, Osorio RW, Minteer WB, et al. Excellent Outcomes of Liver Transplantation Following Down-Staging of Hepatocellular Carcinoma to Within Milan Criteria: A Multicenter Study. Clin Gastroenterol Hepatol. 2018;16(6):955-64.
37. Metha N. Liver Transplantation Criteria for Hepatocellular Carcinoma, Including Posttransplant Management. Clinical Liver Disease: Wileyonlinelibrary.org; 2020.
38. James T, Hill J, Fahrbach T, Collins Z. Differences in Radiation Activity Between Glass and Resin 90Y Microspheres in Treating Unresectable Hepatic Cancer. Health physics. 2017;112(3):300-4.
39. Lewandowski RJ, Geschwind JF, Liapi E, Salem R. Transcatheter intraarterial therapies: Rationale and overview. Radiology. 2011; 259(3):641-57.
40. Memon K, Lewandowski RJ, Kulik L, Riaz A, Mulcahy MF, Salem R. Radioembolization for Primary and Metastatic Liver Cancer. Seminars in Radiation Oncology. 2011;21(4):294-302.
41. Molvar C, Lewandowski RJ. Intra-Arterial Therapies for Liver Masses. Data Distilled. Radiologic Clinics of North America. 2015;53(5):973-84.
42. Sacco R, Mismas V, Marceglia S, Romano A, Giacomelli L, Bertini M, et al. Transarterial radioembolization for hepatocellular carcinoma: An update and perspectives. World Journal of Gastroenterology. 2015; 21(21):6518-25.
43. Emami B, Lyman J, Brown A, Coia L, Goitein M, Munzenrider JE, et al. Tolerance of normal tissue to therapeutic irradiation. International Journal of Radiation Oncology Biology Physics. 1991;21(1):109-22.
44. Van Hazel GA, Heinemann V, Sharma NK, Findlay MPN, Ricke J, Peeters M, et al. SIRFLOX: Randomized phase III trial comparing first-line mFOLFOX6 (Plus or Minus Bevacizumab) versus mFOLFOX6 (Plus or Minus Bevacizumab) plus selective internal radiation therapy in patients with metastatic colorectal cancer. Journal of Clinical Oncology. 2016;34(15):1723-31.

45. Khatib J, Kainthla R. Optimal Use of FOLFOXIRI Plus Bevacizumab as First-Line Systemic Treatment in Metastatic Colorectal Cancer. Current Colorectal Cancer Reports. 2020;16(4):89-95.
46. Levi Sandri GB, Ettorre GM, Giannelli V, Colasanti M, Sciuto R, Pizzi G, et al. Trans-arterial radio-embolization: a new chance for patients with hepatocellular cancer to access liver transplantation, a world review. Transl Gastroenterol Hepatol. 2017;2:98.
47. Ahn JC, Lauzon M, Luu M, Friedman ML, Kosari K, Nissen N, et al. Transarterial radioembolization versus systemic treatment for hepatocellular carcinoma with macrovascular invasion: Analysis of the US National Cancer Database. J Nucl Med. 2021;62(12):1692-701.
48. Mehta N, Heimbach J, Harnois DM, Sapisochin G, Dodge JL, Lee D, et al. Validation of a Risk Estimation of Tumor Recurrence After Transplant (RETREAT) Score for Hepatocellular Carcinoma Recurrence After Liver Transplant. JAMA Oncol. 2017;3(4):493-500.
49. Halazun KJ, Najjar M, Abdelmessih RM, Samstein B, Griesemer AD, Guarrera JV, et al. Recurrence After Liver Transplantation for Hepatocellular Carcinoma: A New MORAL to the Story. Ann Surg. 2017;265(3):557-64.
50. Rajendran L, Ivanics T, Claasen MP, Muaddi H, Sapisochin G. The management of post-transplantation recurrence of hepatocellular carcinoma. Clin Mol Hepatol. 2022;28(1):1-16.
51. Kim Y-s, Lim HK, Rhim H, Lee WJ, Joh JW, Park CK. Recurrence of Hepatocellular Carcinoma After Liver Transplantation: Patterns and Prognostic Factors Based on Clinical and Radiologic Features. American Journal of Roentgenology. 2007;189(2):352-8.
52. Guerrini GP, Berretta M, Tarantino G, Magistri P, Pecchi A, Ballarin R, et al. Multimodal oncological approach in patients affected by recurrent hepatocellular carcinoma after liver transplantation. Eur Rev Med Pharmacol Sci. 2017;21(15):3421-35.
53. Chok K. Management of recurrent hepatocellular carcinoma after liver transplant. World J Hepatol. 2015;7(8):1142-8.
54. Geissler EK, Schnitzbauer AA, Zülke C, Lamby PE, Proneth A, Duvoux C, et al. Sirolimus Use in Liver Transplant Recipients With Hepatocellular Carcinoma: A Randomized, Multicenter, Open-Label Phase 3 Trial. Transplantation. 2016;100(1):116-25.
55. Woerner AJ, Johnson GE. Advances in Y-90 radioembolization for the treatment of hepatocellular carcinoma.
56. Salem R, Lewandowski RJ, Kulik L, Wang E, Riaz A, Ryu RK, et al. Radioembolization results in longer time-to-progression and reduced

toxicity compared with chemoembolization in patients with hepatocellular carcinoma. Gastroenterology. 2011;140(2):497-507.e2.
57. Casadei Gardini A, Tamburini E, Iñarrairaegui M, Frassineti GL, Sangro B. Radioembolization versus chemoembolization for unresectable hepatocellular carcinoma: a meta-analysis of randomized trials. Onco Targets Ther. 2018;11:7315-21.
58. Cappelli A, Sangro P, Mosconi C, Deppe I, Terzi E, Bilbao JI, et al. Transarterial radioembolization in patients with hepatocellular carcinoma of intermediate B2 substage. Eur J Nucl Med Mol Imaging. 2019;46(3):661-8.
59. Goswami P, Adeniran OR, K. Frantz S, Matsuoka L, Du L, Gandhi RT, et al. Overall survival and toxicity of Y90 radioembolization for hepatocellular carcinoma patients in Barcelona Clinic Liver Cancer stage C (BCLC-C).
60. Salem R, Padia SA, Lam M, Chiesa C, Haste P, Sangro B, et al. Clinical, dosimetric, and reporting considerations for Y-90 glass microspheres in hepatocellular carcinoma: updated 2022 recommendations from an international multidisciplinary working group. European Journal of Nuclear Medicine and Molecular Imaging. 2022.
61. Entezari P, Riaz A. Intrahepatic Cholangiocarcinoma. Semin Intervent Radiol. 2020;37(5):475-83.
62. Valle J, Wasan H, Palmer DH, Cunningham D, Anthoney A, Maraveyas A, et al. Cisplatin plus gemcitabine versus gemcitabine for biliary tract cancer. N Engl J Med. 2010;362(14):1273-81.
63. Buettner S, Braat A, Margonis GA, Brown DB, Taylor KB, Borgmann AJ, et al. Yttrium-90 Radioembolization in Intrahepatic Cholangiocarcinoma: A Multicenter Retrospective Analysis. J Vasc Interv Radiol. 2020; 31(7):1035-43.e2.
64. Wright GP, Perkins S, Jones H, Zureikat AH, Marsh JW, Holtzman MP, et al. Surgical Resection Does Not Improve Survival in Multifocal Intrahepatic Cholangiocarcinoma: A Comparison of Surgical Resection with Intra-Arterial Therapies. Ann Surg Oncol. 2018;25(1):83-90.
65. Edeline J, Touchefeu Y, Guiu B, Farge O, Tougeron D, Baumgaertner I, et al. Radioembolization Plus Chemotherapy for First-line Treatment of Locally Advanced Intrahepatic Cholangiocarcinoma: A Phase 2 Clinical Trial. JAMA Oncology. 2020;6(1):51-9.
66. Park SY, Kim JH, Yoon HJ, Lee IS, Yoon HK, Kim KP. Transarterial chemoembolization versus supportive therapy in the palliative treatment of unresectable intrahepatic cholangiocarcinoma. Clin Radiol. 2011;66(4):322-8.

67. Malone CD, Gibby W, Tsai R, Kim SK, Lancia S, Akinwande O, et al. Outcomes of Yttrium-90 Radioembolization for Unresectable Combined Biphenotypic Hepatocellular-Cholangiocarcinoma. J Vasc Interv Radiol. 2020;31(5):701-9.
68. Renzulli M, Ramai D, Singh J, Sinha S, Brandi N, Ierardi AM, et al. Locoregional Treatments in Cholangiocarcinoma and Combined Hepatocellular Cholangiocarcinoma. Cancers (Basel). 2021;13(13).
69. Chan LS, Sze DY, Poultsides GA, Louie JD, Abdelrazek Mohammed MA, Wang DS. Yttrium-90 Radioembolization for Unresectable Combined Hepatocellular-Cholangiocarcinoma. Cardiovasc Intervent Radiol. 2017;40(9):1383-91.
70. Huang Y-H, Park BV, Chen Y-F, Gaba RC, Guzman G, Lokken RP. Locoregional Therapy of Hepatocellular-Cholangiocarcinoma versus Hepatocellular Carcinoma: A Propensity Score–Matched Study. Journal of Vascular and Interventional Radiology. 2019.
71. Aguado A, Dunn SP, Averill LW, Chikwava KR, Gresh R, Rabinowitz D, et al. Successful use of transarterial radioembolization with yttrium-90 (TARE-Y90) in two children with hepatoblastoma. Pediatr Blood Cancer. 2020;67(9):e28421.
72. Balli HT, Aikimbaev K, Guney IB, Piskin FC, Yagci-Kupeli B, Kupeli S, et al. Trans-Arterial Radioembolization with Yttrium-90 of Unresectable and Systemic Chemotherapy Resistant Hepatoblastoma in Three Toddlers. Cardiovasc Intervent Radiol. 2022;45(3):344-8.
73. Core JM, Frey GT, Sharma A, Bussone ST, Legout JD, McKinney JM, et al. Increasing Yttrium-90 Dose Conformality Using Proximal Radioembolization Enabled by Distal Angiosomal Truncation for the Treatment of Hepatic Malignancy. Journal of Vascular and Interventional Radiology. 2020;31(6):934-42.
74. Morán V, Prieto E, Sancho L, Rodríguez-Fraile M, Soria L, Zubiria A, et al. Impact of the dosimetry approach on the resulting 90Y radioembolization planned absorbed doses based on 99mTc-MAA SPECT-CT: is there agreement between dosimetry methods? EJNMMI Physics. 2020;7(1).
75. Abbott E, Young RS, Hale C, Mitchell K, Falzone N, Vallis KA, et al. Stereotactic Inverse Dose Planning After Yttrium-90 Selective Internal Radiation Therapy in Hepatocellular Cancer. Advances in Radiation Oncology. 2021;6(2).
76. Mok GSP, Dewaraja YK. Recent advances in voxel-based targeted radionuclide therapy dosimetry. Quantitative Imaging in Medicine and Surgery. 2021;11(2):483-9.

77. Kafrouni M, Allimant C, Fourcade M, Vauclin S, Delicque J, Ilonca AD, et al. Retrospective voxel-based dosimetry for assessing the ability of the body-surface-area model to predict delivered dose and radioembolization outcome. Journal of Nuclear Medicine. 2018;59(8):1289-95.
78. Salem R, Lewandowski R, Roberts C, Goin J, Thurston K, Abouljoud M, et al. Use of Yttrium-90 Glass Microspheres (TheraSphere) for the Treatment of Unresectable Hepatocellular Carcinoma in Patients with Portal Vein Thrombosis. Journal of Vascular and Interventional Radiology. 2004;15(4):335-45.
79. Ibrahim SM, Nikolaidis P, Miller FH, Lewandowski RJ, Ryu RK, Sato KT, et al. Radiologic findings following Y90 radioembolization for primary liver malignancies. Abdominal Imaging. 2009;34(5):566-81.
80. Kennedy AS, Salem R. Radioembolization (yttrium-90 microspheres) for primary and metastatic hepatic malignancies. Cancer Journal. 2010;16(2):163-75.
81. DeBacker S JJ, Vavricek J, Iqbal S, Hunt SL, et al. Retrospective Review of Survival Outcomes in Glass and Resin Y-90 Microsphere Treatment of Hepatic Malignancies. Journal of Interventional Radiology Nuclear Medicine. 2018:1-9.
82. Haverkamp BT, Pedersen WR, Hunt S, Walter C, Hill JD, Collins ZC. Tumor response, time to progression, and progression-free survival in glass versus resin radioembolization of hepatocellular cancer. Journal of Vascular and Interventional Radiology. 2017;28(2):e22.
83. Chiesa C, Mira M, Maccauro M, Romito R, Spreafico C, Sposito C, et al. A dosimetric treatment planning strategy in radioembolization of hepatocarcinoma with90Y glass microspheres. Quarterly Journal of Nuclear Medicine and Molecular Imaging. 2012;56(6):503-8.
84. Vente MAD, Wondergem M, van der Tweel I, van den Bosch MAAJ, Zonnenberg BA, Lam MGEH, et al. Yttrium-90 microsphere radioembolization for the treatment of liver malignancies: A structured meta-analysis. European Radiology. 2009;19(4):951-9.
85. Biederman DM, Titano JJ, Bishay VL, Durrani RJ, Dayan E, Tabori N, et al. Radiation segmentectomy versus Tace combined with Microwave ablation for Unresectable solitary hepatocellular carcinoma Up to 3 cm: A Propensity Score Matching Study. Radiology. 2017;283(3):895-905.
86. Medical S. A Prospective, Multicenter, Open-label Single Arm Study Evaluating the Safety & Efficacy of Selective Internal Radiation Therapy Using SIR-Spheres® Y-90 Resin Microspheres on DoR & ORR in Unresectable Hepatocellular Carcinoma Patients clinicaltrials.gov2021 [updated March 23, 2021.

87. Rizzo S, Botta F, Raimondi S, Origgi D, Fanciullo C, Morganti AG, et al. Radiomics: the facts and the challenges of image analysis. European radiology experimental. 2018;2(1):36.
88. Creasy JM, Cunanan KM, Chakraborty J, McAuliffe JC, Chou J, Gonen M, et al. Differences in Liver Parenchyma are Measurable with CT Radiomics at Initial Colon Resection in Patients that Develop Hepatic Metastases from Stage II/III Colon Cancer. Annals of Surgical Oncology. 2021;28(4):1982-9.
89. Wei L, Cui C, Xu J, Kaza R, El Naqa I, Dewaraja YK. Tumor response prediction in 90Y radioembolization with PET-based radiomics features and absorbed dose metrics. EJNMMI Physics. 2020;7(1).
90. Eisenhauer EA, Verweij J. New response evaluation criteria in solid tumors: RECIST guideline version 1.1. European Journal of Cancer, Supplement. 2009;7(2-3):5.
91. Dohan A, Gallix B, Guiu B, Le Malicot K, Reinhold C, Soyer P, et al. Early evaluation using a radiomic signature of unresectable hepatic metastases to predict outcome in patients with colorectal cancer treated with FOLFIRI and bevacizumab. Gut. 2020;69(3):531-9.
92. Shur J, Orton M, Connor A, Fischer S, Moulton CA, Gallinger S, et al. A clinical-radiomic model for improved prognostication of surgical candidates with colorectal liver metastases. Journal of Surgical Oncology. 2020;121(2):357-64.
93. ABK Biomedical I, editor Eye90 microspheres. CIRSE; 2022; Barcelona, Spain.
94. Henry EC, Strugari M, Mawko G, Brewer K, Liu D, Gordon AC, et al. Precision dosimetry in yttrium-90 radioembolization through CT imaging of radiopaque microspheres in a rabbit liver model. EJNMMI Physics. 2022;9(1):21.
95. Stella M, Braat AJAT, van Rooij R, de Jong HWAM, Lam MGEH. Holmium-166 Radioembolization: Current Status and Future Prospective. CardioVascular and Interventional Radiology. 2022; 45(11):1634-45.
96. Radosa CG, Radosa JC, Grosche-Schlee S, Zöphel K, Plodeck V, Kühn JP, et al. Holmium-166 Radioembolization in Hepatocellular Carcinoma: Feasibility and Safety of a New Treatment Option in Clinical Practice. Cardiovasc Intervent Radiol. 2019;42(3):405-12.
97. Reinders MTM, Smits MLJ, van Roekel C, Braat A. Holmium-166 Microsphere Radioembolization of Hepatic Malignancies. Semin Nucl Med. 2019;49(3):237-43.

98. Worlikar T, Zhang M, Ganguly A, Hall TL, Shi J, Zhao L, et al. Impact of Histotripsy on Development of Intrahepatic Metastases in a Rodent Liver Tumor Model. Cancers (Basel). 2022;14(7).
99. Xu Z, Hall TL, Vlaisavljevich E, Lee FT, Jr. Histotripsy: the first noninvasive, non-ionizing, non-thermal ablation technique based on ultrasound. Int J Hyperthermia. 2021;38(1):561-75.
100. Vidal-Jove J, Serres X, Vlaisavljevich E, Cannata J, Duryea A, Miller R, et al. First-in-man histotripsy of hepatic tumors: the THERESA trial, a feasibility study. Int J Hyperthermia. 2022;39(1):1115-23.

CHAPTER 8

OVERVIEW OF METASTATIC DISEASE APPLICATIONS

AARON ROHR MD, MS, JOLEY BEELER MD

Introduction

More than half of patients with metastatic cancer have liver metastases (1,2). Further, liver failure is the most common cause of death in patients with metastatic disease (3). Control of metastatic disease in the liver is paramount in improving patient prognosis and symptomatic management.

Treatment of liver metastases with curative intent, such as surgical resection, provides the best overall survival outcomes (4). However, few patients with metastatic disease are eligible for resection due to the distribution of hepatic disease, extrahepatic disease, comorbidities, and resultant surgical candidacy. Systemic chemotherapy has traditionally been the most available option for unresectable hepatic metastases. With the development of locoregional therapies such as ablation and catheter-based intervention, new treatment options continue to be made available for hepatic metastases and have become a mainstay in treatment regimens.

Unlike primary hepatocellular cancer for which treatment strategies are linked to clinical staging systems, for example, Barcelona Clinic Liver Cancer classification (5), the appropriateness and timing of locoregional therapy for metastatic liver disease has not been well defined and its use is highly variable.

Image guided percutaneous tumor ablation can be utilized to destroy unresectable liver metastases while minimizing damage to normal liver tissue. Tumor ablation has the potential for curative treatment, making it a favorable choice for unresectable disease. The most common ablation techniques used for hepatic metastases include microwave ablation and

RFA, with modality choice based on tumor burden/location and provider preference, which was previously discussed in detail. For liver-dominant, unresectable metastases <3 cm in patients with acceptable labs and performance status, ablation is considered a primary treatment (6).

For patients with liver-dominant, unresectable metastases greater than 3 cm or diffuse disease not amenable to ablation, transcatheter arterial chemoembolization and radioembolization therapies (TACE and TARE, respectively) may be performed. These locoregional therapies are generally applied to one or more segments of the liver and are indicated for more diffuse disease. The goals of care are to slow down tumor progression and prolong survival. These therapies can also be combined with ablation, such as in patients with oligometastatic liver metastases greater than 3 cm. In treatment of HCC, combination of ablation and TACE has demonstrated significantly higher OS rate and recurrence-free survival rate over ablation alone (7).

Colorectal cancer metastases

Metastatic colorectal adenocarcinoma is the most common hepatic malignancy. In 2021, there were approximately 150,000 new cases of colorectal cancer diagnosed, resulting in an estimated 52,000 annual deaths, the 2nd leading cause of cancer deaths in the US (8). Further, 10-25% of patients with colorectal carcinoma present with synchronous liver metastases at time of primary diagnosis, and another 20-25% develop metachronous liver metastases during the course of the disease (9). The liver is the first and most common site of metastases due to drainage of the colorectal region by the portal system into the liver.

Surgical resection of hepatic metastases remains the first-choice treatment and may result in improved long term survival, but only 25% of patients with colorectal liver metastases are candidates for liver resection (9). For the 75% of patients who are not resectable, palliative treatment to delay cancer progression is the standard of care, as half of patients die from liver failure (10). Historically, systemic chemotherapy was the only treatment for patients with unresectable distant metastases. With the implementation of ablation, TACE, and TARE, newer promising therapeutic options continue to emerge.

The vast majority of patients with hepatic metastases will receive systemic chemotherapy in addition to liver directed therapy, and it is important for the interventionalist to have a basic knowledge of the regimens as well as associated toxicities. First line systemic chemotherapy consists of 5-fluorouracil or capecitabine combined with leucovorin and either irinotecan (FOLFIRI) or oxaliplatin (FOLFOX). If the patient develops progression or intolerance, the other triplet combination is initiated (FOLFIRI or FOLFOX) (9). KRAS and BRAF status are also reviewed, as KRAS wild-type tumors have demonstrated some response to anti EGFR antibodies, and BRAF mutations confer an aggressive subtype that typically calls for an aggressive first-line regimen (11). Carcinoembryonic antigen (CEA) is the most common tumor blood marker evaluated in colorectal carcinoma, used in screening, initial staging, and response assessment.

Evaluation for treatment options in a patient with colorectal carcinoma hepatic metastases includes assessment of performance status, review of labs and imaging, and collaboration with surgical and medical oncology. In a patient with unresectable disease, review of imaging is paramount to analyze size, location, and distribution of hepatic metastases as well as evaluate for variant arterial anatomy, status of bile ducts, portal venous involvement, presence of ascites and extrahepatic disease.

Percutaneous ablation can be performed for colorectal carcinoma hepatic metastases with the same technique as described previously for primary hepatic disease. Aggressive local treatment of liver metastases with ablation prolongs overall survival in patients with unresectable metastases (12). Compared with systemic chemotherapy, patients who underwent local ablation had far more quality-adjusted life years (13). In patients with lesions less than 3 cm, patient survival and local recurrence rate are similar after percutaneous ablation as compared with surgical resection (14-17).

For patients with larger or more diffuse hepatic metastases from colorectal carcinoma, locoregional therapy such as transarterial chemoembolization (TACE) is preferred to ablation. Embolization slows the passage of chemotherapy through the hepatic circulation, increasing drug concentrations in the tumor and retention within tumor cells for as long as 1 month after infusion. Embolization also causes tumor ischemia, increasing the effects of the cytotoxic drugs by increasing their uptake and retention in tumor cells (18).

Patient workup, indications, and contraindications for TACE are similar to those described for primary liver malignancies. The ideal candidate for TACE has liver metastases only. However, patients with mild extrahepatic disease may also benefit from liver directed therapy when survival is driven by degree of liver involvement. Patients with disease burden >75% of liver volume are unlikely to derive long term benefits from chemoembolization (19). For patients with a singular hepatic lesion of intermediate size (3-6 cm), chemoembolization followed by ablation may be effective.

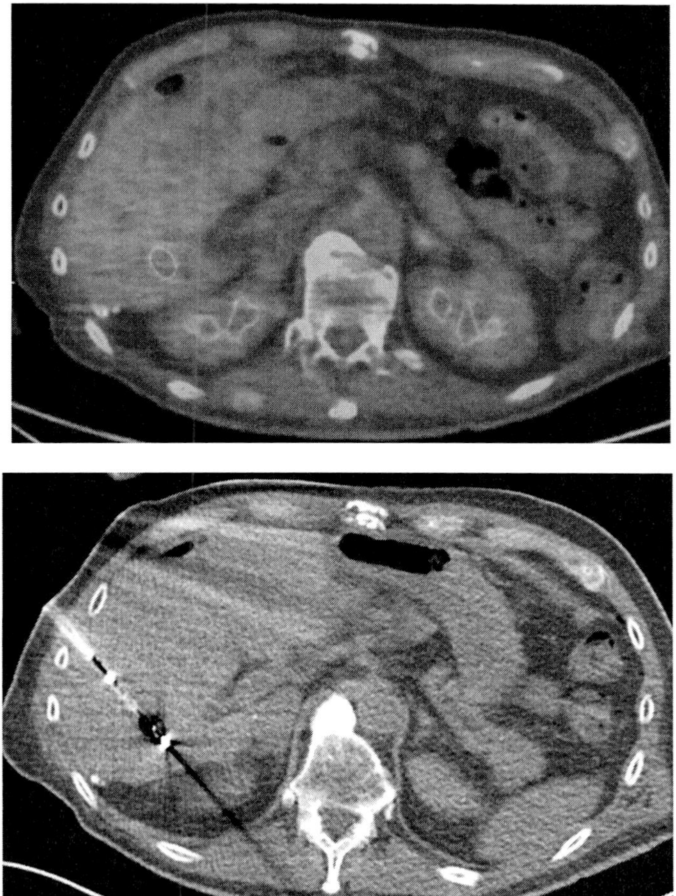

A)

B)

C) 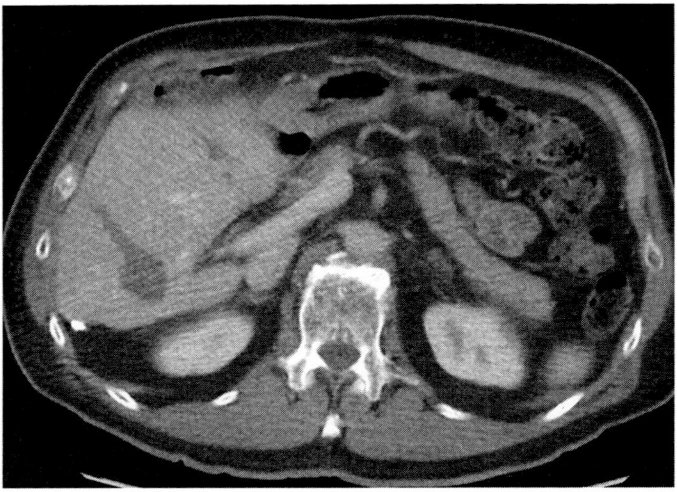

Figure 1. 66-year-old male with metastatic colon cancer. PET (A) demonstrates a hypermetabolic liver metastasis. Limited CT during microwave ablation (B) shows gas within the lesion. Contrast-enhanced CT (C) 1-month post-ablation demonstrates ablation cavity without enhancement.

TACE for colorectal adenocarcinoma differs from TACE for primary liver malignancies in the chemotherapeutic agents utilized. Chemoembolization regimens vary widely. The most commonly used drugs include a combination of cisplatin, doxorubicin, and mitomycin C (9). Embolization agents also vary, including polymeric microspheres, gelatin sponge, starch microspheres, and collagen particles. Conventional regimens include lipiodol. Drug eluting microspheres, an embolic agent which serves as carrier of chemotherapeutic drugs, may also be used. Adjuvant TACE offers higher objective response rates and longer hepatic progression-free survival than systemic therapy alone (20).

Transarterial radioembolization (TARE) is another option for locoregional treatment of liver metastases. As with TARE of primary liver malignancies, glass or resin microspheres incorporating 90Y are utilized to deliver high doses of beta radiation selectively into liver tumors. Compared with TACE, TARE causes less alteration in vascularity and embolic phenomena. Thus, it can be administered over large areas to patients with multiple and large-volume liver metastases. While portal vein thrombosis without cavernous transformation and hepatopetal flow is a well-accepted relative contraindication for TACE, TARE is usually well tolerated in patients with portal vein thrombus (21, 22). Pretreatment workup including vascular mapping and careful patient selection is similar to patients with primary hepatic malignancy. Patients with limited hepatic reserve and clearly reduced performance status are at higher risk of developing severe side effects, such as radiation-induced liver disease. Currently, evidence suggests greater utility of TARE in the salvage setting as opposed to in combination with first-line chemotherapy (11). The addition of TARE to systemic chemotherapy in patients with liver-dominant or liver-only metastatic colorectal cancer significantly delays disease progression in the liver, increases treatment related response, and increases survival (23, 24).

Neuroendocrine tumor metastases

Second to colorectal carcinoma in prevalence, neuroendocrine tumors (NET) are another malignancy with a propensity for hepatic metastases. NETs have increased in prevalence rapidly, with a nearly 7-fold increase in incidence in the USA over the last few decades. Because NETs are frequently indolent in nature, they often grow undetected for several years before being diagnosed (25). The liver is the most frequent site of metastasis and the prognosis for metastatic disease is poor (26). NETs are comprised of a spectrum of epithelial neoplasms that originate from cells which synthesize peptide hormones released in response to a neuronal stimulus. If functional, these tumors can secrete a variety of vasoactive or hormonal substances, such as serotonin, glucagon, gastrin, or insulin. The development of hepatic metastases from functional NETs causes release of these hormonal substances into the systemic circulation, resulting in symptoms such as flushing, hypertension, diarrhea, and electrolyte disorders, collectively known as carcinoid syndrome. Nonfunctional NETs are often diagnosed incidentally or when hepatic metastases cause symptoms related to hepatic tumor burden such as abdominal pain. The majority of patients express somatostatin receptors and can be treated with long-acting somatostatin analogue (SSA), which acts as a cytostatic agent as well as controls hormonal symptoms (27). However, patients often become refractory to this treatment over time, necessitating locoregional treatments for hepatic metastatic disease.

Since NETs are often indolent and there are many targeted systemic therapies, locoregional treatment for hepatic metastases is usually palliative or for more aggressive/recurrent diseases. Ablation can be used for palliation of carcinoid symptoms or management of recurrent disease in patients with fewer than 4-5 metastases less than 3 cm in maximum diameter.

Indications for TACE in hepatic NET metastases include palliation for hormone-related symptoms that are uncontrolled with somatostatin analogs, palliation of symptoms related to tumor bulk, and progression of unresectable hepatic metastases that threaten liver function (27). Two of the most commonly reported TACE regimens include doxorubicin alone or a combo of cisplatin, adriamycin, and mitomycin C (9). Intra-arterial therapy can be first-line therapy for unresectable liver-dominant low-grade NETs and has demonstrated a significantly better 5-year survival rate than medical therapies (28, 29). Intra-arterial intervention may be withheld in asymptomatic patients with normal liver function until tumor burden reaches 25-50% of liver volume, as embolization therapies can only be applied a finite number of times and slow growing disease may take years before it threatens liver function. DEB-TACE has demonstrated higher complication rates for metastatic NETs and is not recommended as first line liver directed therapy (30, 31).

TARE has also demonstrated effectiveness as treatment for hepatic NET metastases, generally performed in patients with more diffuse disease or in those who have failed TACE, resulting in high response rates and increased rates of survival (32, 33).

A)
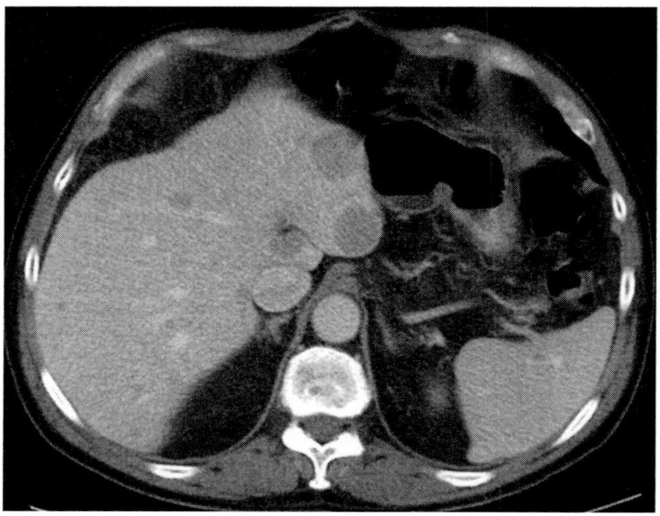

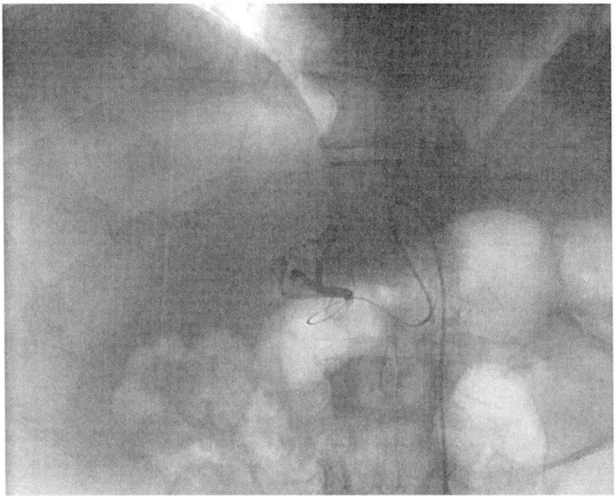

B)

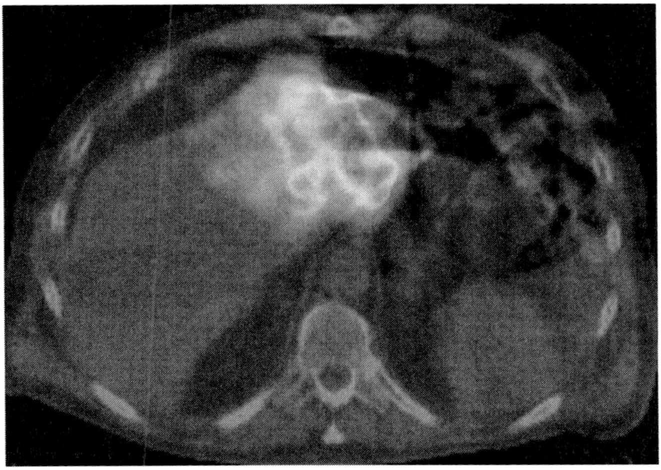

C)

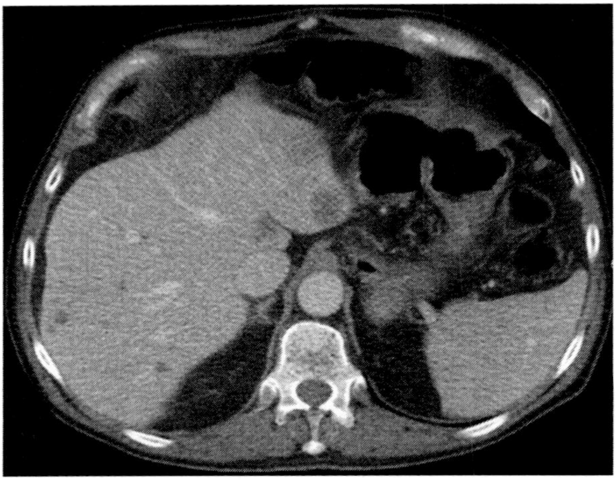
D)

Figure 2. 61 year old male with metastatic neuroendocrine carcinoma. Contrast-enhanced CT (A) shows multiple low-density liver metastases. Intra-procedure fluoro spot image (B) shows a catheter in the left hepatic artery after injection of Y90 microspheres. C) Post-procedure spect CT demonstrates heterogeneous deposition of microspheres within the left lobe of the liver. D) Follow-up contrast-enhanced CT 2 months later shows decreased size of the left hepatic lesions.

Breast cancer metastases

Another common cause of hepatic metastatic disease is breast cancer. Breast cancer is the leading cause of cancer in the US with approximately 284,000 new cases in 2021 and 44,000 annual deaths (34). More than half of patients with breast cancer will develop hepatic metastases, and development of hepatic metastatic disease portends a poorer diagnosis, with hepatic failure causing death in 20% of patients. In addition, liver compromise necessitates chemotherapy dosing modifications, limiting its antitumor effectiveness. Similar to other etiologies of hepatic metastases, surgical resection may play a role, but less than 1% of patients are resection candidates. The ideal resection candidate has a solitary lesion (<4-5cm), stable disease following neoadjuvant systemic therapy, and at least two years between development of primary lesions and metastases (a marker of favorable biology). Even in the ideal candidate, results are mixed, with 5-year overall survival rates from 12-75% and recurrence in 60% of patients (35, 36).

Given the limitations of resection, locoregional therapies play a large part in treatment of hepatic metastases from breast cancer. Ablation can be considered in patients with small solitary lesions, metachronous lesions, and unresectable lesions that demonstrate partial response following neoadjuvant chemotherapy. Microwave and radiofrequency ablation have demonstrated similar results, with local tumor response rates of 63 to 97% (37).

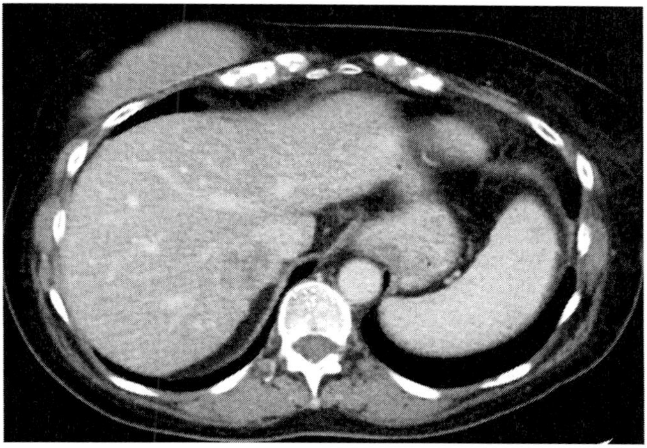

A)

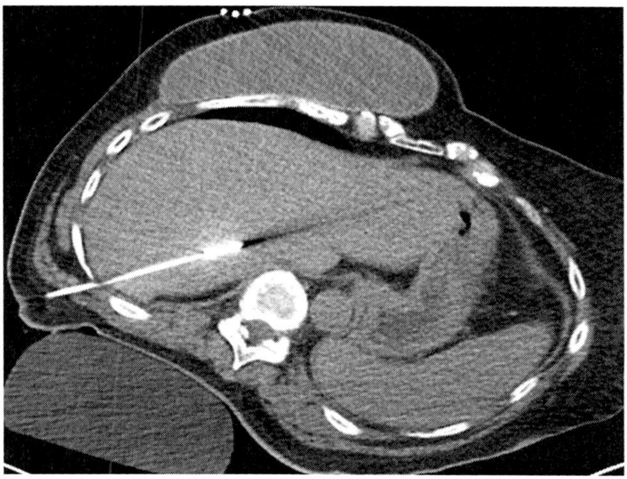

B)

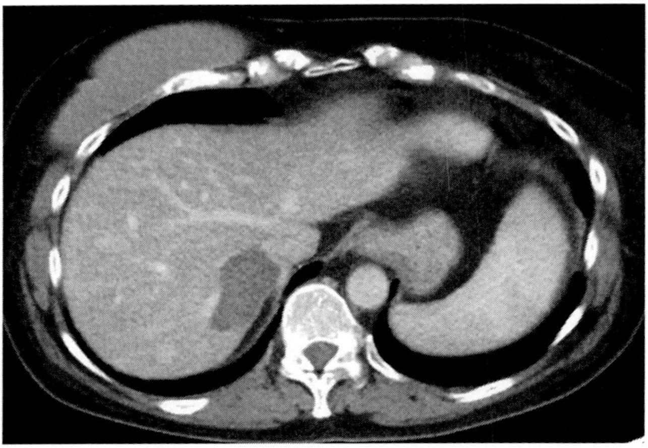

C)

Figure 3. 61 year old female with metastatic breast cancer. Contrast-enhanced CT (A) demonstrates a peripherally enhancing metastatic segment 7 lesion. Intra-procedural CT (B) shows the microwave ablation probe within the lesion. C) One month follow-up contrast-enhanced CT shows ablation cavity without residual enhancement.

TACE

Unfortunately, many patients present with tumor burden not amenable to ablation due to diffuse nature or location. Intra-arterial therapies are often utilized for hepatic metastatic breast cancer patients with limited systemic options or during systemic chemotherapy holidays. TACE considerations are generally tailored to patients with limited extrahepatic disease. The overarching goals are to target the hepatic disease burden while preserving hepatic function and to offer palliation of abdominal pain caused by large hepatic masses.

TACE with mitomycin C and gemcitabine has been shown effective in patients with metastatic breast cancer, with partial response by RECIST criteria in 13% and stable disease in 50% (38). Drug-eluting chemoembolization with doxorubicin has demonstrated partial imaging response in 26-58% (39). Systemic chemotherapy combined with TACE has demonstrated increased survival over chemotherapy alone (40).

Similar results have been demonstrated with TARE in patients with hepatic metastases from breast cancer. Partial response has been observed in 25-

61% of patients, the majority who had undergone multiple prior treatments with systemic chemotherapy. Negative prognostic factors for survival after TARE include hepatic tumor burden greater than 25% and serum bilirubin greater than 1.1 mg/dL (41).

Uveal melanoma

Uveal melanoma is the most common primary intraocular malignant tumor in adults. Up to 50% of patients will develop metastases, and the liver is involved in more than 90% of those patients (42). There is no standard of care for patients with systemic metastases, and no adjuvant chemotherapy has been shown to improve outcomes in patients at high risk for metastatic disease. For most patients, survival is determined by hepatic tumor burden and its response to treatment, thus liver-directed therapies play a key role in treatment.

Thermal ablation can be used as an alternative or adjunct to surgery. Similar to other etiologies of hepatic metastatic disease, ablation and surgical resection demonstrate equivalent overall survival and progression free survival in patients with tumors < 3 cm (43). Local ablation with the ability to spare surrounding normal liver is key in this disease with limited systemic treatment options.

In patients with tumors >5 cm or more than 50% of the liver parenchyma replaced by tumor, TACE is utilized. TACE can also be used in the salvage setting with patients who progress following immunoembolization or TARE. Chemoembolization regimens for uveal melanoma liver metastases vary and no one regimen has shown to be superior (44). A significant increase in survival has been shown with adjuvant TACE compared with systemic chemotherapy alone (45). DEB-TACE utilizing both doxorubicin and irinotecan has been effective in treating uveal melanoma liver metastases (44).

For tumors not amenable to resection or ablation with less than 50% of the liver replaced by tumor, immune- or radioembolization is initiated. TARE is used as salvage therapy and has demonstrated effective local tumor control in the majority of patients after failing first line therapy (46, 47).

Immunoembolization

Despite control of hepatic metastases with chemoembolization, progression of extrahepatic metastases is seen in two thirds of patients (48).

Immunoembolization is a newer regimen that has shown promise in controlling growth of liver metastases and delaying or preventing the development of systemic metastases (49). Immunoembolization utilizes selective hepatic arterial injection of ethiodized oil and granulocyte-macrophage colony stimulating factor (GM-CSF) to induce ischemia of the local tumor tissue, attract and stimulate antigen presenting cells to uptake antigen released from necrotic tumor cells, and induce systemic immunity against melanoma cells which can delay development of remote systemic metastases (48).

References

1. Benson AB, Al-Hawary MM, Arain MA. et al. NCCN Guidelines Version 4.2020 Colon Cancer Continue NCCN Guidelines Panel Disclosures. 2020.
2. Cummings MC, Simpson PT, Reid LE, Jayanthan J, Skerman J, Song S, McCart Reed AE, Kutasovic JR, Morey AL, Marquart L, O'Rourke P, Lakhani SR. Metastatic progression of breast cancer: insights from 50 years of autopsies. J Pathol. 2014 Jan;232(1):23-31. doi: 10.1002/path.4288. PMID: 24122263; PMCID: PMC4288974.
3. Field KM, Dow C, Michael M. Part I: Liver function in oncology: biochemistry and beyond. Lancet Oncol 2008; 9 (11) 1092-1101.
4. Aloia TA, Vauthey JN, Loyer EM, Ribero D, Pawlik TM, Wei SH, Curley SA, Zorzi D, Abdalla EK. Solitary colorectal liver metastasis: resection determines outcome. Arch Surg. 2006 May;141(5):460-6; discussion 466-7. doi: 10.1001/archsurg.141.5.460. PMID: 16702517.
5. Forner A, Llovet JM, Bruix J. Hepatocellular carcinoma. Lancet. 2012 Mar 31;379(9822):1245-55. doi: 10.1016/S0140-6736(11)61347-0. Epub 2012 Feb 20. PMID: 22353262.
6. Shamimi-Noori S, Gonsalves CF, Shaw CM. Metastatic Liver Disease: Indications for Locoregional Therapy and Supporting Data. Semin Intervent Radiol 2017;34:145-166.
7. Liu Z, Gao F, Yang G, Singh S, Lu M, Zhang T, Zhong Z, Zhang F, Tang R. Combination of radiofrequency ablation with transarterial chemoembolization for hepatocellular carcinoma: an up-to-date meta-analysis. Tumour Biol. 2014 Aug;35(8):7407-13. doi: 10.1007/s13277-014-1976-z. Epub 2014 Apr 29. PMID: 24777334.
8. American Cancer Society. Cancer Facts & Figures 2021. Atlanta, Ga: American Cancer Society; 2021.

9. Geschwind JH, Soulen MC. Interventional Oncology: Principles and Practice of Image-Guided Cancer Therapy. Cambridge University Press, 2016.
10. Wagner JS, Adson MA, Van Heerden JA, Adson MH, Ilstrup DM. The natural history of hepatic metastases from colorectal cancer. A comparison with resective treatment. Ann Surg. 1984 May;199(5):502-8. doi: 10.1097/00000658-198405000-00002. PMID: 6721600; PMCID: PMC1353475.
11. Marsala A, Lee EW, Padia SA. Yttrium-90 Radioembolization for Metastatic Colorectal Cancer: Outcomes by Number of Lines of Therapy. Semin Intervent Radiol. 2017 Jun;34(2):116-120. doi: 10.1055/s-0037-1602711. Epub 2017 Jun 1. PMID: 28579679; PMCID: PMC5453784.
12. Ruers T, Van Coevorden F, Punt CJ, Pierie JE, Borel-Rinkes I, Ledermann JA, Poston G, Bechstein W, Lentz MA, Mauer M, Folprecht G, Van Cutsem E, Ducreux M, Nordlinger B; European Organisation for Research and Treatment of Cancer (EORTC); Gastro-Intestinal Tract Cancer Group; Arbeitsgruppe Lebermetastasen und tumoren in der Chirurgischen Arbeitsgemeinschaft Onkologie (ALM-CAO); National Cancer Research Institute Colorectal Clinical Study Group (NCRI CCSG). Local Treatment of Unresectable Colorectal Liver Metastases: Results of a Randomized Phase II Trial. J Natl Cancer Inst. 2017 Sep 1;109(9):djx015. doi: 10.1093/jnci/djx015. PMID: 28376151; PMCID: PMC5408999.
13. Ruers TJ, Joosten JJ, Wiering B, Langenhoff BS, Dekker HM, Wobbes T, Oyen WJ, Krabbe PF, Punt CJ. Comparison between local ablative therapy and chemotherapy for non-resectable colorectal liver metastases: a prospective study. Ann Surg Oncol. 2007 Mar;14 (3):1161-9. doi: 10.1245/s10434-006-9312-5. Epub 2006 Dec 31. PMID: 17195903.
14. Mulier S, Ruers T, Jamart J, Michel L, Marchal G, Ni Y. Radiofrequency ablation versus resection for resectable colorectal liver metastases: time for a randomized trial? An update. Dig Surg. 2008;25(6):445-60. doi: 10.1159/000184736. Epub 2009 Feb 12. PMID: 19212117.
15. Solbiati L, Ahmed M, Cova L, Ierace T, Brioschi M, Goldberg SN. Small liver colorectal metastases treated with percutaneous radiofrequency ablation: local response rate and long-term survival with up to 10-year follow-up. Radiology. 2012 Dec;265(3):958-68. doi: 10.1148/radiol.12111851. Epub 2012 Oct 22. PMID: 23091175.

16. Kim KH, Yoon YS, Yu CS, Kim TW, Kim HJ, Kim PN, Ha HK, Kim JC. Comparative analysis of radiofrequency ablation and surgical resection for colorectal liver metastases. J Korean Surg Soc. 2011 Jul;81(1):25-34. doi: 10.4174/jkss.2011.81.1.25. Epub 2011 Jul 11. PMID: 22066097; PMCID: PMC3204557.
17. Tanis E, Nordlinger B, Mauer M, Sorbye H, van Coevorden F, Gruenberger T, Schlag PM, Punt CJ, Ledermann J, Ruers TJ. Local recurrence rates after radiofrequency ablation or resection of colorectal liver metastases. Analysis of the European Organisation for Research and Treatment of Cancer #40004 and #40983. Eur J Cancer. 2014 Mar;50(5):912-9. doi: 10.1016/j.ejca.2013.12.008. Epub 2014 Jan 7. PMID: 24411080.
18. Nakamura H, Hashimoto T, Oi H, Sawada S. Transcatheter oily chemoembolization of hepatocellular carcinoma. Radiology. 1989 Mar;170(3 Pt 1):783-6. doi: 10.1148/radiology.170.3.2536946. PMID: 2536946.
19. Kamat PP, Gupta S, Ensor JE, Murthy R, Ahrar K, Madoff DC, Wallace MJ, Hicks ME. Hepatic arterial embolization and chemoembolization in the management of patients with large-volume liver metastases. Cardiovasc Intervent Radiol. 2008 Mar-Apr;31(2):299-307. doi: 10.1007/s00270-007-9186-3. Epub 2007 Oct 6. PMID: 17922160.
20. Nanashima A, Takeshita H, Abo T, Tou K, Tanaka K, Fukuda D, Kunizaki M, Hidaka S, Sawai T. Recent advances and significance of intra-arterial infusion chemotherapy in non-resectable colorectal liver metastasis. J Gastrointest Oncol. 2013 Jun;4(2):164-72. doi: 10.3978/j.issn.2078-6891.2013.005. PMID: 23730512; PMCID: PMC3635182.
21. Kulik LM, Carr BI, Mulcahy MF, Lewandowski RJ, Atassi B, Ryu RK, Sato KT, Benson A 3rd, Nemcek AA Jr, Gates VL, Abecassis M, Omary RA, Salem R. Safety and efficacy of 90Y radiotherapy for hepatocellular carcinoma with and without portal vein thrombosis. Hepatology. 2008 Jan;47(1):71-81. doi: 10.1002/hep.21980. PMID: 18027884.
22. Salem R, Lewandowski R, Roberts C, Goin J, Thurston K, Abouljoud M, Courtney A. Use of Yttrium-90 glass microspheres (TheraSphere) for the treatment of unresectable hepatocellular carcinoma in patients with portal vein thrombosis. J Vasc Interv Radiol. 2004 Apr;15(4):335-45. doi: 10.1097/01.rvi.0000123319.20705.92. PMID: 15064336.
23. Van Hazel G, Blackwell A, Anderson J, Price D, Moroz P, Bower G, Cardaci G, Gray B. Randomised phase 2 trial of SIR-Spheres plus fluorouracil/leucovorin chemotherapy versus fluorouracil/leucovorin

chemotherapy alone in advanced colorectal cancer. J Surg Oncol. 2004 Nov 1;88(2):78-85. doi: 10.1002/jso.20141. PMID: 15499601.
24. van Hazel GA, Heinemann V, Sharma NK, Findlay MP, Ricke J, Peeters M, Perez D, Robinson BA, Strickland AH, Ferguson T, Rodríguez J, Kröning H, Wolf I, Ganju V, Walpole E, Boucher E, Tichler T, Shacham-Shmueli E, Powell A, Eliadis P, Isaacs R, Price D, Moeslein F, Taieb J, Bower G, Gebski V, Van Buskirk M, Cade DN, Thurston K, Gibbs P. SIRFLOX: Randomized Phase III Trial Comparing First-Line mFOLFOX6 (Plus or Minus Bevacizumab) Versus mFOLFOX6 (Plus or Minus Bevacizumab) Plus Selective Internal Radiation Therapy in Patients With Metastatic Colorectal Cancer. J Clin Oncol. 2016 May 20;34(15):1723-31. doi: 10.1200/JCO.2015.66.1181. Epub 2016 Feb 22. Erratum in: J Clin Oncol. 2016 Nov 20;34(33):4059. PMID: 26903575.
25. Simoneaux R. A Look at the Increasing Incidence of Neuroendocrine Tumors. Oncology Times. 2020;42(6):1-4. doi: 10.1097/01.COT.0000658812.91924.c3
26. Yao JC, Hassan M, Phan A, et al. One hundred years after "carcinoid": epidemiology of and prognostic factors for neuroendocrine tumors in 35,825 cases in the United States. J Clin Oncol. 2008;26:3063–3072.
27. Gandhi RT, Ganguli S. Interventional Oncology: Practical Guides in Interventional Radiology. Thieme, 2016.
28. Roche A, Girish BV, de Baère T, Baudin E, Boige V, Elias D, Lasser P, Schlumberger M, Ducreux M. Trans-catheter arterial chemoembolization as first-line treatment for hepatic metastases from endocrine tumors. Eur Radiol. 2003 Jan;13(1):136-40. doi: 10.1007/s00330-002-1558-0. Epub 2002 Jul 23. PMID: 12541121.
29. Touzios JG, Kiely JM, Pitt SC, Rilling WS, Quebbeman EJ, Wilson SD, Pitt HA. Neuroendocrine hepatic metastases: does aggressive management improve survival? Ann Surg. 2005 May;241(5):776-83; discussion 783-5. doi: 10.1097/01.sla.0000161981.58631.ab. PMID: 15849513; PMCID: PMC1357132.
30. Gaur SK, Friese JL, Sadow CA, Ayyagari R, Binkert CA, Schenker MP, Kulke M, Baum R. Hepatic arterial chemoembolization using drug-eluting beads in gastrointestinal neuroendocrine tumor metastatic to the liver. Cardiovasc Intervent Radiol. 2011 Jun;34(3):566-72. doi: 10.1007/s00270-011-0122-1. Epub 2011 Mar 24. PMID: 21431978.
31. Guiu B, Deschamps F, Aho S, Munck F, Dromain C, Boige V, Malka D, Leboulleux S, Ducreux M, Schlumberger M, Baudin E, de Baere T. Liver/biliary injuries following chemoembolisation of endocrine tumours and hepatocellular carcinoma: lipiodol vs. drug-eluting beads.

J Hepatol. 2012 Mar;56(3):609-17. doi: 10.1016/j.jhep.2011.09.012. Epub 2011 Oct 23. PMID: 22027582.
32. Devcic Z, Rosenberg J, Braat AJ, Techasith T, Banerjee A, Sze DY, Lam MG. The efficacy of hepatic 90Y resin radioembolization for metastatic neuroendocrine tumors: a meta-analysis. J Nucl Med. 2014 Sep;55(9):1404-10. doi: 10.2967/jnumed.113.135855. Epub 2014 Jul 10. PMID: 25012459.
33. Kennedy AS, Dezarn WA, McNeillie P, Coldwell D, Nutting C, Carter D, Murthy R, Rose S, Warner RR, Liu D, Palmedo H, Overton C, Jones B, Salem R. Radioembolization for unresectable neuroendocrine hepatic metastases using resin 90Y-microspheres: early results in 148 patients. Am J Clin Oncol. 2008 Jun;31(3):271-9. doi: 10.1097/COC.0b013e31815e4557. PMID: 18525307.
34. American Cancer Society. Cancer Facts & Figures 2021. Atlanta, Ga: American Cancer Society; 2021
35. Golse N, Adam R. Liver Metastases From Breast Cancer: What Role for Surgery? Indications and Results. Clin Breast Cancer. 2017 Jul;17(4):256-265. doi: 10.1016/j.clbc.2016.12.012. Epub 2017 Jan 9. PMID: 28196771.
36. Elsberger B, Roxburgh CS, Horgan PG. Is there a role for surgical resections of hepatic breast cancer metastases? Hepatogastroenterology. 2014 Jan-Feb;61(129):181-6. PMID: 24895817.
37. Vogl TJ, Farshid P, Naguib NN, Zangos S. Thermal ablation therapies in patients with breast cancer liver metastases: a review. Eur Radiol. 2013 Mar;23(3):797-804. doi: 10.1007/s00330-012-2662-4. Epub 2012 Oct 13. PMID: 23064713.
38. Vogl TJ, Naguib NN, Nour-Eldin NE, Eichler K, Zangos S, Gruber-Rouh T. Transarterial chemoembolization (TACE) with mitomycin C and gemcitabine for liver metastases in breast cancer. Eur Radiol. 2010 Jan;20(1):173-80. doi: 10.1007/s00330-009-1525-0. Epub 2009 Aug 6. PMID: 19657653.
39. Martin RC, Robbins K, Fagés JF, Romero FD, Rustein L, Tomalty D, Monaco R. Optimal outcomes for liver-dominant metastatic breast cancer with transarterial chemoembolization with drug-eluting beads loaded with doxorubicin. Breast Cancer Res Treat. 2012 Apr;132(2):753-63. doi: 10.1007/s10549-011-1926-z. Epub 2011 Dec 27. PMID: 22200868.
40. Li XP, Meng ZQ, Guo WJ, Li J. Treatment for liver metastases from breast cancer: results and prognostic factors. World J Gastroenterol. 2005 Jun 28;11(24):3782-7. doi: 10.3748/wjg.v11.i24.3782. PMID: 15968739; PMCID: PMC4316035.

41. Mouli SK, Gupta R, Sheth N, Gordon AC, Lewandowski RJ. Locoregional Therapies for the Treatment of Hepatic Metastases from Breast and Gynecologic Cancers. Semin Intervent Radiol. 2018 Mar;35(1):29-34. doi: 10.1055/s-0038-1636518. Epub 2018 Apr 5. PMID: 29628613; PMCID: PMC5886768.
42. Spagnolo F, Caltabiano G, Queirolo P. Uveal melanoma. Cancer Treat Rev. 2012 Aug;38(5):549-53. doi: 10.1016/j.ctrv.2012.01.002. Epub 2012 Jan 24. PMID: 22270078.
43. Mariani P, Almubarak MM, Kollen M, Wagner M, Plancher C, Audollent R, Piperno-Neumann S, Cassoux N, Servois V. Radiofrequency ablation and surgical resection of liver metastases from uveal melanoma. Eur J Surg Oncol. 2016 May;42(5):706-12. doi: 10.1016/j.ejso.2016.02.019. Epub 2016 Feb 23. PMID: 26968227.
44. Shamimi-Noori S, Gonsalves CF, Shaw CM. Metastatic Liver Disease: Indications for Locoregional Therapy and Supporting Data. Semin Intervent Radiol. 2017;34(2):145-166. doi:10.1055/s-0037-1602712
45. Bedikian AY, Legha SS, Mavligit G, Carrasco CH, Khorana S, Plager C, Papadopoulos N, Benjamin RS. Treatment of uveal melanoma metastatic to the liver: a review of the M. D. Anderson Cancer Center experience and prognostic factors. Cancer. 1995 Nov 1;76(9):1665-70. doi: 10.1002/1097-0142(19951101)76:9<1665::aid-cncr2820760925> 3.0.co;2-j. PMID: 8635073.
46. Gonsalves CF, Eschelman DJ, Sullivan KL, Anne PR, Doyle L, Sato T. Radioembolization as salvage therapy for hepatic metastasis of uveal melanoma: a single-institution experience. AJR Am J Roentgenol. 2011 Feb;196(2):468-73. doi: 10.2214/AJR.10.4881. PMID: 21257902.
47. Schelhorn J, Richly H, Ruhlmann M, Lauenstein TC, Theysohn JM. A single-center experience in radioembolization as salvage therapy of hepatic metastases of uveal melanoma. Acta Radiol Open. 2015 Apr 6;4(4):2047981615570417. doi: 10.1177/2047981615570417. PMID: 25922690; PMCID: PMC4406923.
48. Valsecchi ME, Terai M, Eschelman DJ, Gonsalves CF, Chervoneva I, Shields JA, Shields CL, Yamamoto A, Sullivan KL, Laudadio M, Berd D, Mastrangelo MJ, Sato T. Double-blinded, randomized phase II study using embolization with or without granulocyte-macrophage colony-stimulating factor in uveal melanoma with hepatic metastases. J Vasc Interv Radiol. 2015 Apr;26(4):523-32.e2. doi: 10.1016/j.jvir.2014.11.037. Epub 2015 Feb 9. PMID: 25678394; PMCID: PMC4417549.

49. Yamamoto A, Chervoneva I, Sullivan KL, Eschelman DJ, Gonsalves CF, Mastrangelo MJ, Berd D, Shields JA, Shields CL, Terai M, Sato T. High-dose immunoembolization: survival benefit in patients with hepatic metastases from uveal melanoma. Radiology. 2009 Jul;252(1): 290-8. doi: 10.1148/radiol.2521081252. PMID: 19561263; PMCID: PMC6944074.

CHAPTER 9

TRANSARTERIAL CHEMOEMBOLIZATION (TACE) FOR SECONDARY LIVER MASSES

STEVE LEMONS MD, BRENT SMITH MD, CAROLINE MUSSATTO MD

Introduction

TACE is also utilized in the treatment of metastatic liver tumors. A significant proportion of these are primary colorectal cancers (CRC) which have metastasized to the liver.[1] Liver metastases are typically associated with extensive underlying disease and/or recurrent disease at diagnosis, making treatment challenging and available options limited. Surgical resection is utilized for management of CRC metastases to the liver when feasible; however, micrometastases undetectable on imaging frequently lead to recurrence despite wide resection margins.[2] TACE directed at secondary liver tumors has been shown to provide survival benefit and symptomatic benefit in certain challenging cases.[1] Selection criteria are similar to those of conventional TACE, with exclusion of patients who have poor performance status, poor underlying liver function, and/or complete portal vein thrombosis. Patients with extrahepatic metastases in addition to secondary liver metastases have also been treated with TACE, though certain research studies exclude these patients. Presence of extrahepatic metastases should be noted when evaluating rates of efficacy and overall survival.[1]

DEBIRI-TACE

TACE with drug-eluting beads coated in irinotecan (DEBIRI-TACE) is a unique modality that has been developed for treatment of unresectable CRC liver metastases, and shown to have survival benefit and potentially improve quality of life.[1, 3] DEBIRI-TACE utilizes the same vascular approach as conventional TACE (c-TACE). DEBIRI-TACE is often delivered in a lobar distribution to aid in treating occult micrometastases, rather than the selective approach utilized in treatment of primary liver tumors.[1, 2]

Summary and Conclusion

DEBIRI-TACE is a viable treatment option for colorectal cancer patients with unresectable metastases to the liver. It may be used in combination with systemic chemotherapy and/or radiation to achieve disease control and improve overall survival while also targeting micrometastases undetectable on imaging.[1, 2] Further research will be helpful to delineate which patient populations receive the most benefit from DEBIRI-TACE.

References

1. Vogl TJ, Lahrsow M. The Role of Conventional TACE (cTACE) and DEBIRI-TACE in Colorectal Cancer Liver Metastases. Cancers (Basel) 2022;14(6).
2. Voizard N, Ni T, Kiss A, et al. Small Particle DEBIRI TACE as Salvage Therapy in Patients with Liver Dominant Colorectal Cancer Metastasis: Retrospective Analysis of Safety and Outcomes. Curr Oncol 2022;29(1):209-20.
3. Aquina CT, Eskander MF, Pawlik TM. Liver-Directed Treatment Options Following Liver Tumor Recurrence: A Review of the Literature. Front Oncol 2022;12:832405.

CHAPTER 10

TRANSARTERIAL RADIOEMBOLIZATION (TARE) FOR SECONDARY HEPATIC TUMORS

ZACHARY S. COLLINS MD, FSIR,
IAN KOZLOWSKI MD, MAXIMILIAN MAYR MS IV

Colorectal cancer is the fourth most common neoplasm that affects both men and women after breast, prostate, and lung cancers [1]. There are slightly greater than 1.5 million people affected by colorectal cancer in the United States with an estimated 106,970 new cases per year [1]. However, these numbers are improving due to advancements in detection methods. It is also the second most common cause of cancer deaths, after lung cancer, resulting in an estimated 52,550 deaths in 2023 [1]. Even with a high number of deaths, the 5-year survival rate is reassuring. Upon diagnosis of localized disease, the 5-year survival rate is 91%. However, upon distant metastasis, such as to the liver, the survival rate drops drastically to approximately 15% [1-3]. An important consideration is that liver metastasis is present in approximately 20-35% of patients at the time of diagnosis [4]. For these reasons, it is important to consider early detection methods but also treatment options.

Before we discuss treatment options, it is important to consider the staging system of colorectal cancer. For the purpose of our discussion here, the utilization of Y90 is for colorectal cancer stage IV and beyond as this is the stage where the cancer has metastasized distally, for instance to the liver. There is currently an abundance of treatment options for metastatic colorectal cancer which include: surgery, chemotherapy, targeted therapies, ablation and embolization, including Y90 TARE, cTACE, and drug-eluting bead transarterial chemoembolization (DEB-TACE), hepatic arterial infusion pump (HAIP) therapy, immunotherapy, stereotactic body radiation therapy, and enrollment in clinical trials. It is important to note that tailoring treatment to the molecular and pathologic features of the tumor is key to long-term survival [2].

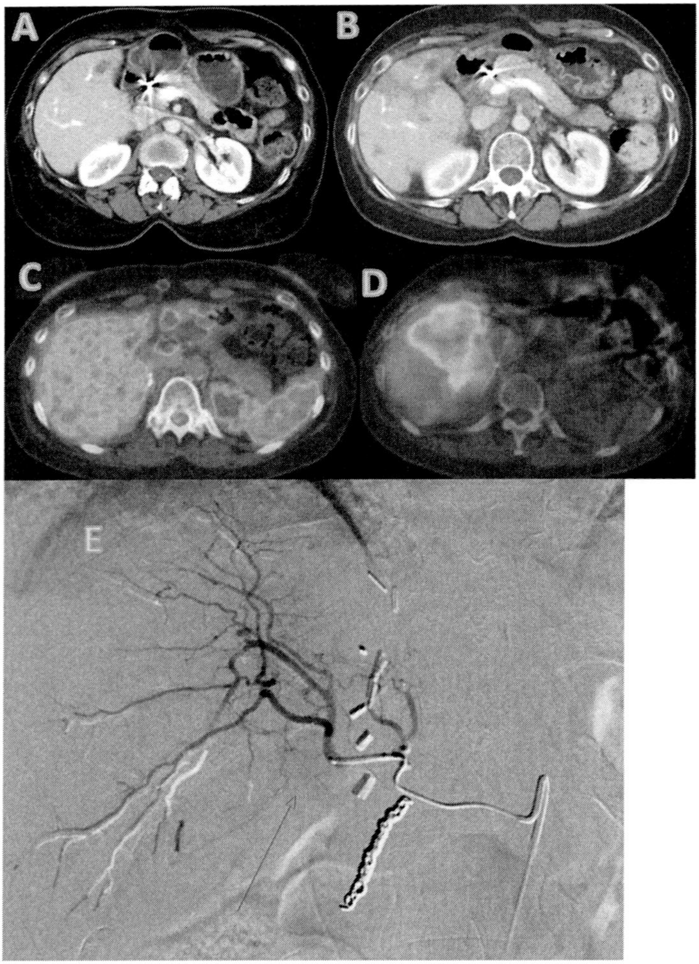

Figure 1 - 57-year-old female with metastatic colorectal cancer to liver with progression on systemic therapy (irinotecan). Multifocal right hepatic disease with dominate segment 4 lesion supplied by right hepatic artery (A/E/C). Patient received right lobar Y-90 treatment with 1.3GBq of activity with Sirpheres (Sirtex, Woburn, MA). Post treatment CT scan two months later shows treatment response, similar to the post deliver SPECT (D).

Now, what is the best treatment for metastatic colorectal cancer you may ask? There is a good amount of data individually demonstrating overall survival of the various treatments described above. Surgery has a high cure rate at approximately 90% when diagnosed early [5]. However, in mCRC, surgical cure is only possible in a fraction of the patients, roughly 10-15%, of those who even meet candidacy due to extent of metastasis. Treatments with Y90 had promising survival outcomes. One study enrolled 442 participants and utilized Y90 as either primary, secondary, or tertiary line of therapy for mCRC [6]. Outcomes demonstrated that median overall survival (OS) was 15 months for the entire cohort [6]. Additional landmark study information regarding Y90 in mCRC can be found in the Y90 chapter under "Y90 in Practical Detail."

Transarterial chemoembolization is another alternative to mCRC treatment. A large prospective study on patients with unresectable mCRC was performed utilizing TACE. These patients also failed systemic therapy and had > 5 cm metastasis at the time of chemotherapy initiation [7]. TACE was performed utilizing mitomycin C alone, mitomycin C with gemcitabine, or mitomycin with irinotecan. Median survival from the start of TACE was 14 months [7]. Most DEB-TACE for mCRC now utilizes irinotecan and also in conjunction with ablation (RFA and MWA). When it comes to the direct comparison of one treatment vs another, additional randomized clinical trials are still required, of which there are several ongoing currently.

The SIRFlox study was a randomized multicenter trial designed to assess the utilization of resin Y90 with standard fluorouracil, leucovorin, oxaplatin (FOLFOX) systemic chemotherapy in patients with untreated mCRC to any metastatic site [8]. They included 530 patients who were randomly assigned to receive either modified FOLFOX, or FOLFOX with Y90 plus or minus bevacizumab to analyze progression-free survival at any site [8]. The study demonstrated that Y90 was not useful in tissues outside of the liver as the median progression free survival at any site was 10.2 and 10.7 months in patients receiving modified FOLFOX compared to FOLFOX plus Y90 [8]. However, progression free survival was significantly improved by addition of Y90 across populations with tumor burden, +/- bevacizumab, with regards to liver metastasis with 12.6 months compared to 20.5 months in controls vs SIRT, respectively [8].

References

1. Siegel, R.L., et al., *Cancer statistics, 2023.* CA: a cancer journal for clinicians, 2023. **73**(1): pp. 17-48.
2. Biller, L.H. and D. Schrag, *Diagnosis and Treatment of Metastatic Colorectal Cancer: A Review.* Jama, 2021. **325**(7): pp. 669-685.
3. Morris, V.K., et al., *Treatment of Metastatic Colorectal Cancer: ASCO Guideline.* J Clin Oncol, 2023. **41**(3): pp. 678-700.
4. Jeyarajah, D.R., et al., *Role of yttrium-90 selective internal radiation therapy in the treatment of liver-dominant metastatic colorectal cancer: an evidence-based expert consensus algorithm.* J Gastrointest Oncol, 2020. **11**(2): pp. 443-460.
5. Bester, L., et al., *Current role of transarterial chemoembolization and radioembolization in the treatment of metastatic colorectal cancer.* Hepat Oncol, 2014. **1**(2): pp. 215-228.
6. Emmons, E.C., et al., *Survival and Toxicities after (90)Y Transarterial Radioembolization of Metastatic Colorectal Cancer in the RESIN Registry.* Radiology, 2022. **305**(1): pp. 228-236.
7. Vogl, T.J., et al., *Repeated transarterial chemoembolization in the treatment of liver metastases of colorectal cancer: prospective study.* Radiology, 2009. **250**(1): pp. 281-9.
8. van Hazel, G.A., et al., *SIRFLOX: Randomized Phase III Trial Comparing First-Line mFOLFOX6 (Plus or Minus Bevacizumab) Versus mFOLFOX6 (Plus or Minus Bevacizumab) Plus Selective Internal Radiation Therapy in Patients With Metastatic Colorectal Cancer.* J Clin Oncol, 2016. **34**(15): pp. 1723-31.

CHAPTER 11

RENAL NEOPLASM

ADAM ALLI MD, BRIAUNA HAWTHORNE MD, MACKENZIE GWINNER MD

Pathophysiology

Renal cell carcinoma (RCC) is classified into clear cell carcinoma, papillary carcinoma, chromophobe carcinoma, Xp11 translocation carcinoma, and collecting duct carcinoma. In this chapter, we will focus on the conventional or clear cell renal subtype, which comprises 70-80% of RCC.[1]

Clear cell RCC arises from the proximal renal tubular epithelium[2]. It is most commonly associated with loss of the short arm of chromosome 3.[3] Inactivation of the Von Hipple-Lindau (VHL) gene occurs, which normally is expressed to yield a protein responsible for destabilization and degradation by ubiquitination of hypoxia inducible factors (HIF) -1α and 2α.[4] Inactivation of the VHL protein leads to overexpression of HIF-1α and 2α which regulate genes involved in angiogenesis (e.g. vascular endothelial growth factor [VEGF]), glucose uptake (e.g. glucose transporter [GLUT]-1), erythropoiesis (e.g. erythropoietin [EPO]), cell proliferation (e.g. transforming growth factor [TGF]-α), and apoptosis[5] (apoptosis repressor with a caspase recruitment domain [ARC]).[4,6]

Imaging

Currently, an abdominal ultrasound with IV contrast, an MRI abdomen without and with IV contrast, and CT abdomen without and with IV contrast are all considered appropriate initial imagining by the American College of Radiology (ACR) for an indeterminate renal mass in a patient without contraindications to iodinated or gadolinium based IV contrast.

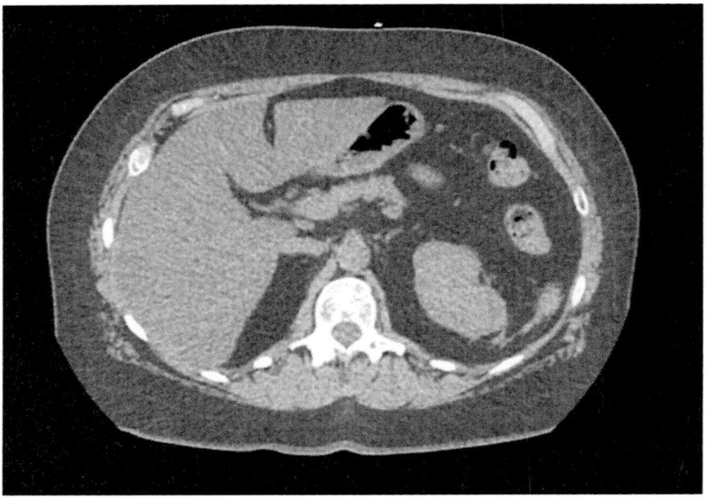

A)

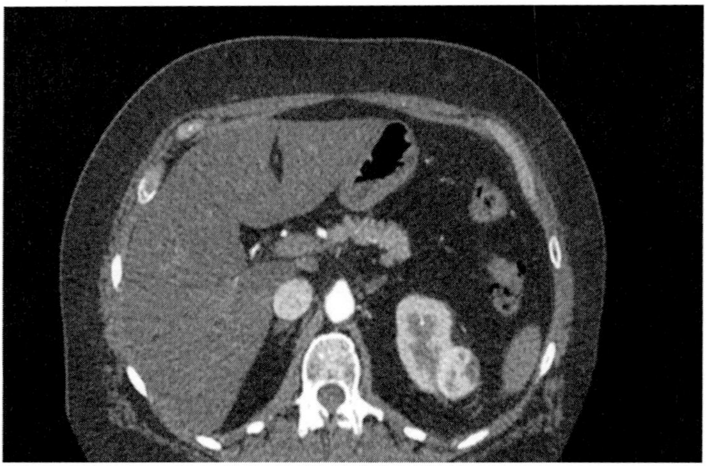

B)

C) 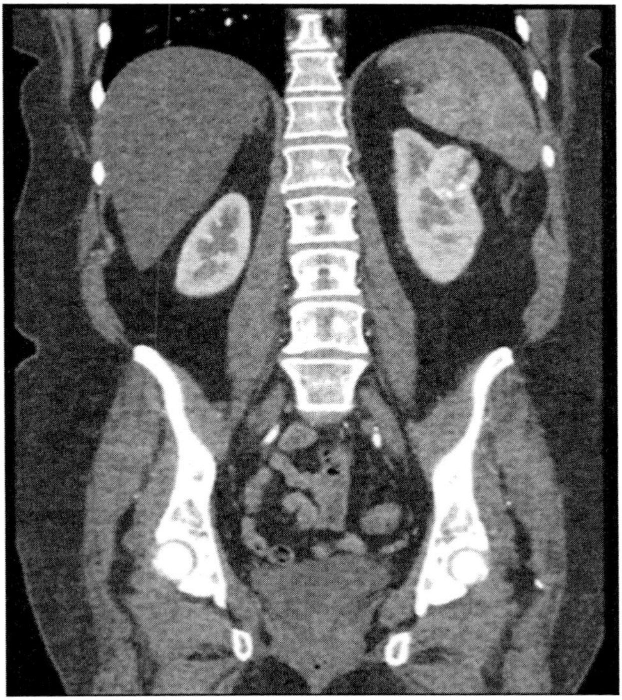

Figure 1: A) Axial non-enhanced CT demonstrating renal cell carcinoma B) Axial contrast enhanced CT demonstrating left renal cell carcinoma C) Coronal contrast enhanced CT demonstrating left renal cell carcinoma.

A nonenhanced image of the renal mass should be obtained to provide a baseline for subsequent images to be compared. RCC displays soft tissue attenuation of between 20-70 HU.[7] Following contrast administration, enhancement greater than 15 HU is suspicious for malignancy.[8] Small lesions are typically homogenous, while larger lesions may be heterogenous with areas of hemorrhage, calcifications, or necrosis.[7]

During the corticomedullary phase, approximately 25-80 seconds after contrast administration, clear cell carcinoma will enhance to around the level of the renal cortex, which is typically greater than the other subtypes of RCC.[9-10] Jeong Kim *et al* found that enhancement to 84 HU during the corticomedullary phase and 44 HU 120 seconds after contrast administration has 100% and 91% specificity for RCC, respectively.

MRI has been found to have a similar sensitivity to CT at detecting renal cell carcinoma.[11] On T1 weighted sequences, RCC will typically be either isointense or hypointense to that of the renal cortex.[11] On T2 weight images, RCC will appear hyperintense in comparison to the renal cortex.[11] Depending on the size of the lesion, it display either homogenous or heterogenous enhancement immediately following gadolinium administration.[11]

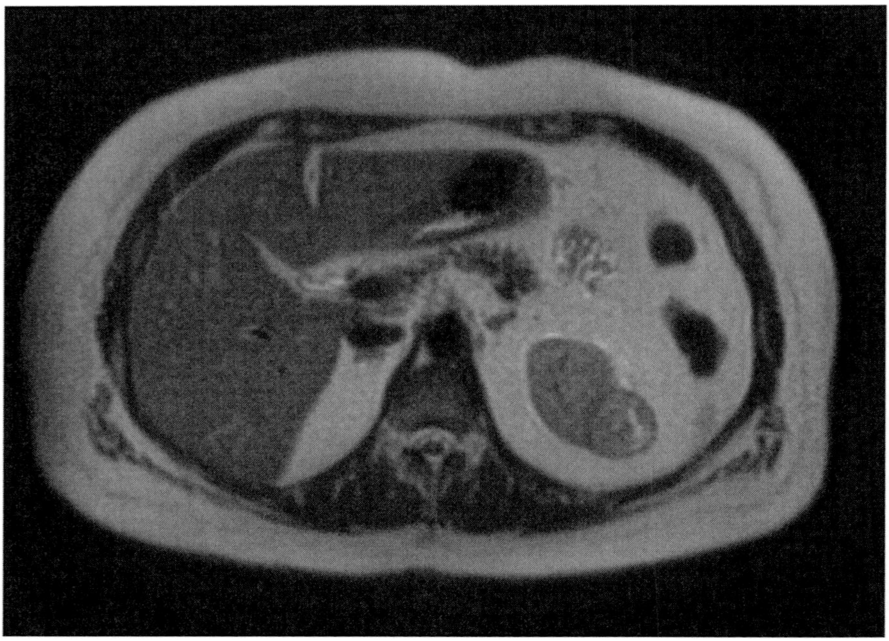

Figure 4: Axial T1 weighted MRI from KU Left Renal Cell Carcinoma

Staging System

The staging systems used for renal cell carcinoma include the TNM and the Robson systems. The TNM staging system utilizes tumor size (T), spread to lymph nodes (N), and metastasis of the cancer elsewhere in the body (M) to standardize characterization of tumor stage. The Robson staging system focuses on localization of the tumor and extension to adjacent structures, such as the renal vein, spread to lymph nodes, and distant metastasis.

<table>
<tr><th colspan="4">TNM System</th></tr>
<tr><td rowspan="14">T</td><td colspan="3"></td></tr>
<tr><td rowspan="3">T1</td><td colspan="2">The tumor is confined to the kidney</td></tr>
<tr><td>T1a</td><td>Tumor is <4cm at greatest dimension</td></tr>
<tr><td>T1b</td><td>Tumor is <4cm but <7cm at greatest dimension</td></tr>
<tr><td rowspan="3">T2</td><td colspan="2">The tumor is confined to the kidney</td></tr>
<tr><td>T2a</td><td>Tumor is >7cm but <10cm at greatest dimension</td></tr>
<tr><td>T2b</td><td>Tumor is >10cm at greatest dimension</td></tr>
<tr><td rowspan="4">T3</td><td colspan="2">Tumor
1)Extends to perirenal fat
2)Does not extend to ipsilateral adrenal gland
3)Is confined by Gerota's fascia</td></tr>
<tr><td>T3a</td><td>Tumor exhibits one of the following characteristics:
- involves renal vein
- involves renal vein segmental branch
- invades perirenal fat
- invades renal sinus fat</td></tr>
<tr><td>T3b</td><td>Tumor involves infra diaphragmatic IVC</td></tr>
<tr><td>T3c</td><td>Tumor exhibits one of the following characteristics:
- involves supra diaphragmatic IVC
- invades the wall of the IVC</td></tr>
<tr><td>T4</td><td colspan="2">Tumor exhibits one of the following characteristics:
- involves ipsilateral adrenal gland
- invades beyond Gerota's fascia</td></tr>
<tr><td rowspan="3">N</td><td colspan="3"></td></tr>
<tr><td>N0</td><td colspan="2">No nodal involvement</td></tr>
<tr><td>N1</td><td colspan="2">Regional lymph node involvement</td></tr>
<tr><td rowspan="3">M</td><td colspan="3"></td></tr>
<tr><td>M0</td><td colspan="2">No distant metastases</td></tr>
<tr><td>M1</td><td colspan="2">Distant metastases present</td></tr>
</table>

Stages by TNM Grouping			
Stage I	T1	N0	M0
Stage II	T2	N0	M0
Stage III	T1	N1	M0
	T2	N1	M0
	T3	N1	M0
	T3	N0	M0
Stage IV	T1	N0	M1
	T1	N1	M1
	T2	N0	M1
	T2	N1	M1
	T3	N0	M1
	T3	N1	M1
	T4	N0	M0
	T4	N1	M1
	T4	N0	M1

Robson Staging		
Stage I	Tumor is limited to the kidney	
Stage II	Tumor involves the perinephric fat, but is limited to Gerota's fascia	
Stage III	IIIa	Tumor involves the renal vein
	IIIb	Tumor involves the lymph nodes
	IIIc	Tumor involves the renal vein and the lymph nodes
Stage IV	Iva	Tumor invades adjacent structures
	IVb	Distant metastases are present

Management

RCC is managed with surgical excision via partial or radical nephrectomy.[12] Thermal ablation is a minimally invasive alternative that may be an especially attractive treatment option for high surgical risk patients, though patients are more likely to experience tumor recurrence compared to surgical excision.[13] Thermal ablation for treatment of renal cell carcinoma will be expounded upon in a later chapter.

Oncocytoma

Pathophysiology

Oncocytoma is a benign tumor that arises from the intercalating cells of the renal collecting ducts.[8] The genetic abnormalities associated with oncocytomas include loss of chromosome 1, rearrangement of 11q13, loss of Y, and deletion of chromosome 14.[14,15] 11q13 is the locus for the CCND1 gene, therefore some oncocytomas are associated with Cyclin D1 rearrangement.[15] Deregulation of Cyclin D1 has been linked to various malignancies.[16] Cyclin D1 forms complexes with kinases to promote cell cycle progression from G1 to S phase by inactivating retinoblastoma protein (RB).[16] Sukov *et al* found that patients with Cyclin D1 overexpression were more likely to have a solitary lesion as opposed to multifocal lesions. Oncocytomas display morphologic features similar to chromophobe renal cell carcinoma, complicating diagnosis.[15,17]

Imaging

Oncocytomas are difficult to distinguish from RCC on imaging.[18] Both oncocytomas and RCC can display central scars. One third of oncocytomas will exhibit a stellate central scar on imaging.[18] Furthermore, oncocytomas can coexist with RCC, so resection of the lesion is currently recommended. A study performed by Gorin *et al* shows promise for using ^{99m}Tc-sestamibi SPECT/CT to diagnose oncocytomas and hybrid oncocytic/chromophobe tumors with a sensitivity of 87.5% and a specificity of 95.2%. In a pilot study, Gorin *et al* found that oncocytomas accumulated the radiotracer at or greater than that of the renal parenchyma compared to renal cell carcinoma which accumulated the radiotracer at much lower levels.[19,20]

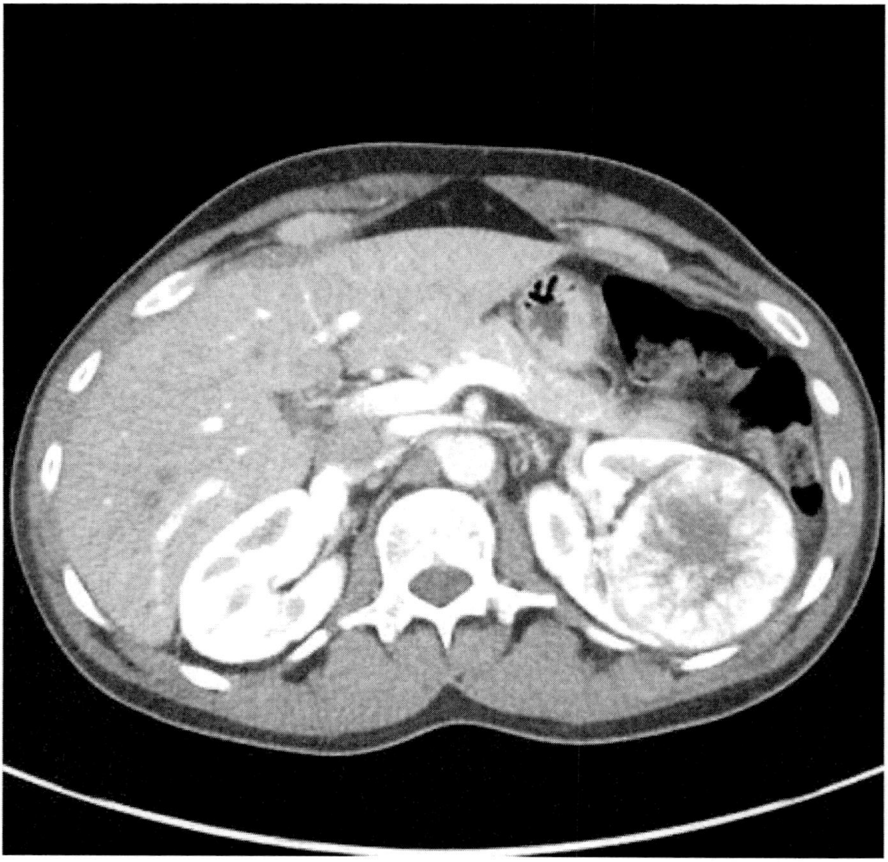

Figure 5: Axial CT L Renal Oncocytoma from Radiopaedia. *Copyright 2023 Paul Simkin. Image courtesy of Paul Simkin and Radiopaedia.org. Used under license.*

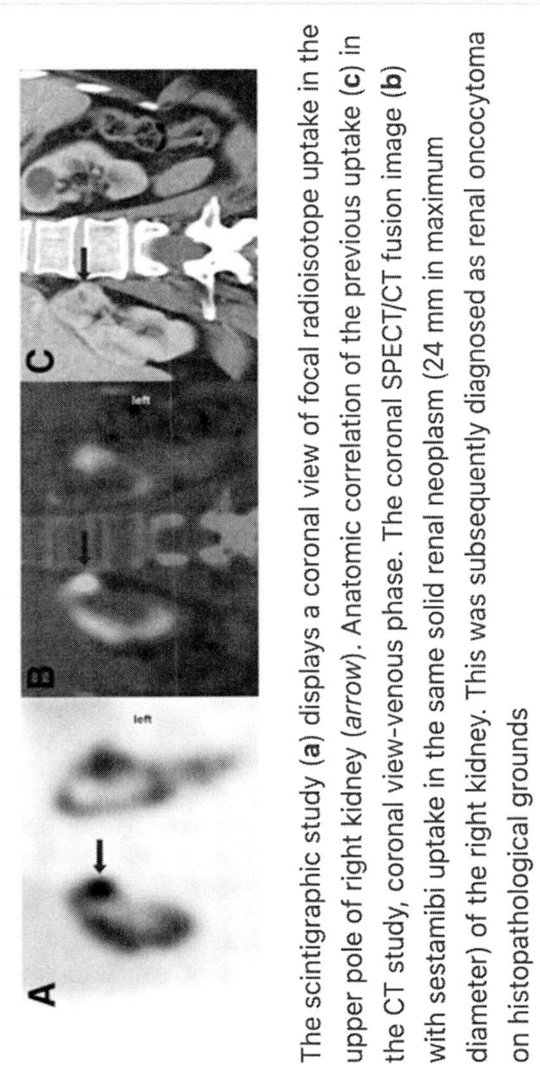

Figure 6: Coronal SPECT/CT R Renal Oncocytoma. Tzortzakakis, A., Gustafsson, O., Karlsson, M. *et al.* Visual evaluation and differentiation of renal oncocytomas from renal cell carcinomas by means of ^{99m}Tc-sestamibi SPECT/CT. *EJNMMI Res* 7, 29 (2017). https://doi.org/10.1186/s13550-017-0278-z.

Management

Oncocytomas are typically managed by radical nephrectomy, partial nephrectomy, or thermal ablation. Due to their benign nature, its debated that renal oncocytomas are being overtreated with surgical resection.[18] Active surveillance may be a safe management option for patients with slow tumor growth rate as well as patient with multiple comorbidities.[18] Arguments against active surveillance cite the capability that an oncocytoma can reach a large size, harm healthy renal tissue, and coexistence with renal cell carcinoma.[18] There is limited data on the use of thermal ablation to treat oncocytomas. Ogan *et al* used radiofrequency ablation as treatment option for patients with small renal masses and found there was low morbidity from the procedure.[21]

Angiomyolipoma

Pathophysiology

Angiomyolipoma (AML) is the most common benign renal tumor and is composed of varying proportions of blood vessels, smooth muscle, and adipose tissue. 80% of AML's arise sporadically, while 20% develop in association with either tuberous sclerosis (TSC), complex or pulmonary lymphangioleimyomatosis. Limited studies have been performed to analyze the genetic basis of the development of AML in patients without TSC or pulmonary lymphangioleimyomatosis.[22] Studies show that sporadic AML is associated with mutations in the TSC2 gene.[22,23] TSC2 is a tumor suppressor gene that encodes the protein tuberin, a GTPase activating protein.[22] Tuberin regulates Rheb, a GTP-binding protein that activates mTOR.[22] mTOR regulates translation of proteins involved in cell growth and proliferation.[22] Loss of function mutations in TSC2 result in overaction of mTOR which leads to cell hyperproliferation.[24]

Imaging

CT can be utilized for definitive diagnosis of AML.[1] Fat containing renal lesions (-20 to -80HU) found on CT imagining strongly suggests AML.[2] Isoattenuating angiomyolipoma attenuates between -10 and 45HU due to adipocytes being scattered amongst the smooth muscle and blood vessels components of the tumor.[25] Hyperattenuating AML's attenuate at a value greater than 45HU and may be preoperatively diagnosed as RCC.[25]

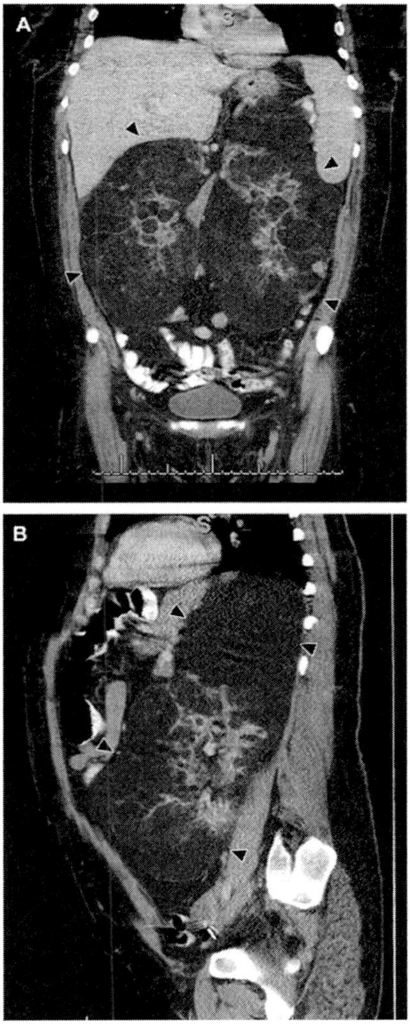

Source: Khaled M. Elsayes, Sandra A. A. Oldham: *Introduction to Diagnostic Radiology*:
www.accessmedicine.com

Figure 7: Coronal (A) and Sagittal (B) CT bilateral angiomyolipomas. Usama Salem; Eduardo J. Matta; Ayda Youssef; Khaled M. Elsayes. Eds. *Introduction to Diagnostic Radiology*. McGraw Hill;2014. Figure C10.2. https://accessmedicine.mhmedical.com/content.aspx?bookid=1562&sectionid=95874457 . Reprinted with permission

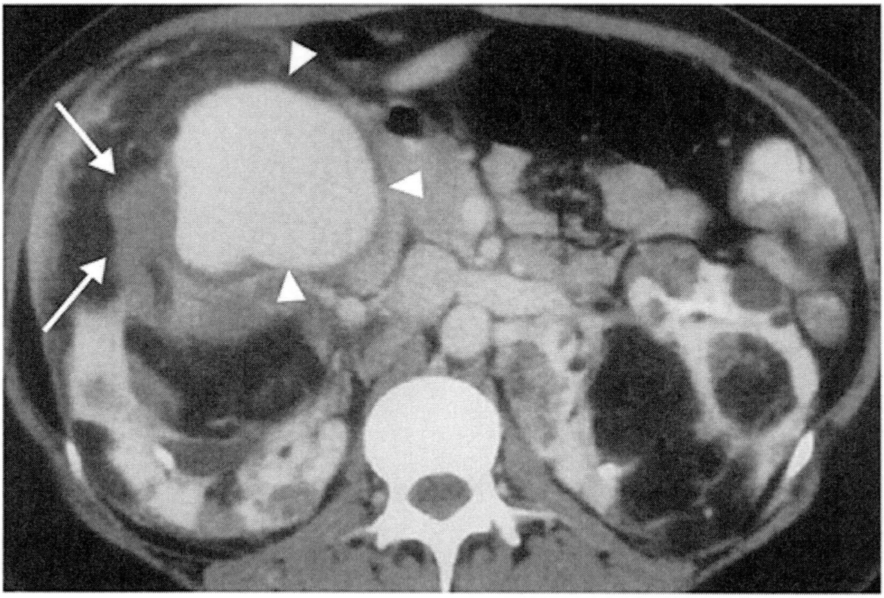

Figure 8: Postcontrast Axial CT with bilateral angiomyolipomas and fatty renal masses. Usama Salem; Eduardo J. Matta; Ayda Youssef; Khaled M. Elsayes. Eds. *Introduction to Diagnostic Radiology*. McGraw Hill;2014. Figure C10.4
https://accessmedicine.mhmedical.com/content.aspx?bookid=1562&sectionid=958 74457 .

Magnetic Resonance Imaging

MRI is advantageous for diagnosing lipid poor or invisible AML.[2] Normally, due to the adipose deposition, it will display a bright signal on non-fat suppressed T1 weighted images that will be lost when observing a fat suppressed sequence.[8] Lipid poor AML displays a tumor-to-spleen ratio (TSR) of <0.71 and a signal intensity index (SII) of $>16.5\%$. Lipid invisible AML is characterized by a TSR of ≥ 0.71 SII of $\leq 16.5\%$.[26]

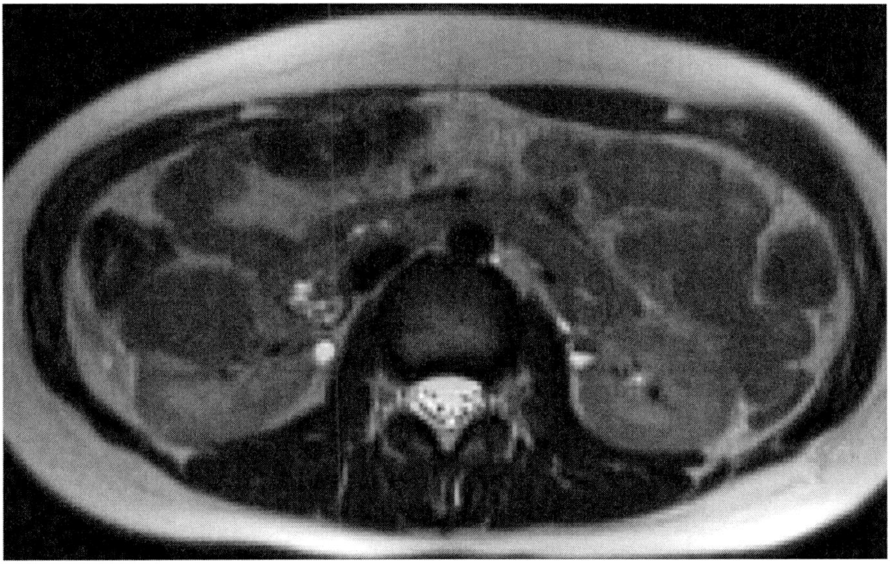

Figure 9: Axial MRI lipid poor angiomyolipoma homogenous signal intensity. Wilson MP, Patel D, Murad MH, McInnes MD, Katlariwala P, Low G. *Diagnostic Performance of MRI in the Detection of Renal Lipid-Poor Angiomyolipomas: A Systematic Review and Meta-Analysis.* 2020. Figure 4a. Copyright Radiological Society of North America.

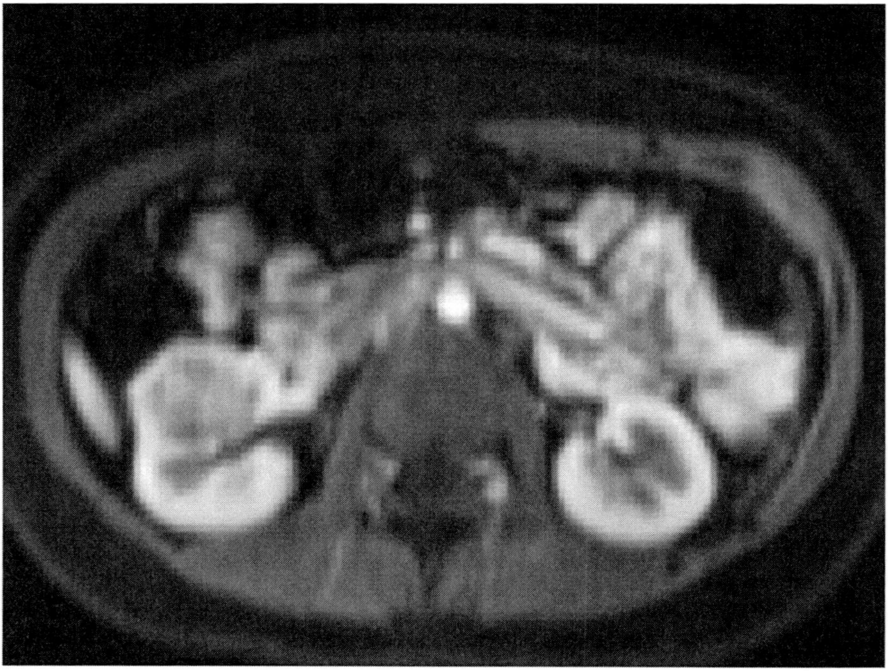

Figure 10: Axial contrast enhanced MRI lipid poor angiomyolipoma with hypervascular enhancement. Wilson MP, Patel D, Murad MH, McInnes MD, Katlariwala P, Low G. *Diagnostic Performance of MRI in the Detection of Renal Lipid-Poor Angiomyolipomas: A Systematic Review and Meta-Analysis.* 2020. Figure 4b. Copyright Radiological Society of North America

Management

Most AML's can be managed conservatively with active surveillance. Historically, the indications for treatment included the patient being symptomatic, presence in a woman of childbearing age, and size >4cm. Using 4cm as a threshold for treating angiomyolipoma is currently being challenged as there is evidence that aneurysm size and vascularity are more significant predictors of the feared complication, retroperitoneal hemorrhage. While there is currently no consensus, AML's <4cm should be surveilled annually by CT or ultrasound, while lesions measuring >4cm should be surveilled semiannually. Treatment options include embolization, partial or radical nephrectomy, and, for smaller lesions, radio or cryoablation.[26]

Renal Metastases

Etiology

Metastases to the kidney occurs more commonly than primary renal malignancies.[1] They are usually asymptomatic and therefore are frequently discovered at autopsy.[11] The most common primary tumor sites that metastasize to the kidney are the lungs, stomach, and breasts.[1] Malignant cells in the primary tumor site most commonly hematogenous spreads to the kidney.[11]

Imaging

Renal metastases are usually isodense or slightly more hypodense than the renal parenchyma. They tend to be hypovascular and thus only marginally enhance upon contrast administration[27]. In contrast to primary malignancies, renal metastases will usually be multifocal or endophytic without calcifications or invasion of the renal vein.[11,27]

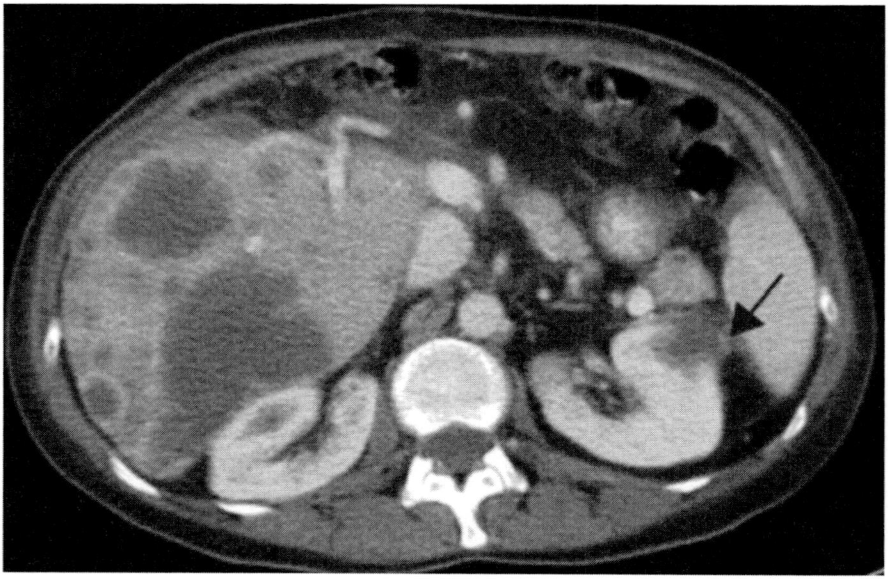

Figure 11: Metastatic Disease to the kidney. Post-contrast CT of metastatic cholangiocarcinoma to liver and left kidney. Reprinted from Grainger & Allison's Diagnostic Radiology Edition 7, Giles Rottenberg, Hema Verma, Renal Masses: Imaging and Biopsy, 791-802, Copyright (2021) with permission from Elsevier

Management

No clear guidelines exist for management of renal metastases. Patients with metastases to the kidney are generally managed with systemic chemotherapy or palliative care.[28] Nephrectomy is typically reserved for circumstances such as patients with hemorrhage refractory to embolization.[28]

References

1. Katz MH, Doherty GM. Urology. In: Doherty GM, editor. Current Diagnosis & Treatment: Surgery, 15e. New York, NY: McGraw Hill LLC; 2020.
2. Odisho AY, Greene KL. Renal Parenchymal Neoplasms. In: McAninch JW, Lue TF, editors. Smith & Tanagho's General Urology, 19e. New York, NY: McGraw Hill; 2020.

3. Nabi S, Kessler ER, Bernard B, Flaig TW, Lam ET. Renal cell carcinoma: a review of biology and pathophysiology. F1000Res 2018;7:307.
4. Cohen HT, McGovern FJ. Renal-cell carcinoma. N Engl J Med 2005;353(23):2477-90.
5. Razorenova OV, Castellini L, Colavitti R, Edgington LE, Nicolau M, Huang X, Bedogni B, Mills EM, Bogyo M, Giaccia AJ. The Apoptosis Repressor with a CARD Domain (ARC) Gene Is a Direct Hypoxia-Inducible Factor 1 Target Gene and Promotes Survival and Proliferation of VHL-Deficient Renal Cancer Cells. Molecular and Cellular Biology 2014;34(4):739-751.
6. Li L, Zhang L, Zhang X, Yan Q, Minamishima YA, Olumi AF, Mao M, Bartz S, Kaelin WG, Jr. Hypoxia-inducible factor linked to differential kidney cancer risk seen with type 2A and type 2B VHL mutations. Mol Cell Biol 2007;27(15):5381-92.
7. Sheth S, Scatarige JC, Horton KM, Corl FM, Fishman EK. Current Concepts in the Diagnosis and Management of Renal Cell Carcinoma: Role of Multidetector CT and Three-dimensional CT. RadioGraphics 2001;21(suppl_1):S237-S254.
8. Salem U, Matta EJ, Youssef A, Elsayes KM. Genitourinary System. In: Elsayes KM, Oldham SAA, editors. Introduction to Diagnostic Radiology. New York, NY: McGraw-Hill Education; 2015.
9. Wolin EA, Hartman DS, Olson JR. Nephrographic and pyelographic analysis of CT urography: principles, patterns, and pathophysiology. AJR Am J Roentgenol 2013;200(6):1210-4.
10. Kim JK, Kim TK, Ahn HJ, Kim CS, Kim K-R, Cho K-S. Differentiation of Subtypes of Renal Cell Carcinoma on Helical CT Scans. American Journal of Roentgenology 2002;178(6):1499-1506.
11. Rottenberg G, Verma H. Renal Masses: Imaging and Biopsy. Grainger & Allison's Diagnostic Radiology. Seventh Edition ed: Elsevier Health Sciences; 2021. p 791-802.
12. Barata PC, Rini BI. Treatment of renal cell carcinoma: Current status and future directions. CA Cancer J Clin 2017;67(6):507-524.
13. Campbell SC, Novick AC, Belldegrun A, Blute ML, Chow GK, Derweesh IH, Faraday MM, Kaouk JH, Leveillee RJ, Matin SF and others. Guideline for Management of the Clinical T1 Renal Mass. The Journal of Urology 2009;182(4):1271-1279.
14. Goldblum JR, Lamps LW, McKenney J, Myers JL. Rosai and Ackerman's Surgical Pathology E-Book. Elsevier Health Sciences; 2017.

15. Wobker SE, Williamson SR. Modern Pathologic Diagnosis of Renal Oncocytoma. J Kidney Cancer VHL 2017;4(4):1-12.
16. Alao JP. The regulation of cyclin D1 degradation: roles in cancer development and the potential for therapeutic invention. Mol Cancer 2007;6:24.
17. Sukov WR, Ketterling RP, Lager DJ, Carlson AW, Sinnwell JP, Chow GK, Jenkins RB, Cheville JC. CCND1 rearrangements and cyclin D1 overexpression in renal oncocytomas: frequency, clinicopathologic features, and utility in differentiation from chromophobe renal cell carcinoma. Hum Pathol 2009;40(9):1296-303.
18. Abdessater M, Kanbar A, Comperat E, Dupont-Athenor A, Alechinsky L, Mouton M, Sebe P. Renal Oncocytoma: An Algorithm for Diagnosis and Management. Urology 2020;143:173-180.
19. Gorin MA, Rowe SP, Baras AS, Solnes LB, Ball MW, Pierorazio PM, Pavlovich CP, Epstein JI, Javadi MS, Allaf ME. Prospective Evaluation of (99m)Tc-sestamibi SPECT/CT for the Diagnosis of Renal Oncocytomas and Hybrid Oncocytic/Chromophobe Tumors. Eur Urol 2016;69(3):413-6.
20. Rowe SP, Gorin MA, Gordetsky J, Ball MW, Pierorazio PM, Higuchi T, Epstein JI, Allaf ME, Javadi MS. Initial experience using 99mTc-MIBI SPECT/CT for the differentiation of oncocytoma from renal cell carcinoma. Clin Nucl Med 2015;40(4):309-13.
21. Ogan K, Jacomides L, Dolmatch BL, Rivera FJ, Dellaria MF, Josephs SC, Cadeddu JA. Percutaneous radiofrequency ablation of renal tumors: technique, limitations, and morbidity. Urology 2002;60(6): 954-8.
22. Rosset C, Netto CBO, Ashton-Prolla P. TSC1 and TSC2 gene mutations and their implications for treatment in Tuberous Sclerosis Complex: a review. Genet Mol Biol 2017;40(1):69-79.
23. Anoshkin K, Vasilyev I, Mosyakova C, Tanas A, Karandasheva K, Bagmet N, Karagyozyan G, Doludin YV, Kuznetsova E, Gurevich L. Mutations in TSC1/TSC2 genes are prevalent in sporadic renal angiomyolipoma and insulinoma tumors, supporting their responsiveness to mTOR inhibitors. Annals of Oncology 2018;29:vi25.
24. Rabenou RA, Charles HW. Differentiation of Sporadic Versus Tuberous Sclerosis Complex–Associated Angiomyolipoma. American Journal of Roentgenology 2015;205(2):292-301.
25. Jinzaki M, Silverman SG, Akita H, Nagashima Y, Mikami S, Oya M. Renal angiomyolipoma: a radiological classification and update on recent developments in diagnosis and management. Abdom Imaging 2014;39(3):588-604.

26. Vos N, Oyen R. Renal Angiomyolipoma: The Good, the Bad, and the Ugly. J Belg Soc Radiol 2018;102(1):41.
27. Cazacu SM, LD SA, Mitroi G, Neagoe DC, Streba C, Albulescu DM. Metastases to the Kidney: A Case Report and Review of the Literature. Curr Health Sci J 2020;46(1):80-89.
28. Campbell SC, Lane BR, Pierorazio PM. Malignant Renal Tumors. Campbell-Walsh-Wein Urology. Twelfth Edition ed2021. p 2133-2184.

CHAPTER 12

RENAL ABLATION

BRANDON CUSTER MD

Introduction

Renal carcinoma is a common malignancy in the aging population with 81,800 new cases diagnosed every year, most presenting in the sixth and seventh decades (1). Incidence has been steadily increasing due to increased detection of asymptomatic, early stage, masses as incidental findings on ultrasound, computed tomography (CT), or magnetic resonance (MR). Historically, the gold standard for management of Renal carcinoma is surgical excision with either radical or partial nephrectomy. However, an elderly population and comorbidities make many patients poor surgical candidates. This necessitated the development of minimally invasive treatment options for small renal masses. Thermal Ablation was first utilized for this purpose in 1998. Beginning in 2017, the American Urological Association has recommended considering percutaneous ablation as a first line treatment in masses less than 3 cm in diameter (2). Thermal ablation offers good outcomes with reduced complications rates, better protection of renal function, and faster recoveries.

The types of thermoablative technology utilized in renal ablation include radiofrequency ablation (RFA), microwave ablation (MWA), and cryoablation. Alternative therapies requiring additional research also include High Intensity Focused Ultrasound (HIFU) and irreversible electroporation. All thermal ablation options have shown safety and efficacy in the treatment of small renal masses, with the most robust data available for RFA. To review the mechanism of action, strengths, and weaknesses of each ablative technology, please refer to the liver ablation chapter.

Indications

Thermal ablation offers a repeatable, effective, low-cost, and safe treatment option for patients with primary renal masses. It is the ideal treatment for patients who are poor surgical candidates, have limited renal reserve (i.e. solitary kidney, renal failure), or patients with a genetic syndrome predisposed to multiple renal masses (von Hippel-Lindau).

Typically, thermal ablation is performed with curative intent for small renal masses. Increasing tumor size has a direct correlation with treatment failure, particularly in masses greater than 5 cm in size. The need for multiple treatments to obtain complete tumor response also increases in masses greater than 3 cm in size. Alternatively, ablation can be used for palliative intent in patients with very large masses or intractable hematuria (3-4).

Contraindications

The only absolute contraindication to percutaneous thermal ablation of renal masses is uncorrectable coagulopathy. Renal ablation is considered a High Bleeding risk procedure in the SIR guidelines, recommending an INR <1.7-2.0 and platelets > 50k for the procedure to be performed (5). Relative contraindications are tumor characteristics that increase procedural risks. This includes proximity of the ablation zone to adjacent vital structures (collecting system, bowel). In these patients, advanced techniques described later in the chapter can be employed to minimize complications.

Outcomes

The most robust data for thermal ablation has been performed on tumors less than 4 cm in size using Radiofrequency Ablation (RFA). Key outcomes evaluated on these studies were 5-year recurrence-free survival (RFS) (93.5-96.1%), Disease-free survival (DFS) (89-91.5%), Metastasis-free survival (MFS) (96-100%), and cancer-specific survival (CSS) (96-100%) (6-8).

One major benefit of ablation compared to surgical treatment options is the sparing of healthy nephrons, which optimizes maintenance of renal function. Studies have shown that 98% of patients have comparable GFR before and after thermal ablation, confirming the renal-protective nature (9).

The greatest predictors of treatment success are small size and posterior, exophytic location of the mass. Tumors bigger than 3 cm have been linked to a higher frequency of recurrence within the T1a classification, with a disease-free survival rate of 68% compared to 97% of tumors 3 cm or smaller (7). Location also has a role on outcomes in masses less than 3 cm in diameter, where exophytic masses have a greater than 95% primary success rate. Conversely, masses centrally located were more likely to require re-treatment due to persistent viable disease (9).

Thermal ablation is still an effective treatment option as masses increase in size, but the likelihood of needing multiple treatments to obtain complete tumor necrosis increases with tumor size. In masses <3 cm in size, studies have shown 100% of tumors reaching complete necrosis with 92% reaching it with only a single ablation session. In masses 3-5 cm in size, 92% of masses with reach complete necrosis with only 53% reaching it after a single session. In masses greater than 5 cm, only 25% will ever reach complete necrosis and none occurred after a single session (Table 1) (10).

Tumor Size	<3 cm	3-5 cm	>5 cm
Complete Tumor necrosis with 1 Treatment	92%	53%	0%
Complete Tumor necrosis after multiple treatment	100%	92%	25%

Table 1: Tumor size is indirectly correlated with treatment response. As tumor size increases, the likelihood of complete tumor necrosis decreases and need for multiple treatments increases.

A large meta-analysis comparing partial nephrectomy and thermal ablation in T1a or T1b renal masses, performed by Chan et al, showed no difference in Cancer specific survival (95% CI). Some prior reports have shown higher recurrence rates in thermal ablation vs partial nephrectomy, but the meta-analysis showed no statistically significant difference between the two groups at the 5-year follow up. There was no difference between metastasis-free or disease-free survival between the two groups (11). In contrast, studies on active surveillance of small renal masses show significantly reduced overall survival compared to intervention groups (Radical Nephrectomy, Partial Nephrectomy, or Ablation) (12). Thermal ablation offers several potential benefits compared to surgical resection. In addition to the preservation of renal function, percutaneous thermal ablation is attractive because of much shorter hospital stay, lower cost, lower blood loss, shorter operative time, and acceptable morbidity in comparison to nephron sparing surgery (13-16).

Comparative studies have shown no statistically significant difference in outcomes or complications between RFA, Cryoablation, and Microwave ablation (17,18). Some studies have suggested improved 10-year outcomes of overall survival and cancer specific survival from Microwave Ablation compared to radiofrequency ablation. However, there are known strengths and weakness for each ablation type (Table 2) (19,20). As overall outcomes are similar, choice of ablative technology will likely come down to provider comfort and experience.

Ablation Technique	Advantages	Disadvantages
Radiofrequency Ablation (RFA)	Lower Cost Abundant research and data Shorter procedure times than Cryoablation	Lower efficacy on masses larger than 3 cm Susceptibility to heat sink No Visualization of ablation zone
Cryoablation (CA)	Visualization of ablation zone Synergy with multiple probes to treat larger masses Potentially more protective of nontarget thermal injury	Long Procedure time leading to prolonged sedation and poor room utilization. Potentially increased bleeding risk
Microwave Ablation (MWA)	Less susceptibility to heat sink Shortest procedure time Largest ablation zones	No real time visualization of ablation zone Potentially higher risk of nontarget thermal injury High Cost

Table 2: Comparison of advantages and disadvantages of radiofrequency ablation (RFA), Cryoablation (CA), and Microwave ablation (MWA)

Complications

Complications can be the result of probe insertion or thermal injury. Overall, complication rates for percutaneous thermal ablation are low, ranging from 3%-14% (21-23). Major complicated rate (Grade II or higher according to the Clavien-Dindo classification) is around 5% and not significantly different between type of thermal ablation. Hemorrhage is the most common major complication. Hemorrhage can present as either hematuria or perinephric hematoma. Hemorrhage is self-limited in most cases and does not require further intervention (24). There is a 2% risk of pneumothorax (25). Tract seeding, while historically thought to be a risk with renal cancer, has been shown to be extremely rare in contemporary research (26). Thermal damage to adjacent structures is an increased risk when the ablation zone is less than 20 mm from the ureter (27) or 5 mm from the bowel (28). Thermal injury can also rarely injure the genitofemoral nerve, which will present with inguinal pain or numbness after the procedure. Advanced technique described later in the chapter can be used to minimize these risks.

Preprocedure

All patients being considered for thermal ablation need to be evaluated in clinic prior to the procedure. The clinic visit should include a full history and physical exam with a focus on renal function and ECOG (Eastern Cooperative Oncology Group) functional status. ECOG status should be less than 3. Relevant information to review includes cardiopulmonary function for anesthesia, renal function testing (Creatinine), laboratory analysis within 30 days (Hgb, Plt, INR), and a full review of medications. Renal ablation is categorized as a high bleeding risk procedure by the society of Interventional radiology (SIR). This means INR should be less than 1.7-2.0, platelets greater than 50k, and all blood thinners should be held for a sufficient amount of time prior to the procedure. If blood thinners cannot be held, bridging with heparin should be considered.

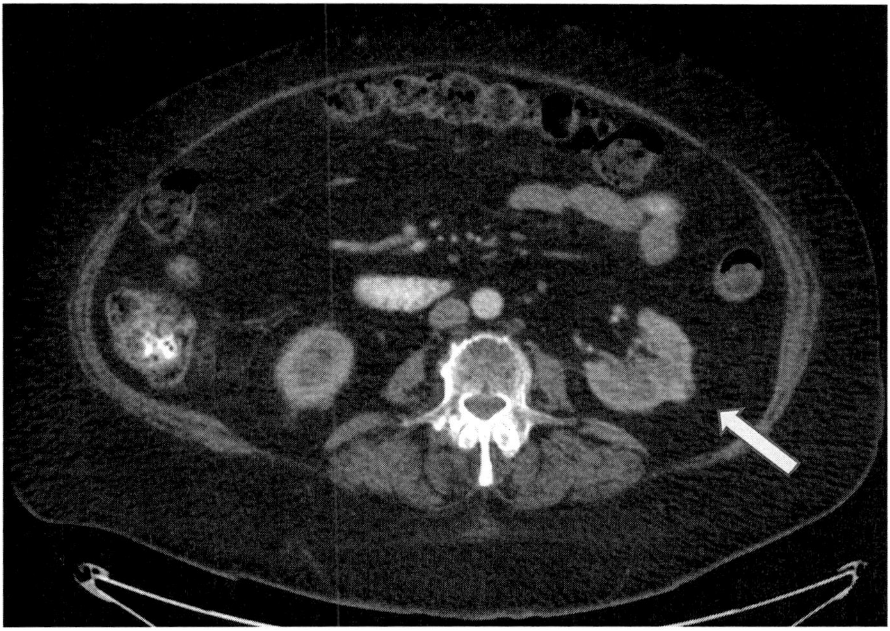

Figure 1: Preprocedural contrast enhanced CT shows an enhancing, exophytic mass (arrow) extending posteriorly from the left midpole, measuring less than 3 cm. This is the ideal appearance for a mass being treated with thermal ablation.

Current cross-sectional imaging within 3 months of the procedure is required (Figure 1). Imaging should be reviewed at the clinic visit to determine tumor size, number, shape, location, and procedural approach. This information is necessary to have an informative discussion with the patient regarding procedural expectation, outcomes, and potential complications. The clinic appointment is also the time to address goals of care, the majority of which is curative in nature.

Procedure

Thermal ablation is performed in the outpatient setting under most circumstances. The patient should arrive to the department at least one hour prior to the procedure start time. This allows time to review all relevant labs and ensure anesthesia adequate time to re-evaluate the patient prior to the procedure.

The Society of Interventional Radiology (SIR) considers kidney ablation to be a "clean contaminated" procedure. As such, it recommends periprocedural antibiotics to cover skin and genito-urinary flora. While there is no consensus on which antibiotic to use, the society recommends 1 g ceftriaxone IV (29).

Conscious Sedation, monitored anesthesia care, and general anesthesia can all be utilized for thermal ablation. The type of anesthesia will be largely driven by local practices and provider comfort. General anesthesia is used for the vast majority of renal thermal ablations at our institution. The risks and benefits of each type of anesthesia must be weighed for each individual patient to determine what type of sedation is best.

Once the patient has been sedated and positioned as desired, thermal ablation antenna placement can be guided by CT (Figure 2). Prone position is most commonly utilized, but for superior pole masses ipsilateral decubitus positioning can also be utilized to minimize risk of pneumothorax (21). MRI can also be used for guidance; however, in practice the availability of interventional MRI units is limited.

A)

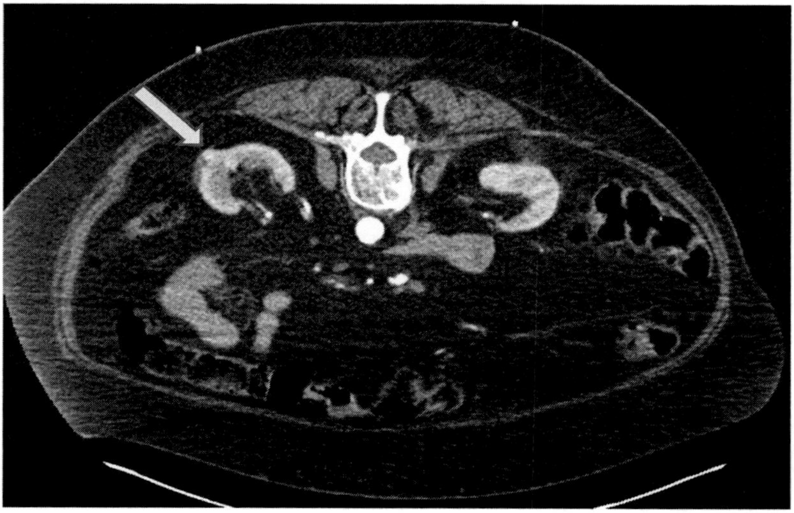

B)

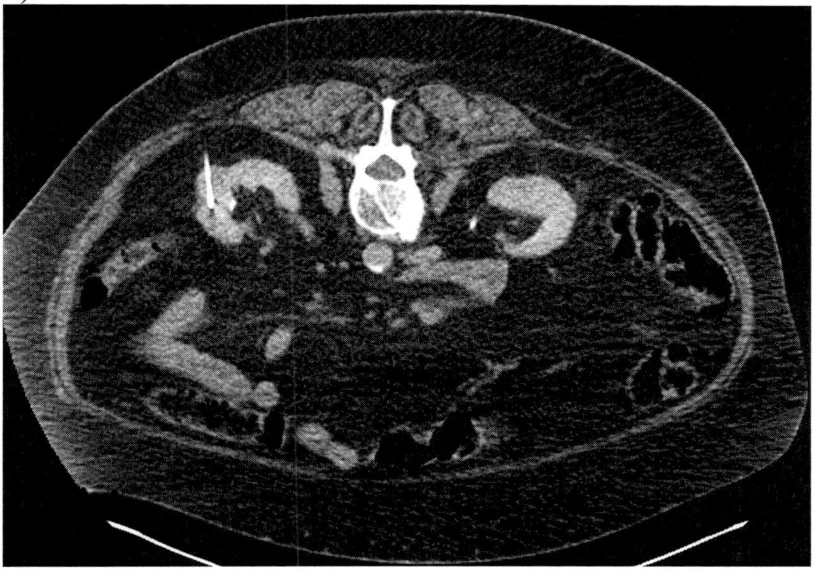

Figure 2: A) Intraprocedural CT with arterial phase contrast in prone position redemonstrates the enhancing left renal mass. (arrow). Posterior exophytic masses are the most easily accessible for ablation while minimizing procedural risks. B) From a posterior approach, a Microwave antenna is shown advanced through the central long axis of the mass. The Tip of the ablation antenna should be advanced to the distal margin of the mass as the ablation zone propagates back along the shaft.

When choosing the optimal trajectory for antenna placement, the goal is creating an ablation zone that covers the mass and a 5-10 mm margin without overtreating healthy kidney. This allows ablation to be the most "nephron-sparing" treatment option for small renal masses. There are several factors to consider. First is determining a safe percutaneous path to the target mass which avoids major vascular structures, the genitofemoral nerve, and surrounding viscera such as colon. One should also minimize length of parenchymal tract and avoids nontarget thermal injury to the collecting system or surrounding organs. Next is determining the size and shape of the target lesion, as it is ideal to position the ablation antenna along the long axis of the mass. Most devices create the largest dimension of extreme temperature along the course of the antenna. Also, if multiple overlapping treatment zones are required, this can easily be performed simply by retracting the antenna.

Once the ablation antenna trajectory is optimized, a safe treatment can be performed. MWA zones are determined by information provided by each specific vendor. Treatment times usually vary between 1-10 minutes with wattages between 60-150 W. Ablation zone size increases as power and duration increase and each power/time combination can create a different size ablation zone. Most modern MWA antennas create ablation zones that are nearly spherical. With cryoablation, the shape of the ablation zone is determined by the type of antenna, with each manufacturer creating antennas of various shapes from spherical to elongated ovoid. The antenna you choose should be guided by the tumor shape and your desired treatment zone. For cryoablation, the antenna is what determines the ablation zone size/shape and all cryoablation requires two cycles of a 10-minute freeze followed by 5-minute thaw, for a total ablation time of approximately 30 minutes.

After completion of the ablation, it is important to scrutinize a final CT with a wide field of view after removal of the ablation antenna. Acute complications to identify are an expanding retroperitoneal hematoma (Figure 3) or pneumothorax (particularly tension pneumothorax). A Small amount of perinephric hematoma is normal after procedure completion. If necessary, serial CT scans can be performed to confirm stability of small hematomas.

A)

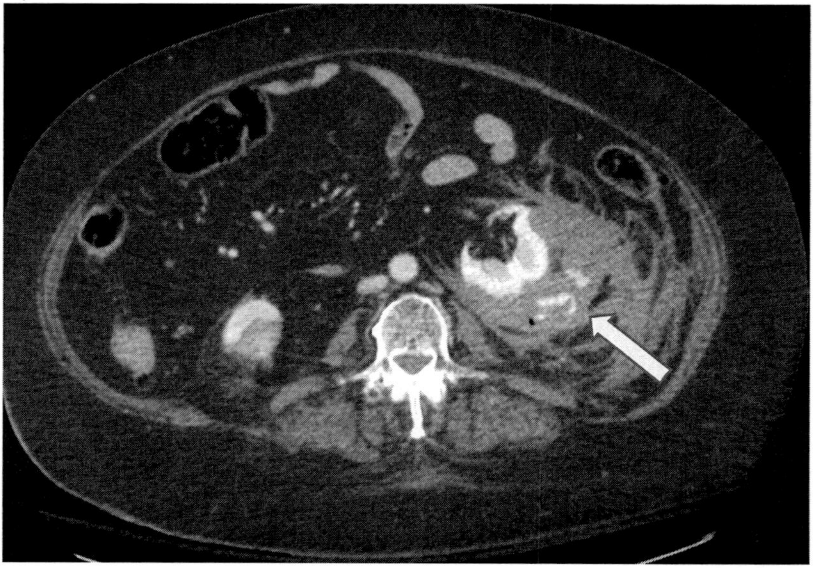

B)

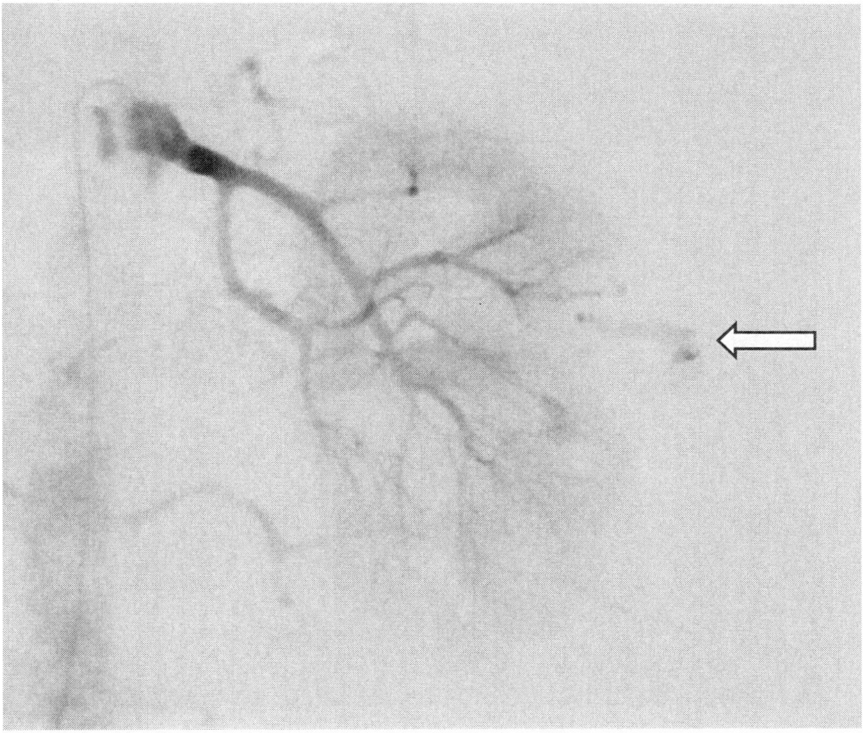

C)

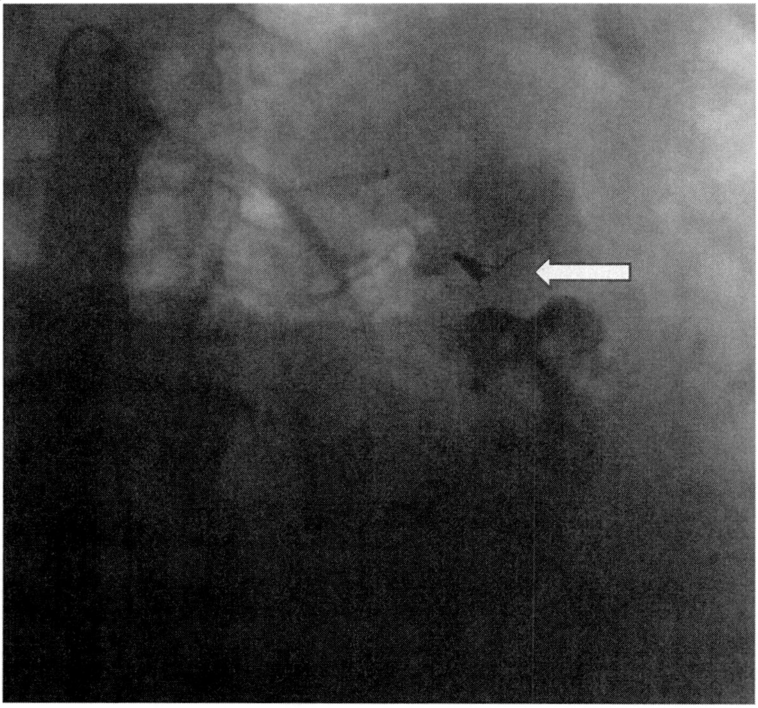

Figure 3: A) Post Procedural CT after removal of the ablation antenna shows a large left perinephric and paranephric hematoma with active extravasation of contrast. B) The patient was immediate taken for angiography which again showed active bleeding from the ablation zone (arrow). C) Selective coil embolization (arrow) through a microcatheter was performed with good stasis in the bleeding vessel. No further extravasation is seen after embolization.

Advanced Techniques

For large renal masses, measuring greater than 5 cm in size, studies have shown improved outcomes with combining thermal ablation therapy with selective endovascular particle embolization. Concurrent particle embolization has shown to have two effects. First, it acts synergistically with the thermal ablation to improve the rates of tumor necrosis on large masses. Second, the preemptive embolization has been shown to reduce bleeding complication, especially on central masses (30,31).

Thermal injury to the renal collecting system increases with mass size and central location. Retrograde pyeloperfusion can be utilized in these patients to avoid ureteral injury or stenosis. Retrograde pyeloperfusion involves the placement of ureteral catheters under cystoscopic guidance into the renal pelvis. During thermal ablation using heat (RFA or MWA), cooled 5% dextrose is infused through the catheters to keep temperatures below cytotoxic levels (32-34).

Commonly, peripheral renal masses come into close proximity with surrounding bowel loops, particularly the colon. Due to its thin wall, the colon is particularly susceptible to thermal injury. In these cases, 5% Dextrose with dilute contrast can be instilled through a needle to displace the bowel and create a safe margin for ablation (Figure 4). Another option for displacing bowel is using a high compliance balloon for displacement (i.e. Fogarty Balloon). The balloon is positioned under CT and then inflated to displace the bowel.

A)

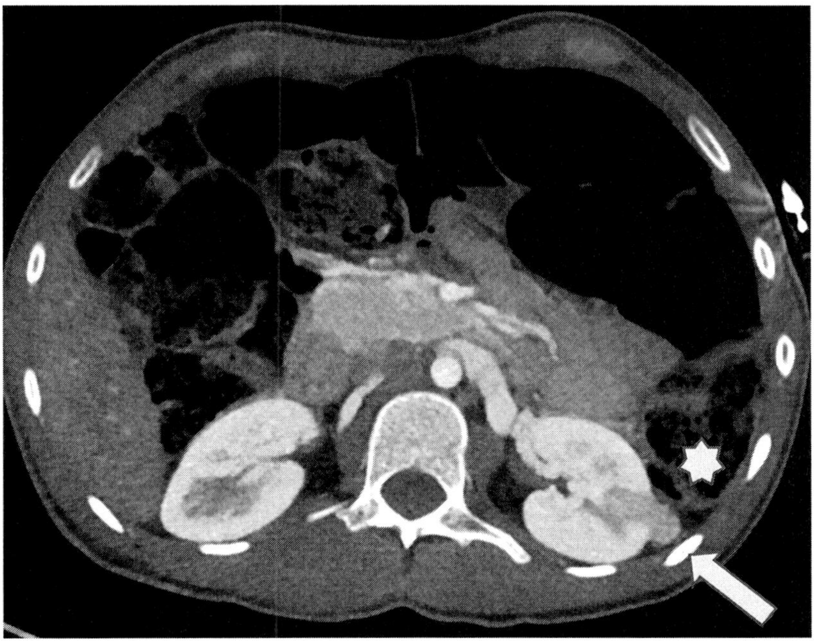

B)

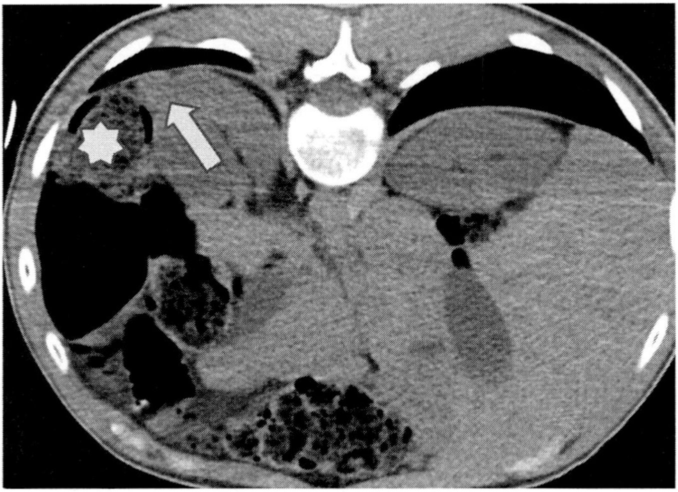

C)

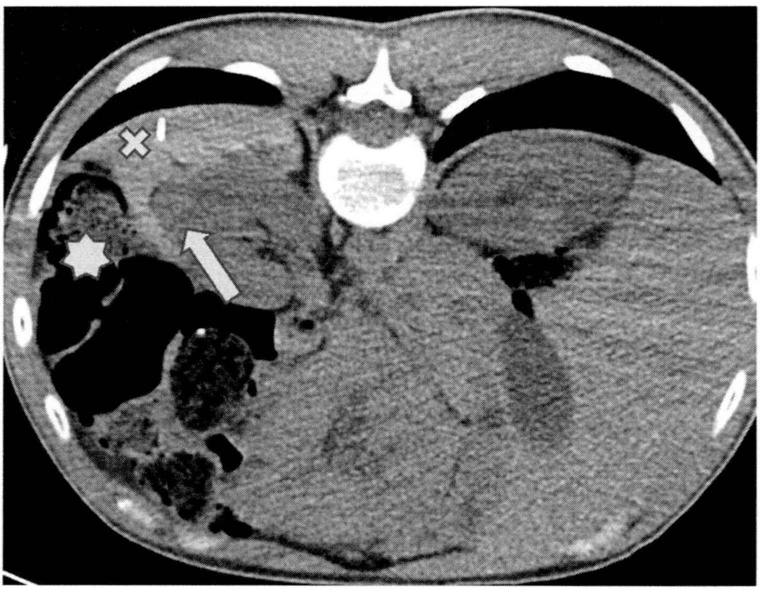

Figure 4: A) Preprocedural contrast enhanced CT shows an enhancing mass in the midpole of the left kidney (arrow). The mass is near the pleural reflexion and abuts the adjacent colon (*). During the clinic visit risks for pneumothorax and non-target thermal injury to bowel should be discussed. B) (upper) Pretreatment

intraprocedural CT in prone position shows the mass (arrow) with adjacent colonic flexure (star). (lower) A 22-Gauge needle has been advanced into the space between the mass (arrow), colon (*) and pleura. Dilute Contrast in D5W (x) in instilled to hydro-dissect vital structures away from the ablation zone. After the hydro-dissection (x), A safe margin has been created around the renal mass (arrow) with the colon (*) and pleural displaced a safe distance.

Rarely, percutaneous access to an upper pole mass with requires and transthoracic/transpleural approach (Figure 5). In this scenario, care should be taken to avoid ablation of the visceral pleura. Iatrogenic pleural effusion or pneumothorax can be performed to displace the lung and visceral pleura during ablation. After ablation is performed, the air or fluid can be aspirated to allow lung re-expansion.

A)

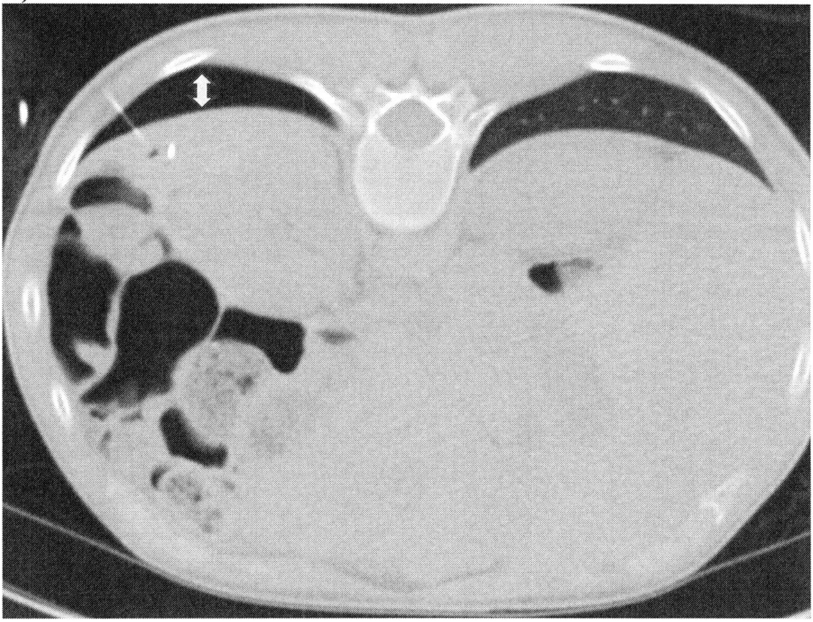

B)

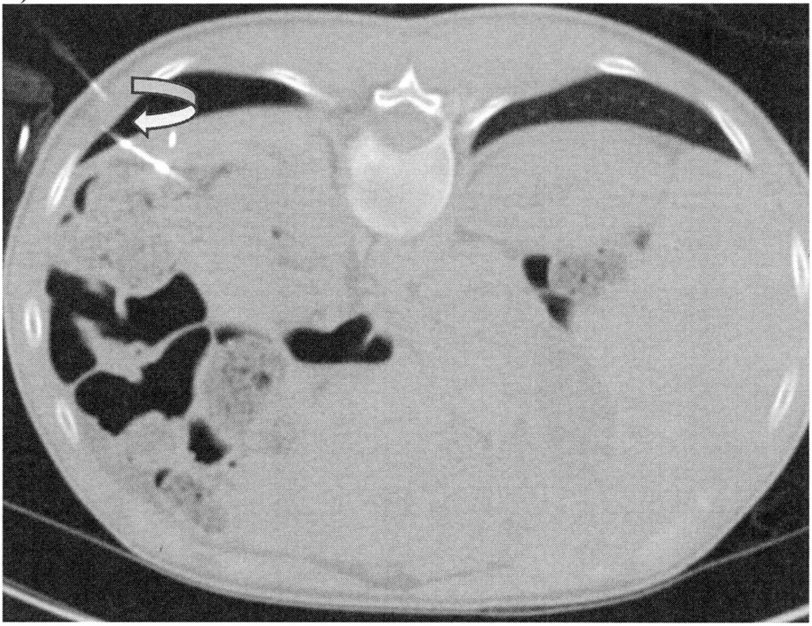

C)

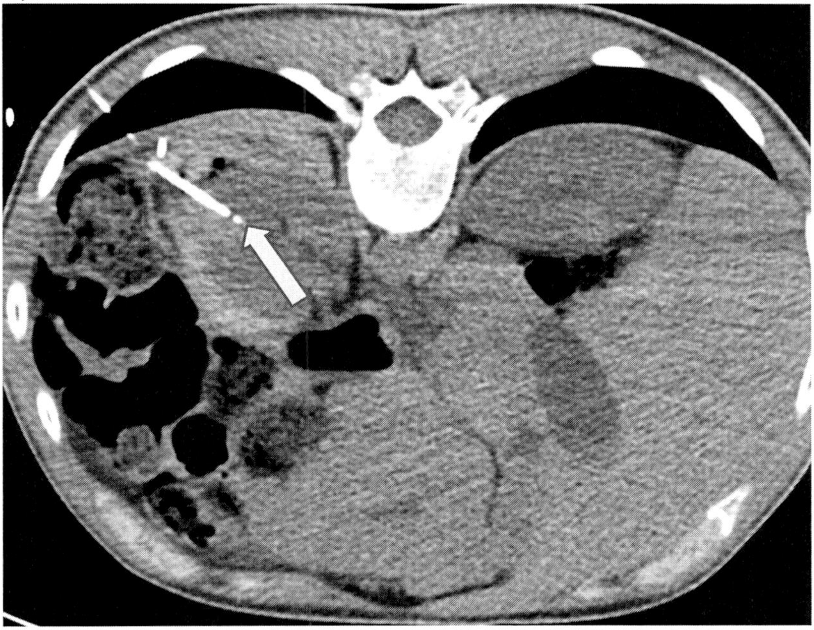

Figure 5: A) During Placement of hydro-dissection needles and the ablation antenna, an iatrogenic pneumothorax (double arrow) is created to prevent injury to the visceral pleural and lung parenchyma. B and C) The ablation antenna is advanced on a trans-pleural approach through the iatrogenic pneumothorax and into the mass along its long axis (arrow).

Post Procedure

Patients are observed in the post procedural area for 2-6 hours following the procedure. In the immediate post-procedural time, bleeding is the most significant complication for which to monitor. During this time, there should be continuous cardiac monitoring and frequent vitals (15-30 minutes). Small perinephric hematomas are common after renal ablation and typically self-limited. If the patient has hemodynamic changes or progressive severe back pain, an expanding hematoma or active hemorrhage is possible and angiographic embolization may be required.

Prior to discharge the patient should meet discharge criteria, which will be institution specific but typically includes the patient being at baseline hemodynamics, tolerating oral intake, pain controlled with oral pain medications, and passing urine. Once meeting discharge criteria, the patient can be discharged home.

Imaging surveillance for treatment response is frequent over the first two years with exact protocol varying between institutions. Most centers perform post-operative imaging every 3-6 months for the first 24 months. High quality cross-sectional imaging with contrast enhanced CT or MRI is paramount for post-procedural surveillance. This should involve noncontrast, corticomedullary, nephrographic, and delayed excretory phases of contrast. On the initial follow-up, the ablation zone may be slightly larger than the original mass and internal hyperdense hemorrhagic material is common on the noncontrast phase or on MRI. This should not be misinterpreted as tumor growth or viability. The ablation zone then serves as a new baseline. The ablation zone should involute over time going forward and any growth on subsequent exams suggests tumor viability and growth (35).

The appearance of a successful ablation on follow is outlined in Table 3. A well-treated tumor appears as a hypodense zone with normal surrounding parenchymal enhancement. 75% of well treated renal masses will develop a thin band, or "halo", of peripheral enhancement. This should be smooth and continuous and is not a sign of residual tumor. On FDG PET, there should be a void of activity within the ablation zone (Figure 6). Hypermetabolic activity on PET or Nodular, discontinuous areas of contrast enhancement on CT is concerning for residual/recurrent disease (Figure 7) (36).

A)

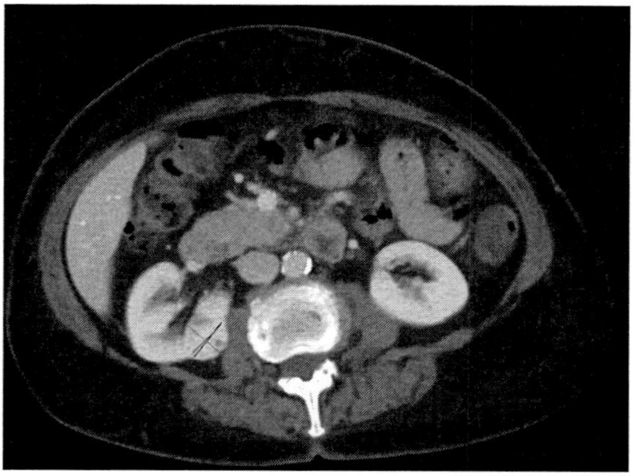

B)

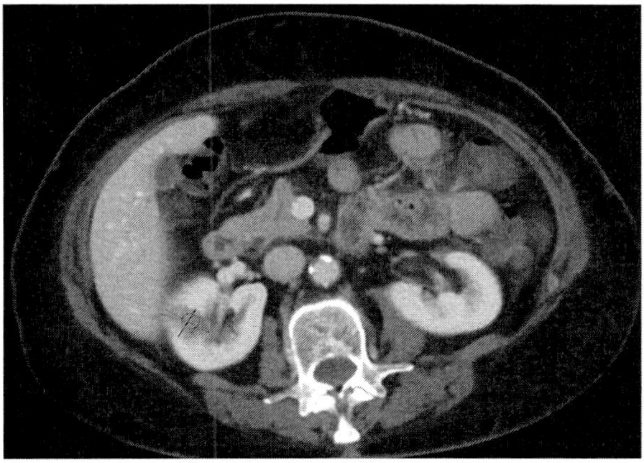

C)

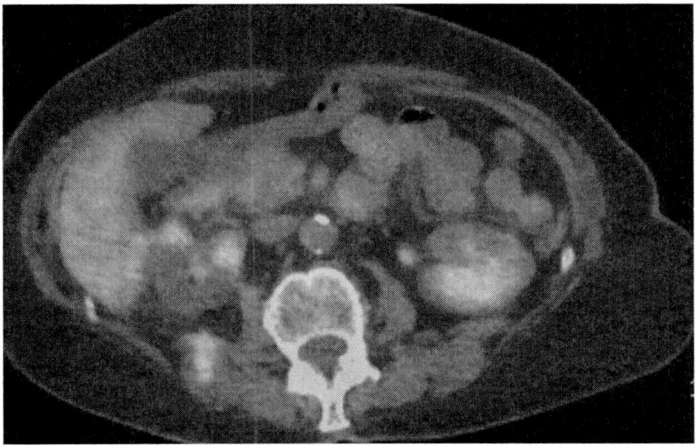

Figure 6: A) Preprocedural contrast enhanced CT shows two posterior right renal masses B) Post Procedural PET-CT shows findings of successful thermal ablation with voids of FDG uptake in the ablation zones.

A)

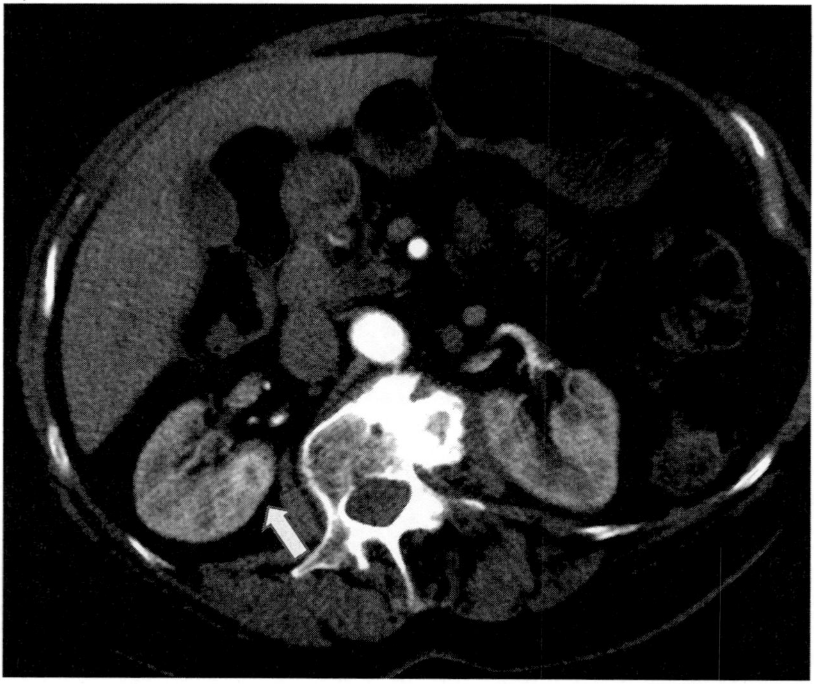

B)

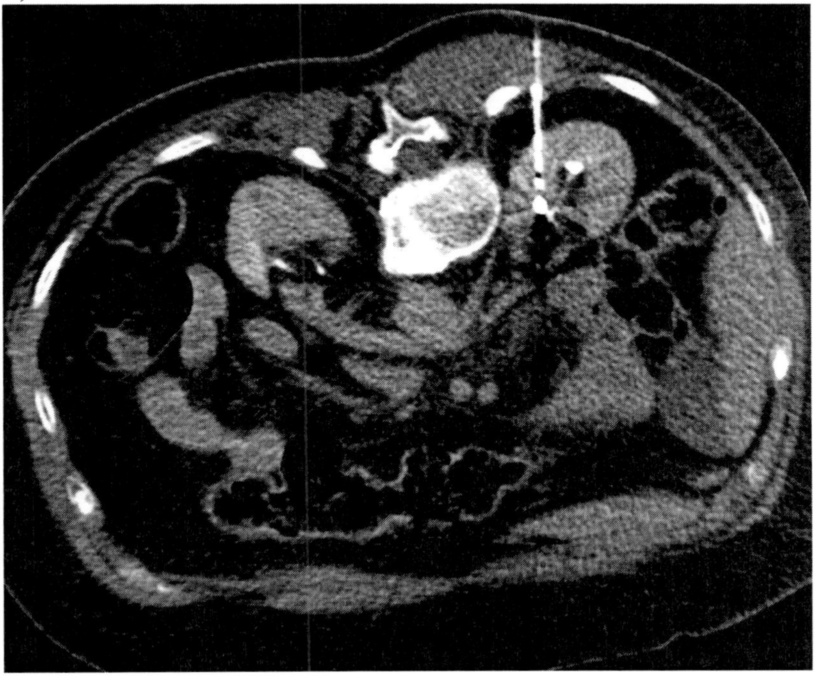

C)

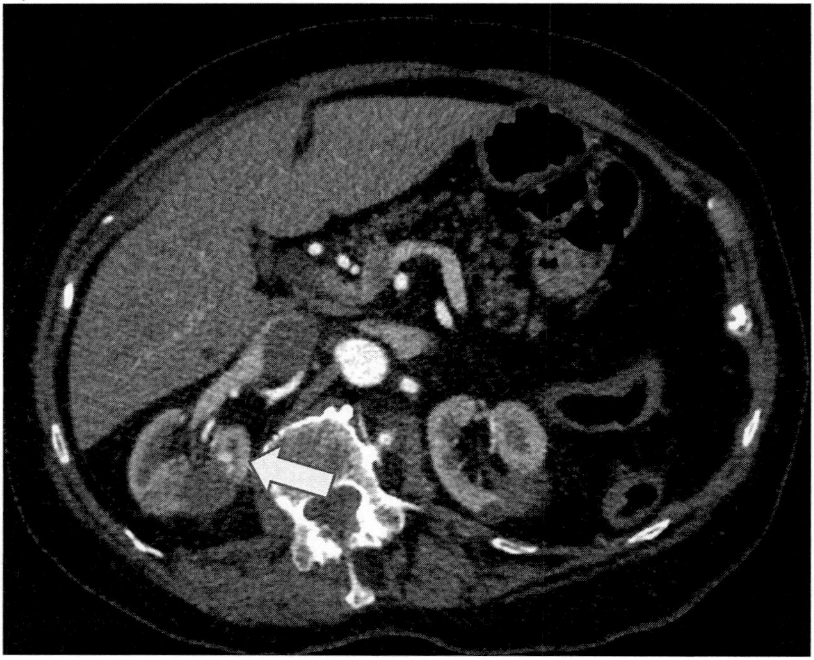

Figure 7: A) Pre-Procedural Contrast enhanced CT Shows an enhancing mass in the medial right kidney (arrow) B) CT Guided Placement of the ablation antenna into the central portion of the right renal mass. C) Follow up contrast enhanced CT shows nodular peripheral enhancement at the margin of the ablation cavity. This appearance is concerning for residual or recurrent malignancy.

Modality	Immediate Post-Procedure Imaging	Follow-Up Surveillance imaging
Computed Tomography (CT)	• Thin halo of enhancing hyperemia. • No Central or Nodular contrast enhancement	• Central High Attenuation (>40 HU) on Pre-contrast Imaging from blood products • "Bull's Eye" or "Halo" of necrotic fat • Fat interposed between ablated mass and normal renal tissue • Dystrophic Calcification
Magnetic Resonance (MRI)	• Loss of T2 Signal • No Central or Nodular Contrast enhancement	• T2 Hypo-intense compared to normal kidney • No central or nodular enhancement on subtracted post contrast T1 Sequences

Table 3: Expected appearance of a successful thermal ablation of renal mass on follow up imaging.

References

1. 8659.00.pdf (cancer.org) (American Cancer Society Website for Kidney Cancer)
2. Campbell S, Uzzo RG, et al: Renal mass and localized renal cancer; AUA guideline. J Urol 198:520-529, 2017
3. Neeman Z, Sarin S, et al: Radiofrequency ablation for tumor-related massive hematuria. J Vasc Interv Radiol 16:417-421, 2005
4. Wood BJ, Grippo J, Pavlovich CP: Percutaneous radio frequency ablation for hematuria. J Urol 166:2303-2304, 2001
5. Patel I, Rahim S, et al: Society of Interventional Radiology Consensus Guidelines for the Periprocedural Management of Thrombotic and Bleeding Risk in Patients Undergoing Percutaneous Image-Guided Interventions—Part II: Recommendations. J Vasc Interv Radiol 30: 1168–1184, 2019
6. Psutka SP, Feldman AS, et al: Long-term oncologic outcomes after radiofrequency ablation for T1 renal cell carcinoma. Eur Urol 63:486-492, 2013

7. Johnson B, Sorokin I, Cadeddu JA: Ten-year outcomes of renal tumor radiofrequency ablation. J Urol 201:251-258, 2019
8. Wah TM, Irving HC, et al: Radiofrequency ablation (RFA) of renal cell carcinoma (RCC): Experience in 200 tumours. BJU Int 113:416-428, 2014
9. Jasinski M, Bielinska M, et al: Ultrasound-Guided Percutaneous Thermal Ablation of Renal Cancers – In Search of the ideal Tumour. Cancers 15:518, 2023.
10. Cantwell C, Gervais D. The Requisites: Image Guided Ablation of Renal Tumors. Elsevier, 2014.
11. Chan V, Abul A, et al: Ablative therapies versus partial nephrectomy for small renal masses – A systamtic review and meta-analysis. Intern Journ of Surgery. 97, 106194, 2022
12. Alam R, Patel H, et al. Comparative effectiveness of management options for patients with small renal masses: a prospective cohort study. British Journ of Urol International. 123: 42-50, 2019
13. Siekiera, J.; Jasinski, M.; Mikołajczak, W. Radiofrequency ablation of small renal masses in comorbid patients. Wideochir Inne Tech. Maloinwazyjne 2018, 13, 212–214.
14. Wo´skowiak, P.; Lewicka, K.; Bureta, A.; Salagierski, M. Active surveillance and focal ablation for small renal masses: A better solution for comorbid patients. Arch. Med. Sci. 2019, 16, 1111–1118.
15. Castle, S.M.; Gorbatiy, V.; Avallone, M.A.; Eldefrawy, A.; Caulton, D.E.; Leveillee, R.J. Cost comparison of nephron-sparing treatments for cT1a renal masses. Urol. Oncol. 2013, 31, 1327–1332.
16. Pandolfo, S.D.; Beksac, A.T.; Derweesh, I.; Celia, A.; Schiavina, R.; Bianchi, L.; Costa, G.; Carbonara, U.; Loizzo, D.; Lucarelli, G.; et al. Percutaneous Ablation Vs Robot-Assisted Partial Nephrectomy for Completely Endophytic Renal Masses: A Multicenter Trifecta Analysis with a Minimum 3-Year Follow-Up. J. Endourol. 2022
17. Georgiades CS, Rodriguez R: Efficacy and safety of percutaneous cryoablation for stage 1A/B renal cell carcinoma: Results of a proscpective, single-arm, 5 year study. Cardiovasc Intervent Radiol 37:1494-1499, 2014
18. Zhou W, Herwald SE, et al: Radiofrequency ablation, cryoablation, and microwave ablation for T1a renal cell carcinoma: A comparative evaluation of therapeutic and renal function outcomes. J Vasc Interv Radiol 30:1035-1042, 2019
19. Shin B, Chick J, et al. Contemporary Status of Percutaneous Ablation for the Small Renal Mass. Curr Urol Rep. 17,23, 2016

20. Regier M, Chun F. Thermal Ablation fo Renal Tumors: Indications, Techniques and Results. Dtsch. Arztebl. Int. 112, 412-418, 2015
21. Abdelsalam M, Ahrar K: Ablation of Small Renal Masses. Tech in Vasc and Interv Radiol 23:100674, 2020
22. Zagoria RJ, Traver MA, et al: Oncologic efficacy of CT-Guided percutaneous radiofrequency ablation of renal cell carcinomas. AJR Am J Roentgenol 189:429-436, 2007
23. Iannuccilli JD, Dupuy DE, et al: Effectiveness and safety of computed tomography-guided radiofrequency ablation of renal cancer: A 14-year single institution experience in 203 patients. Eur Radiol 26: 1656-1664, 2016.
24. Atwell TD, Schmit GD, et al: Percutaneous ablation of renal masses measuring 3.0 cm and smaller: Comparative local control and complications after radiofrequency ablation and cryoablation. AJR Am J Roentgenol 200: 461-466, 2013
25. Ahrar K, Matin S, et al: Percutaneous transthoracic radiofrequency ablation of renal tumors using an iatrogenic pneumothorax. AJR Am J Roentgenol 185:86-88, 2005
26. Mayo-Smith WW, Dupuy DE, et al: Imaging-guided percutaneous radiofrequency ablation of solid renal masses: Techniques and outcomes of 38 treatment sessions in 32 consecutive patients. AJR Am J Roentgenol 180: 1503-1508, 2003
27. McDougal WS, Gervais DA, et al: Long-term followup of patients with renal cell carcinoma treated with radiofrequency ablation with curative intent. J Urol 174:61-63, 2005
28. Ginat DT, Saad WE, Bowel displacement and protection techniques during percutaneous renal tumor thermal ablation. Tech Vasc Interv Radiol 13: 66-74, 2010
29. Chehab M, Thakor A, et al. Adult and Pediatric Antibiotic Prophylaxis during Vascular and IR Procedures: A Society of Interventional Radiology Practice Parameter Update Endorsed by the Cardiovascular and Interventional Radiological Society of Europe and the Canadian Association for Interventional Radiology. 29, 1483-1501, 2018
30. Yamakado K, Nakatsuka A, et al: Radiofrequency ablation combined with renal arterial embolization for the treatment of unresectable renal carcinoma larger than 3.5 cm: Initial experience. Cardiovasc Interven Radiol 29:389-394, 2006
31. Woodrum DA, Atwell TD, et al: Role of intraarterial embolization before cryoablation of large renal tumors: A pilot study. J Vasc Interv Radiol 21: 930-936, 2010

32. Wah TM, Koenig P, et al: Radiofrequency ablation of a central renal tumor: Protection of the collecting system with a retrograde cold dextrose pyeloperfusion technique. J Vasc Interv Radiol 16:1551-1555, 2005
33. Rouviere O, Badet L, et al: Radiofrequency ablation of renal rumors with an expandable multitoned electrode: Results, complications, and pilot evaluation of colled pyeloperfusion for collecting system protection. Cardiovasc Intervent Radiol 31:595-603, 2008
34. Cantwell CP, Wah TM, et al: Protecting the ureter during radiofrequency ablation of renal cell cancer: A pilot study of retrograde pyeloperfusion with cooled dextrose 5% in water. J Vasc Interv Radiol 19:1034-1040, 2008
35. Hegarty NJ, Gill IS, et al: Probe-ablative nephron-sparing surgery: Cryoablation versus radiofrequency ablation. Urology 68(1 Suppl): 7-13, 2006
36. Wile GE, Leyendecker JR, et al: CT and MR imaging after imaging-guided thermal ablation of renal neoplasms. Radiographics 27:325-339, 2007

CHAPTER 13

OSSEOUS THERMAL ABLATION

BRANDON CUSTER MD

Introduction

Thermal ablation is a treatment option for patients with bone lesions of both benign and malignant etiologies. Among malignant lesions, the vast majority represent metastatic spread and frequently are associated with pain. The most commonly treated and abundantly researched benign bone lesion is symptomatic osteoid osteoma. The goal of therapy in both treatment groups is palliation for symptomatic bone pain, preservation of function, and ultimately optimizing quality of life.

Some estimates report bone metastases in up to 84% of patients with underlying cancer (1). Bone metastases can lead to pain, pathologic fracture, and nerve injury. As primary treatments for malignancy improve survival rates, the prevalence of bone metastases increases. After bisphosphonate therapy or targeted bone chemotherapies, radiation therapy is considered standard of care for palliation of these lesions. This therapy is prolonged with multiple treatment sessions and delayed pain relief which can take as long as 6 weeks to be effective (2). Surgical options also exist with reconstructions designed to treat pain and strengthen skeletal stability; however, these procedures have high morbidity/mortality rates and prolonged recovery time (3,4,5).

Osteoid osteoma is a benign bone tumor composed of a nidus of woven bone and osteoid surrounded by osteoblasts, reactive changes, cortical thickening and loose fibrovascular tissue (6). These lesions most commonly occur in the lower extremity of long bones in children and young adults. The classic presentation is pain that worsens at night and is improved with nonsteroidal anti-inflammatory drugs (NSAIDS). If untreated, this can lead to growth disturbances, scoliosis, arthritis, joint swelling, and contracture (7). Traditional treatment is long term analgesia with Ibuprofen or other nonsteroidal anti-inflammatory agents (NSAIDS). These therapies alone can be ineffective at pain control, particularly in periarticular osteoid osteomas (8). Historically, lesions refractory to medical therapy underwent en-bloc surgical excision. Other minimally invasive treatment options include ethanol instillation, laser interstitial therapy, and cryotherapy. Since 1992 when Rosenthal et al (9) reported the safety and efficacy of minimally invasive thermal ablation, particularly RFA, it has become the standard of care.

Minimally invasive thermal ablation procedures have been shown in randomized controlled trials to be safe and effective at treating painful bone metastases and primary benign bone masses. The most well studied ablation modality for bone masses is RFA, but there is growing evidence for the safety and efficacy of MWA and cryoablation as well. To review the mechanism of action, strengths, and weakness of each ablation modality please refer to the liver thermal ablation chapter.

Indications

Up to 85% of patients with cancer will develop bone metastases with 60% of cancer patients developing pain associated with metastases, making it the most common cause for cancer related pain. Management requires a multidisciplinary approach with medical oncology, radiation oncology, and interventional radiology. Intervention is warranted for two possible reasons: palliation of painful lesion or local tumor control for oligometastatic disease. Of these, palliation for pain control is much more common. Ablation is indicated in patients with moderate to severe (pain scale >4/10) pain that correlates with 1 or 2 bone lesions. Mild pain should be managed with oral pain medications. Pain from diffuse bone metastases requires a systemic treatment in most cases. Masses can be targeted for treatment regardless of being lytic, blastic, mixed, or soft tissue masses.

Most patients with benign bone lesions develop mild symptoms that can be controlled medically. With osteoid osteoma specifically, the majority of patients can tolerate the associated pain with or without the help of NSAIDS. However, a subset of patients develop progressive pain which leads to insomnia and significant adverse events effecting quality of life. These patients are typically offered more definitive treatment with thermal ablation.

Contraindications

Contraindications for percutaneous thermal ablation are similar for both benign and malignant bone masses. These include location of lesion within 1 cm of vital structures (particularly nerves and major vessels), pregnancy, active infections, or uncorrectable coagulopathy. Advanced techniques with hydro-dissection of vital structures can be performed to create a safe margin if necessary. In patients with metallic surgical hardware in the treatment zone, Radiofrequency ablation should be avoided for the risk of heat conduction along the hardware and nontarget thermal injury (other ablation modalities are still safe).

Outcomes

Multiple different ablative technologies have been utilized to treat symptomatic bone metastases including RFA, cryoablation, MWA, laser ablation, and focused ultrasound. Of these, the most studied are RFA and cryoablation, with growing evidence for MWA. Technical success is extremely high for all three at approximately 90%, with the most common reason for technical failure being densely sclerotic bone preventing antenna placement (7). All three thermal ablation modalities have been shown to be effective, with no studies showing statistically significant differences in outcomes between them. Patients should expect at least a 2-4 point drop in pain scale rating within one week of treatment and this should be durable with 80% of patient reporting decreased pain at 6 months (18). It is common that mild pain persists after ablation, which can be managed with oral pain medications. Studies have also showed significant reduction in pain medication requirement and improvement in quality of life after treatment (19).

Standard of care for malignant bone pain is narcotic medications and radiation. Radiation therapy has certain limitations with only 60-70% of patient reporting adequate analgesia after the treatment and a delay in treatment response which can take up to 12 weeks (14, 15,16). Percutaneous thermal ablation offers a treatment with similar if not better pain control, with patient's reporting pain improvement by three days post ablation. Percutaneous thermal ablation should be viewed as a safe treatment option with rapid and long-lasting pain relief which can be used alone or in combination with radiation therapy.

Clinical success in the treatment of the underlying bone pain for thermal ablation in benign osteoid osteoma is well documented. Studies show complete pain relief with no further need for analgesics in 86% of patients after a single RF ablation session. In patients with persistent/recurrent pain repeat thermal ablation is warranted and is usually successful. The overall success rate of thermal ablation after 1-2 sessions is 96.5% (7). Most patients who responded to treatment had complete resolution of pain within 1 month, with some taking 6-8 weeks. Technical success is also high for benign bone lesions at 90%. Importantly, technical failure due to suboptimal needle positioning through the nidus has a high correlation with clinical treatment failure, up to 100% in some studies (7). In fact, suboptimal needle positioning is the only factor found to be statistically significant in predicting clinical outcomes for failure.

For osteoid osteoma, en-bloc surgical resection has been the traditional treatment modality. Treatment success was seen in 88-97% of patients (10,11); however, there were several draw backs to the surgical approach. First, open localization was often difficult. When precise localization could be performed, bone defects from resection were vulnerable to fracture and sometimes required internal fixation or bone grafting. Surgical procedures also had longer hospital stays of 3-5 days and longer periods of postoperative limitations to weight baring (10). Comparatively, image guided thermal ablation has become the treatment of choice as it allows easy localization, similar treatment success, less complications, shorter recovery, and shorter hospital stays.

RFA is well studied and documented as a safe and effective treatment modality. More recently, there has been increasing interest in MWA in the treatment of both malignant and benign bone masses. MWA has potential advantages over RFA with less heat loss, faster ablation times, and larger treatment zones. Early studies with MWA in osteoid osteoma have been encouraging with clinical success of 100% (12,13), as determined by cessation of pain at 3 months. Microwave technologies are therefore being increasingly utilized for bone lesions. We almost exclusively utilize microwave ablation for bone lesions at our institution. The major drawback of microwave ablation is its high cost compared to RFA.

Complications

The risk profile is similar for both benign and malignant bone masses. Complications from thermal ablation are rare but include skin burns with thermal necrosis, neurovascular injury, bleeding, and infection. To avoid nontarget thermal injury to the skin or neurovascular structures, it is best to maintain a 5-10 mm margin between the treatment zone and these structures. Intraarticular bone masses have been associated with increased risks of infections as well. Bleeding risk remains very low, but if the lesion is extremely hypervascular, pre-ablation endovascular embolization can be considered to reduce this risk. Diligent preprocedural planning for percutaneous access is vital to avoid complications. If necessary, a safe ablation zone can be created using hydro-dissection.

If thermal injury to the skin occurs, it is evident at the first follow up clinic visit, typically as a non-healing wound or blister. Most skin wounds are self-limited and can be managed with wet to dry dressing changes and topical sulfazadine or bacitracin. If wounds fail to improve, dermatology or plastic surgery consults may be necessary.

Post-operative recovery should include a neurological exam in the region ablated. If there is mild/moderate motor deficit but preserved sensation, it is possible that there is simply acute treatment related inflammation and nerve compression. This can be managed with 20 mg dexamethasone intravenously x 1 followed by 4 mg q6h for 24 hours. If there is a complete motor and/or sensory deficit, a thermal injury has likely occurred, and neurology consult for nerve conduction studies is often necessary (17).

Pre-procedure

The patient should be seen and evaluated in clinic prior to any ablation procedure for a full history and physical. The history should include a pain severity assessment to quantify treatment results. Preprocedural workup should ensure the patient is within coagulation parameters for a high-risk bleeding procedure by SIR or institution specific guidelines. This includes platelet count, International normalized ratio (INR), and prothrombin time. A review of medications for appropriate holds of antiplatelet and anticoagulant medications should also occur. Procedure risks, complication, alternatives, and procedural/post-procedural expectations should be discussed.

Malignant bone masses are commonly identified on CT, MRI, and PET/CT (Figure 1). One should pay attention to the distribution of bone metastases for clinical correlation to the pain symptoms prior to performing ablation.

A)

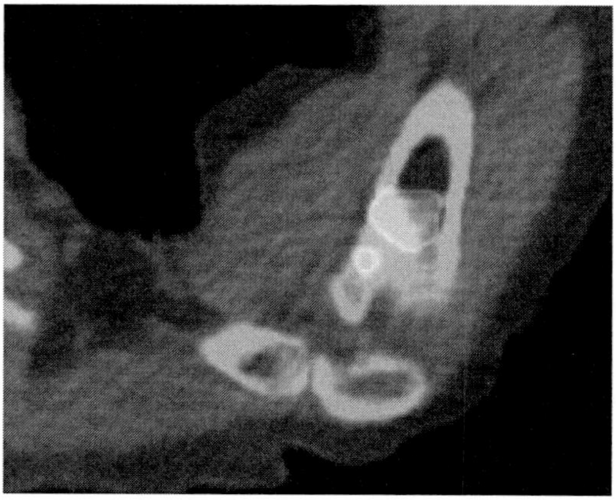

B)

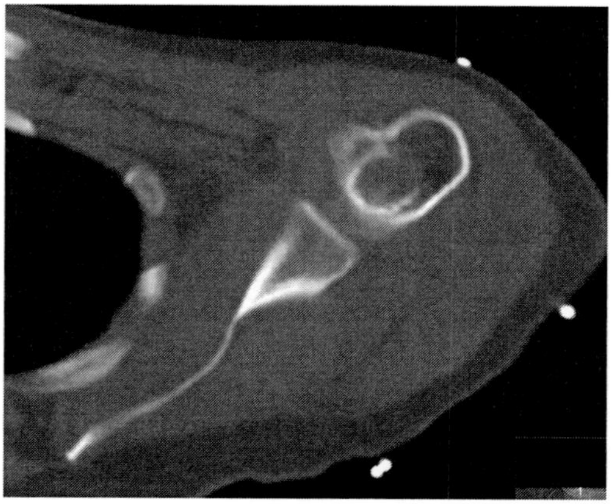

Figure 1: Hypermetabolic metastatic bone mass on PET (A) and CT (B) in a patient with history of melanoma.

CT is the modality of choice for diagnosing osteoid osteoma (Figure 2). The classic radiographic appearance is a central radiolucent nidus with a surrounding zone of sclerotic dense cortical thickening sub-periosteal bone formation. In the correct patient population, these findings are pathognomonic. They will also demonstrate intense radiotracer uptake at the nidus and surrounding bone on Tc 99 HDP Bone scan. MRI is typically only used in cases with inconclusive CT findings.

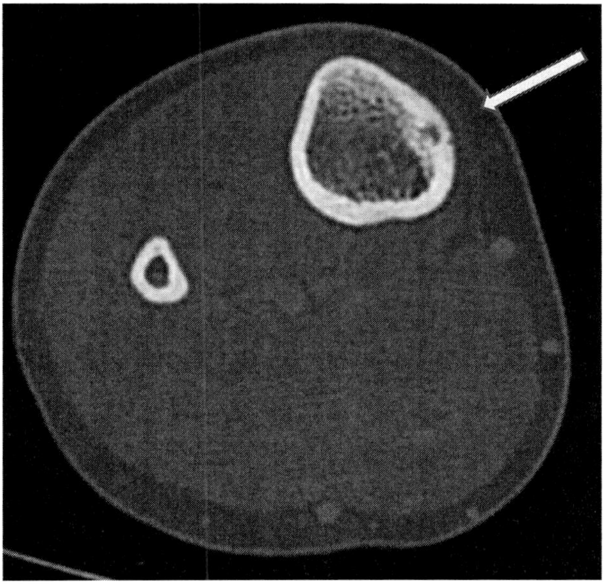

Figure 2: Classic CT appearance of osteoid osteoma showing the characteristic radiolucent central nidus (arrow) measuring <2 cm surrounded by reactive sclerotic bone formation.

CT is used to plan the percutaneous access, ablation modality, treatment zone, and determine number of probes required. The objective of the ablation will differ between indication. For osteoid osteoma, the goal is simply to treat the radiolucent nidus. For palliation of painful metastasis, the goal is ablation of the bone-mass interface. When treating oligometastatic disease, a 5-10 mm treatment margin extending beyond the tumor margin is ideal.

Procedure

Thermal ablation is performed in the outpatient setting under most circumstances. The patient should arrive to the department at least one hour prior to the procedure start time. This allows time to review all relevant labs and ensure anesthesia adequate time to re-evaluate the patient prior to the procedure. SIR considers thermal ablation of bone to be a clean-contaminated procedure. While there is no consensus for antibiotic use, there is a soft recommendation for 1-2 g Cefazolin IV within 2 hours of the ablation procedure.

Conscious sedation, monitored anesthesia care, spinal anesthesia, and general anesthesia can all be utilized for thermal ablation. The type of anesthesia will be largely driven by local practices and provider comfort. General anesthesia is used for most bone thermal ablations at our institution. The risks and benefits of each type of anesthesia must be weighed for each individual patient to determine what type of sedation is best. Ablation of osteoid osteomas is often performed on pediatric patients and providers specifically trained in pediatric sedation/anesthesia are necessary.

Procedural approach and patient positioning is determined at the clinic visit. Once the patient is sedated and appropriately positioned, lesion localization is performed with thin slice CT and skin marking aided by radio-opaque skin strips. The ideal percutaneous approach is perpendicular to the cortical surface of the involved bone with a route planned to avoid surrounding neurovascular structures. Occasionally, an approach through the normal contralateral cortex is required to avoid neurovascular structures or thermal injury to the skin. Another option to avoid thermal injury to the skin is hydro-dissection by creating a large subcutaneous wheal using 5% dextrose in water (D5W).

A core bone biopsy system (bone drill or manual systems) is used to create a channel through the nidus of an osteoid osteoma, or through the central aspect of sclerotic malignant bone mass. The biopsy device should remove a core that extends 5 mm distal to the target lesion to create a channel that correctly positions the center of the treatment zone (Figure 3). This core biopsy can also be used for further diagnostic information. Lytic bone lesions typically do not require creating this channel and the ablation probes can be directly advanced though the mass if there is cortical disruption.

A)

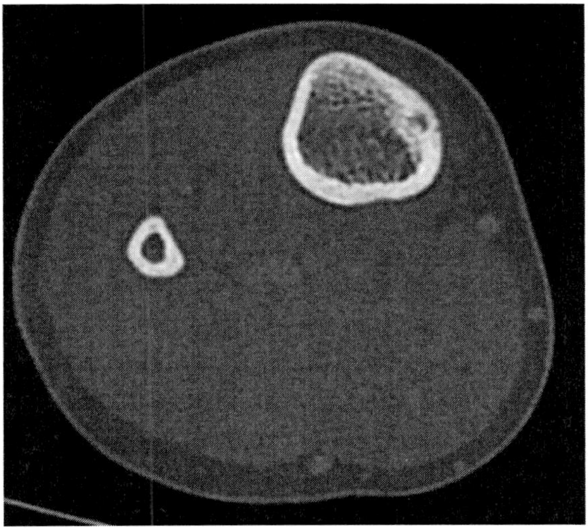

B)

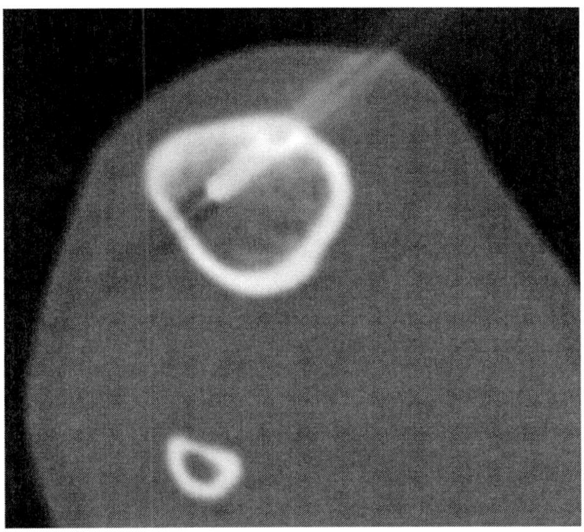

C)

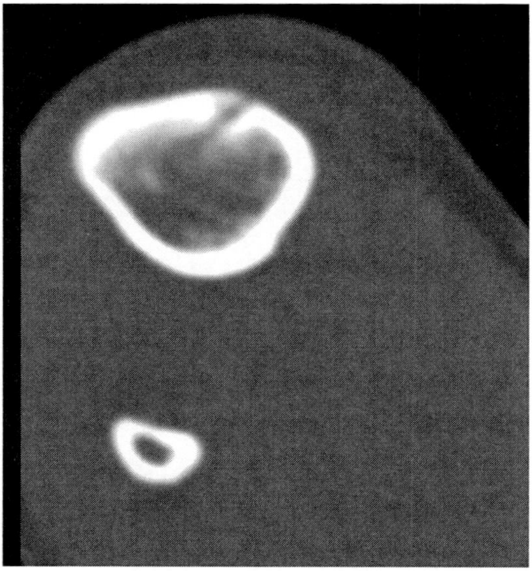

D)

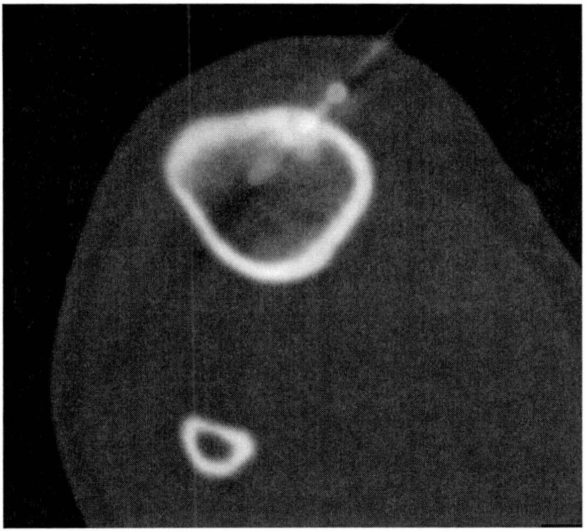

Figure 3: A) A preprocedural diagnostic CT showing classic appearance of osteoid osteoma with radiolucent nidus and surrounding sclerotic new bone formation. B) Core bone biopsy directly through the nidus provides both diagnostic yield and creates a tract for antenna positioning. C) After removal of the core biopsy needle, the tract is confirmed to pass directly through the nidus. The tract should extend 5 mm distal to the target to correction position the ablation zone. D) Ablation antenna positioned for treatment with tip just distal the target nidus. Hydro-dissection (Arrows) was used to displace the skin surface from the ablation zone and avoid thermal skin injury.

The thermal ablation antenna can be advanced de-novo, through the dermatotomy and positioned in the channel using CT. Alternatively, a coaxial introducer can be used for both the biopsy and positioning of the antenna (Figure 4). If a coaxial approach is chosen, the introducer needs to be retracted outside of the anticipated ablation zone prior to treatment. This avoids heat propagation along the introducer needle which can lead to non-target thermal injury to the skin.

A)

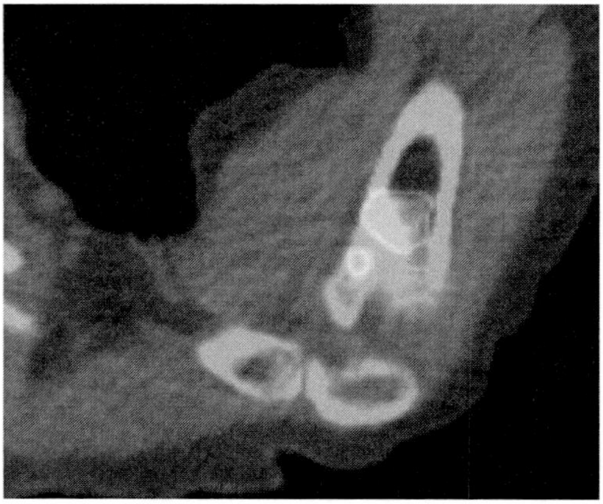

B)

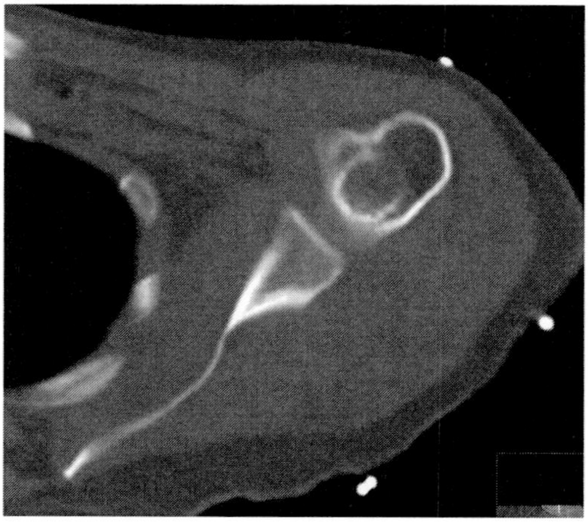

C)

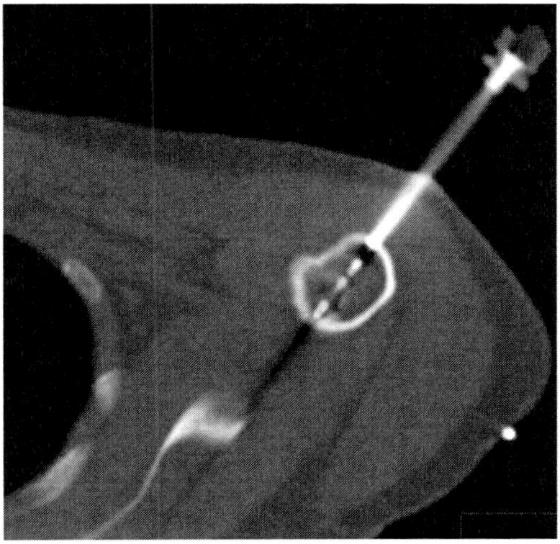

Figure 4: Redemonstration of the previously seen hypermetabolic melanoma metastasis in the proximal left humerus on PET (A) and CT (B). C) The thermal ablation antenna has been coaxially advanced through an introducer needle through a tunnel created through the central aspect of the mass. The introducer needle is then retracted prior to ablation to prevent skin injury.

Once position of the ablation antenna is confirmed with CT, ablation is performed with a target temperature of 90 degrees Celsius. For osteoid osteoma, RF ablation is typically performed for 4-6 minutes. Microwave ablation is performed with three separate 30 second ablations, maintaining ablation temperatures 60-90 degrees C (necessitating varying wattage application). Ablation times for metastatic bone lesions is based on tumor size. The ablation zone is guided by information provided by each specific manufacturer for reach the tumor-bone interface.

Following ablation, the antenna is removed. Hemostasis is achieved with manual pressure and a sterile dressing is applied. Post-treatment CT scan should be performed to evaluate for any acute complications.

Post-procedure

Patients are observed in the post procedural area for 2-6 hours following the procedure. In the immediate post-procedural time, bleeding is the most significant complication for which to monitor. During this time, there should be continuous cardiac monitoring and frequent vitals (15-30 minutes). Prior to discharge the patient should meet discharge criteria which will be institution specific but typically includes the patient being at baseline hemodynamics, tolerating oral intake, pain controlled with oral pain medications, and passing urine. Once meeting criteria, the patient may be discharged home as outpatient. The expectation is that these are outpatient procedures, but rarely patients will require overnight admission for pain control.

Patients should be informed that some post-procedure pain is expected but is typically controlled with oral pain medications. Pain typically is worst in the first 48 hours and then steadily improves but may be present for up to 1 month. All daily activities may be resumed immediately without the use of a case, splint, or other support devices.

Follow up is dependent on indication. For pain palliation (both benign and malignant), follow up is entirely clinical. The patient should be seen for follow up after 1-3 months to evaluate for expected improvement/resolution of pain. Imaging surveillance is typically not utilized in the patients if pain is controlled. If a CT is obtained, a treated osteoid osteoma may show replacement of the nidus with sclerotic bone which occurs between 2 months and two years after the ablation. After 2 years, a treated lesion may no longer be visible on imaging. A persistent lucent nidus, arterial enhancement, or marrow edema are signs of treatment failure and repeat ablation is warranted (8).

For the less common indication of tumor control in the setting of oligometastatic disease, imaging surveillance is typically utilized. There is no consensus imaging guideline, but the treated lesions should be monitored closely over the first year. A reasonable surveillance schedule would be contrast enhanced CT or MRI at 1, 3, 6, and 12 months after treatment. If the disease is controlled, imaging can be less frequent after one year.

References

1) Schulman KL, Kohles J. Economic burden of metastatic bone disease in the US. Cancer 2007; 109:2334-2342
2) Johnstone C, Lutz ST. External beam radiotherapy and bone metastases. Ann Palliat Med 2014; 3:114-122
3) Levy J, Hopkins T, et al. Radiofrequency Ablation for the palliative treatment of Bone Metastases: OPutcomes from the Multicenter OsteoCool Tumor Ablation Post-Market Study (OPuS One Study) in 100 Patients. J Vasc Interv Radiol. 2020; 31:1745-1752

4) Hoffmann RT, Jakobs TF, et al. Radiofrequency ablation in combination with osteoplasty in the treatment of painful metastatic bone disease. J Vasc Interv Radiol 2008; 19:419-421
5) Jacofsky DJ, Papagelopoulos PJ, et al. Advances and challenges in the surgical treatment of metastatic bone disease. Clin Orthop Relat Res 2003; 415(suppl); S14-S18
6) O'Connell JX, Nanthakumar SS, et al. Osteoid osteoma: The uniquely innervated bone tumor. Mod Pathol 1998; 11:175-180.
7) Chahal A, Rajalakshmi P, et al. CT-Guided percutaneous radiofrequency ablation of osteoid osteoma: Our experience in 87 patients. Indian J Radiol Imaging 2017; 27: 207-2015
8) Motamedi D, Learch TJ, et al. Thermal Ablation of Osteoid Osteoma: Overview and Step-by-Step Guide. RadioGraphics 2009; 29:2127-2141
9) Rosenthal DI, Alexander A, et al. Ablation of osteoid osteomas with a percutaneously placed electrode: A new procedure. Radiology 1992; 183: 29-33
10) Rosenthal DI, Hornicek FJ, et al. Percutaneous radiofrequency coagulation of osteoid osteoma compared with operative treatment. J Bone Joint Surg Am 1998; 80: 815-821
11) Sans N, Galy-Fourcade D, et al. Osteoid osteoma: CT-Guided percutaneous resection and follow-up in 38 patients, Radiology 1999; 212: 687-692.
12) Rinzler ES, Shivaram GM, et al. Microwave ablation of osteoid osteoma: Initial experience and efficacy. Pediatr Radiol 2019, 49, 566-570
13) Reis J, Chang Y, et al Radiofrequency ablation vs microwave ablation for osteoid osteomas: Long-term results. Skeletal Radiol. 2020, 49, 1995-2000.
14) Callstrom MR, Charboneau JW. Image-Guided palliation of painful metastases using percutaneous ablation. Tech Vasc Interv Radiol 10:120-131, 2007
15) Agarawal JP, Swangsilpa T, et al. The role of external beam radiotherapy in the management of bone metastases. Clin Oncol 18: 747-760, 2006
16) Tong D, Gillick L, et al. The palliation of symptomatic osseous metastases: final results of the study by the radiation therapy oncology group. Cancer 50:893-899, 1982
17) Nazario J, Hernandez J, Tam A. Thermal Ablation of Painful Bone Metastases. Tech in Vasc and Interv Radiology. 2011 14: 150-159

18) Dupuy DE, Liu D, et al. Percutaneous radiofrequency ablation of painful osseous metastases: A multifcenter American College of Radiology Imaging Network Trial. Cancer 2010. 116:989-997
19) Levy J, Hopkins T, et al. Radiofrequency Ablation for the Palliative Treatment of Bone Metastases: Outcomes from the Multicenter OsteoCool Tumor Ablation Post-Market Study (OPuS One Study) in 100 Patients. J Vasc Interv Radiol 2020; 31:1745-1752

CHAPTER 14

PULMONARY ABLATION

BRANDON CUSTER MD

Introduction

Lung cancer is the leading cause of cancer related mortality for both men and women in the United States and worldwide at 21.7% of all cancer related deaths (1). The lungs also represent a common site of metastatic spread. The gold standard for management of early-stage lung malignancy is surgical resection; however, because of poor cardiopulmonary reserve, only around 15-30% of patients are surgical candidates. Alternative therapies have typically included systemic chemotherapy, immunotherapy, and external radiation therapy, but these are rarely successful at achieving complete tumor remission (2).

Image guided thermal ablation has shown promise as an alternative treatment option for lung cancer since its introduction 2 decades ago (3). This intervention offers several benefits over alternative therapies including reduced procedural morbidity/mortality, conservation of normal lung tissue, lower procedural costs, outpatient setting, safety with underlying interstitial lung disease, repeatability, and use in high risk surgical candidates.

The types of thermo-ablative technology utilized in pulmonary ablation include radiofrequency ablation (RFA), microwave ablation (MWA), and cryoablation. All thermal ablation options have shown safety and efficacy in the treatment of early-stage primary and oligometastatic pulmonary malignancy, with the most robust data available for RFA. To review the mechanism of action, strengths, and weaknesses of each ablative technology, please refer to the liver ablation chapter.

Indications

Thermal ablation offers a repeatable, effective, low-cost, and safe treatment option for nonsurgical patients with both small primary lung cancer and oligometastatic disease. The goal of therapy is typically palliative but in some cases ablation can be performed with curative intent in early stage primary lung cancers (4).

Thermal ablation is recommended for patients with early-stage primary lung cancer that are not candidates for radical surgery (5). Severe comorbidities, poor performance status, limited lung function, and/or unwillingness to undergo surgery are common reasons that a patient is unable to undergo surgery (6).

The lungs represent a common site of metastatic spread from distant malignancies. There is growing evidence suggesting a role for thermal ablation in patients with limited sites of metastasis (oligometastatic disease) regardless of primary disease process. Commonly this is used in combination with or after failure of chemotherapy, radiation therapy, or immunotherapy.

Based on the most recent National Comprehensive Cancer Network Guidelines, thermal ablation is indicated in nonsurgical patients with up to 5 pulmonary masses measuring up to 3 cm in diameter in select patients.

Treatment decision making is difficult in this complex patient population. Discussions in multidisciplinary conferences including interventional radiology, diagnostic radiology, medical oncology, radiation oncology, and thoracic surgery are often necessary to obtain optimal patient outcomes. There are no definitive guidelines regarding size, number, or location of lesions that can be treated with thermal ablation. Data supports good tumor control with masses up to 3 cm in diameter. At larger tumor sizes, recurrence rates start to climb (5).

Absolute contraindication to pulmonary ablation includes uncorrectable coagulopathy, bacteremia, or active infection. Relative contraindications include close proximity to major blood vessels, mediastinum, or chest wall.

Outcomes

Jiang et al performed a large meta-analysis of thermal ablations for lung malignancies. Clinical results showed all thermal ablation to be effective, with slightly improved outcomes for RFA and MWA over cryoablation. No significant differences were described in outcomes between MWA and RFA with average 1,2,3,4, and 5 year-weighted survival rates of 84.3%, 66.8%, 62.4%, 55.1%, and 43.5% respectively (4). Major contributing factors in prognosis and overall survival include: tumor size < 3 cm, ECOG Status, number of disease sites, target lesion within 5 mm of bronchus or blood vessel, and complete coverage of tumor with ablation zone margin of 5-10 mm (7,8).

RFA is the most well studied thermal ablation modality with safety and efficacy proven on masses measuring up to 3 cm in size. As discussed in the previous chapter, RF is limited by poor heat conduction in lung tissue which limits ablation zone size. RF is also susceptible to "heat sink" when the ablation zone abuts vessels greater than 4 mm in size (9). Microwave ablation is a technologic advancement that allows larger ablation zones in less time, as heat production is less dependent on tissue conduction and less susceptible to heat sink. While there are theoretical advantages for MWA over RFA, most studies have shown no significant differences in overall survival between the two modalities (Table 1) (10). Strong evidence is lacking for cryoablation, although early evidence has shown safety and efficacy. The major drawback to cryoablation is procedure time and reduced room efficiency (11,12).

Comparison Between RFA, MWA, and Cryoablation		
	Advantages	Disadvantages
Radiofrequency Ablation	Robust Research/Publications Most Physician Experience Least Expensive	Heat Sink Skin Burns Limited ablation Zone Size Interacts with Cardiac Devices

Microwave Ablation	Low Sensitivity to Heat Sink Easy Set Up Large Ablation zone Shorter Procedure Time	Highest Cost Non-target thermal injury
Cryoablation	Low Sensitivity to Heat Sink Abscopal Immune Effect Synergy using multiple Probes	Least Robust Data Long Procedure Duration Complex set up

Table 1: Comparison of strengths and weaknesses of each thermal ablation modality for treated of pulmonary malignancy (12).

Head to head studies have been performed comparing treatment outcomes and complications between percutaneous thermal ablation and radiation therapy (SBRT). In this propensity matched cohort, median overall survival was not significantly different in the Thermal Ablation and SRT subgroups at 34.4 and 33.7 months, respectively. Additionally, no significant differences in outcomes were seen in comparison of the two modalities for oligometastatic disease (13). Both groups had periprocedural mortality of 0%, but thermal ablation showed higher morbidity as measured by 30-day hospital readmission rate (3.7%) which is likely due to the more invasive nature of the treatment. Adverse events after radiation therapy tend to present over a prolonged treatment phase with severe pulmonary toxicity occurring in up to 20% of patients (14-16).

Compared to surgery, thermal ablation offers high local control rates, shorter hospital stays, lower cost and better patient tolerance. National Comprehensive Cancer Networks guidelines recommend that SBRT should be first considered because of its possible better outcomes (17). Future prospective randomized controlled trials comparing the two options are still necessary to reach a clear conclusion. Ultimately the choice of second-line treatment will be guided by locoregional comfort levels of referrers, as well as interventionalist experience and workflows.

Complications

Overall, image guided thermal ablation has a very good safety profile. Morbidity and mortality is low with an in-hospital mortality of 1.3% (18). By far the most common complication is pneumothorax which occurs in up to 40% of cases (18). A very small number (2%) of the pneumothorax cases required further intervention with chest tube or surgery (19). More severe complications occur at much lower rates and include bronchopleural fistula, parenchymal hemorrhage, hemothorax, pleural effusion, air embolus and abscess.

Careful procedure planning can help reduce complication rates. Factors that increase the likelihood of complications include small lesions, lesions located in the basal and middle lung zones, long parenchymal track, traversing vessels, coagulation disorders, and the use of multiple antennae (20). Risk factors for bronchopleural fistula formation include emphysema, postprocedural infection, and an ablation zone which included a pleural surface (21).

For early-stage lung cancer, surgical resection is the gold standard of treatment with improved overall survival compared to both SBRT and Ablation. Results comparing SBRT and percutaneous thermal ablation have produced heterogeneous results in the literature, with many studies demonstrating no significant difference in survival outcomes but some showing higher survival rates with SBRT (22). Other factors to consider are risk profile of each treatment. Thermal ablation is minimally invasive and optimizes preservation of lung parenchyma, allowing it to be utilized in patients with inadequate pulmonary function for surgery or radiotherapy. Thermal ablation is performed in a single session, reducing hospital visits and morbidity for the patient. Also, thermal ablation can be repeated in case of recurrence without adverse effects on the surrounding parenchyma. Thermal ablation has been shown to improve quality of life by allowing a pause in chemotherapy (7,23,24).

Pre-procedure

All patients being considered for thermal ablation need to be evaluated in clinic prior to the procedure. The clinic visit should include a full history and physical exam with a focus on pulmonary function and ECOG (Eastern Cooperative Oncology Group) functional status. ECOG status should be less than 3. Relevant information to review includes pulmonary function testing, laboratory analysis within 30 days (Hgb, Plt, INR), and a full review of medications. Pulmonary ablation is categorized as a high bleeding risk procedure by the society of Interventional radiology (SIR). This means INR should be less than 1.7-2.0, platelets greater than 50k, and all blood thinners should be held for a sufficient amount of time prior to the procedure. If blood thinners cannot be held, bridging with heparin should be considered.

Current cross-sectional imaging within 3 months of the procedure is required. Imaging should be reviewed at the clinic visit to determine tumor size, number, shape, location, and procedural approach. This information is necessary to have an informative discussion with the patient regarding procedural expectation, outcomes, and potential complications. The clinic appointment is also the time to address goals of care, the majority of which is palliative in nature.

Procedure

Thermal ablation is performed in the outpatient setting under most circumstances. The patient should arrive to the department at least one hour prior to the procedure start time. This allows time to review all relevant labs and ensure anesthesia adequate time to re-evaluate the patient prior to the procedure.

SIR considers lung ablation to be a "clean contaminated" procedure. As such, it recommends periprocedural antibiotics to cover skin and respiratory flora. While there is no consensus on which antibiotic to use, the society recommends 1-2 g cefazolin IV (25).

Conscious Sedation, monitored anesthesia care, and general anesthesia can all be utilized for thermal ablation. The type of anesthesia will be largely driven by local practices and provider comfort. General anesthesia is used for the vast majority of pulmonary thermal ablations at our institution. The risks and benefits of each type of anesthesia must be weighed for each individual patient to determine what type of sedation is best.

Once the patient has been sedated and positioned as desired, thermal ablation antenna placement can be guided by CT (Figure 1). When choosing the optimal trajectory for antenna placement, the goal is creating an ablation zone that covers the mass with a 5 mm-1 cm margin without overtreating healthy lung. There are several factors to consider. First is determining a safe percutaneous path to the target lesion minimizing the number of times traversing pleura, avoiding major vascular structures, and minimizing length of parenchymal tract. Determining the size and shape of the target lesion is necessary, as it is ideal to position the ablation antenna along the long axis of the mass. Most devices create the largest dimension of extreme temperature along the course of the antenna. Also, if multiple overlapping treatment zones are required, this can easily be performed simply by retracting the antenna. Consideration must be given to the size of the anticipated treatment zone and the risk for bronchopleural fistula; if at all possible, you want to avoid ablating the pleural surface to minimize this risk.

Once the ablation antenna trajectory is optimized, a safe treatment can be performed. MWA zones are determined by information provided by each specific vendor. Treatment times usually vary between 1-10 minutes with wattages between 60-100 W. Ablation zone size increases as power and duration increase and each power/time combination can create a different size ablation zone. Most modern MWA antennas create ablation zones that are nearly spherical. With cryoablation, the shape of the ablation zone is determined by the type of antenna, with each manufacturer creating antennas of various shapes from spherical to elongated ovoid. The antenna you choose should be guided by the tumor shape and your desired treatment zone. For cryoablation, the antenna is what determines the ablation zone size/shape and all cryoablation requires two cycles of a 10-minute freeze followed by 5-minute thaw, for a total ablation time of approximately 30 minutes.

After completion of the ablation, it is important to scrutinize a final CT with a wide field of view after removal of the ablation antenna. Acute complications to identify are pneumothorax (particularly tension pneumothorax), massive parenchymal hemorrhage, or rapidly enlarging hemothorax. Vagus nerve stimulation during the procedure can also lead to a vagal response in the patient which may require treatment with atropine.

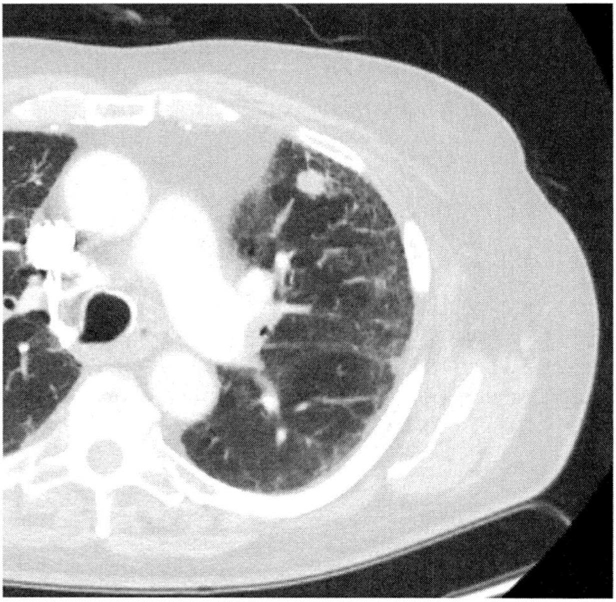

A)

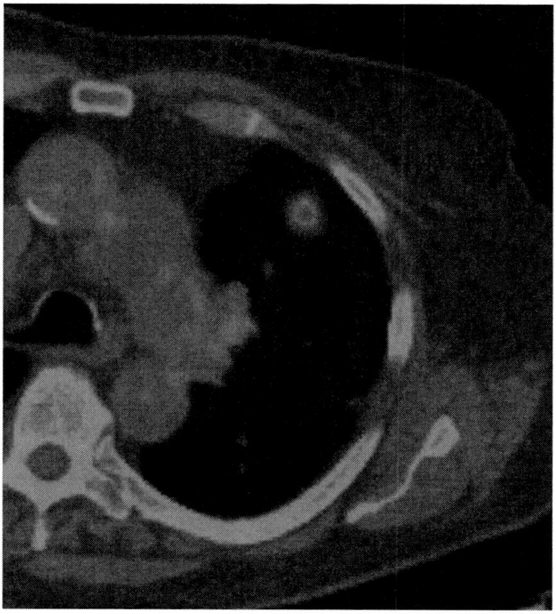

B)

C)

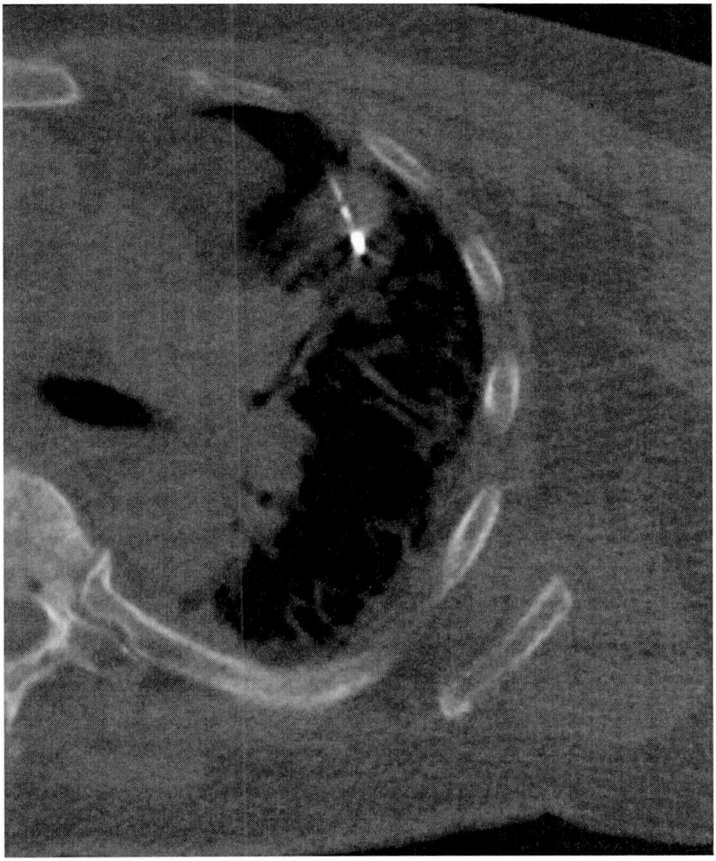

Figure 1: Preprocedural computed tomography (CT) (A) and positron emission tomography. (PET) (B) showing a hypermetabolic solitary pulmonary mass in the left lung. (C) Procedural CT showing thermal ablation antenna placement through the center of the mass prior for ablation.

Post-procedure

Patients are observed in the post procedural area for 2-6 hours following the procedure. In the immediate post-procedural time, bleeding is the most significant complication for which to monitor. During this time, there should be continuous cardiac monitoring and frequent vitals (15-30 minutes). Immediate and one-hour post-procedure chest radiographs should be obtained to monitor for expanding pneumothorax or enlarging hemothorax. Small, stable, asymptomatic pneumothorax can be discharged home with instructions to proceed to the ER if they experience worsening chest pain, shortness of breath, or dizziness. If the pneumothorax is expanding, the patient is symptomatic, or there is evidence of tension, a chest tube should be placed for decompression and the patient observed overnight as an inpatient.

If the patient has massive parenchymal hemorrhage identified at the termination of the procedure, the first step is positioning in a lateral position with the effected side down. This helps isolate the parenchymal hemorrhage to a single lung, maintaining aeration of the unaffected side. If the hemoptysis does not subside in the post procedural bay or the patient develops oxygen desaturation, selective intubation of the unaffected side with endobronchial blocking of the hemorrhagic lung may be necessary.

Prior to discharge the patient should meet discharge criteria, which will be institution specific but typically includes the patient being at baseline hemodynamics, tolerating oral intake, pain controlled with oral pain medications, and passing urine. Once meeting discharge criteria, the patient can be discharged home.

Imaging surveillance for treatment response is frequent over the first two years with exact protocol varying between institutions. Most centers perform post-operative imaging at 3, 6, 9, 12, 18, and 24 months using a combination of non-contrast CT and PET/CT. There is no societal consensus for modality of post procedural imaging. It is expected for the target lesion to appear larger in size on initial post treatment scan due to the treatment margin and surrounding ground glass opacities, which are common. The first post-procedural CT serves as a new baseline and subsequent imaging should show continued reduction in size of the target mass. PET imaging should show no FDG uptake in a well-treated mass (Figure 2). Other expected post-procedural findings are outline in Table 2 (26).

Likelihood of Post Operative Imaging Features Following Pulmonary Thermal Ablation at different time points					
CT Feature (% Present)	Immediate Post Op	< 4w	5-24 w	25-52 w	>52 w
Consolidation	81%	77%	73%	52%	22%
Ground-Glass Opacities	96%	91%	40%	26%	22%
Hyperdensity	68%	18%	4%	0%	0%
Cavitation	6%	54%	29%	13%	11%
Pneumatocele	27%	32%	13%	6%	5%
Parenchymal Bands	26%	54%	91%	90%	94%
Pleural Effusion	43%	32%	11%	10%	5%
Pleural Thickening	26%	77%	64%	52%	39%
Pneumothorax	29%	27%	4%	0%	0%

Table 2: Likelihood of common post-ablation imaging findings based on time since procedure.

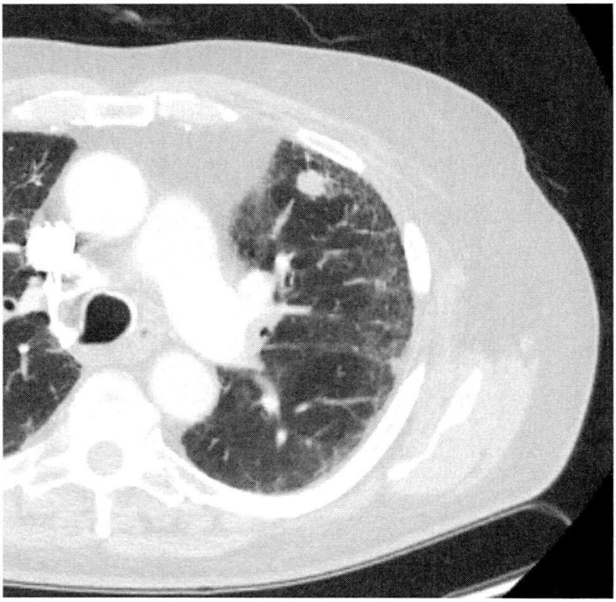

A)

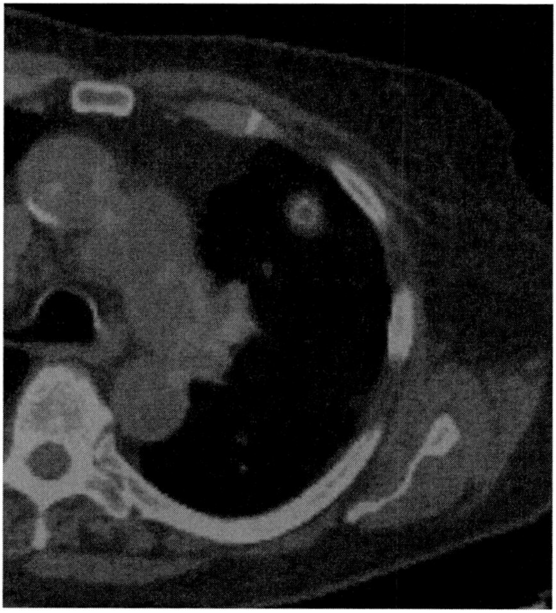

B)

C) 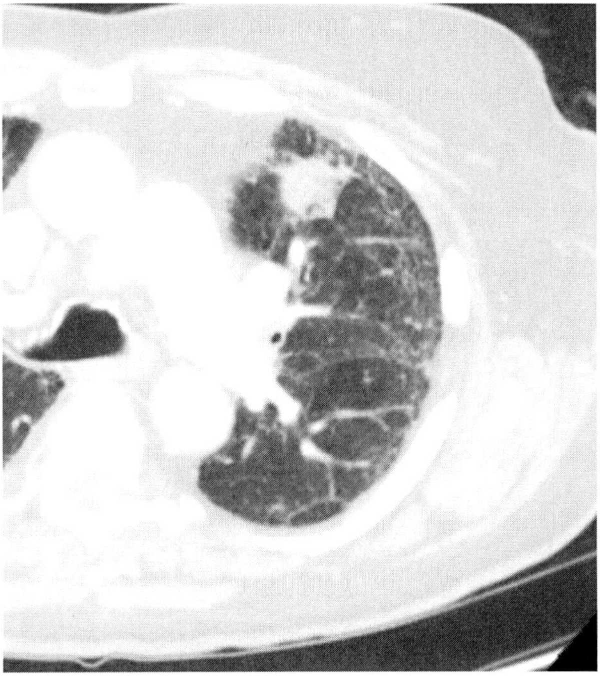

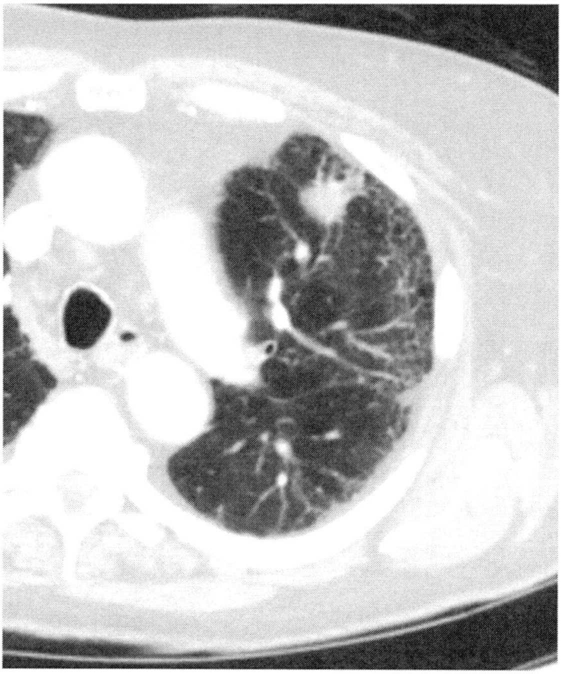
D)

E) 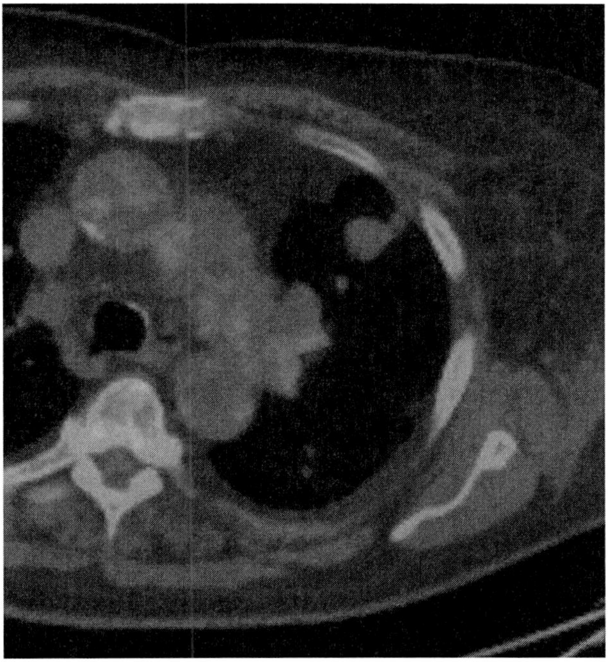

Figure 2: A) and B) Preprocedural chest CT and PET/CT show a small hypermetabolic mass in the left upper lobe. C) Three month post procedural CT shows mild enlargement of the target lesion with surrounding ground glass. Typical appearance of a well-treated mass at the 3-month time point and serves as a new baseline going forward. D) Six-month postprocedural CT shows reduction of size of the treated mass with reduced surrounding ground glass opacity. E) PET/CT at 9 months post procedure shows continued reduction in size of the mass and a complete lack of FDG uptake.

References

1. National cancer Institute. Lung and Bronchus Cancer. Cancer Stat Facts: Lung and Bronchus Cancer. https://seer.cancer.gov/statfacts/html/lungb.html. Accessed 2/18/2022.
2. Reck M, Heigener DF, et al. Management of non-small-cell lung cancer: Recent developments. Lancet. 2013; 382:709-19
3. Dupuy DE, Zagoria RJ, et al. Percutaneous radiofrequency ablation of malignancies in the lung. Am J Roentgenol 2000; 174: 57-9

4. Jiang B, Mcclure MA, et al. Efficacy and safety of thermal ablation of lung malignancies: A Network meta-analysis. Ann Thorac Med 2018;13:243-50.
5. De Baere T, Tselikas L, et al. Percutaneous thermal ablation of primary lung cancer. Diagn Interv Imaging 2016; 97:1019-24
6. Lin M, Eiken P, et al. Image guided thermal ablation in lung cancer treatment. J Thoracic Dis 2020; 12(11):7039-7047
7. Ghosn M, Solomon S. Current Management of Oligometastatic Lung Cancer and Future Perspective: Results of Thermal Ablation as a Local Ablative Therapy. Cancers 2021; 13:5202
8. Venturini M, Cariati M, et al. CIRSE Standards of Practice on Thermal Ablation of Primary and Secondary Lung Tumours. Cardiovasc Interv Radiol 2020; 43: 667-83
9. Lu DS, Raman SS, et al. Effect of vessel size on creation of hepatic radiofrequency lesions in pigs: assessment of the "heat sink" effect. AJR Am J Roentgenol 2002; 178:14-51
10. Macchi M, Belfiore MP, et al. Radiofrequency versus microwave ablation for treatment of the lung tumours: LUMIRA (lung microwave radiofrequency) randomized trial. Med Oncol 2017;34:96
11. Brace CL, Laeseke PF, et al. Microwave ablation with a single small-gauge triaxial antenna: in vivo porcine liver model. Radiology 2007; 242:435-40
12. Wright AS, Sampson LA, et al. Radiofrequency versus microwave ablation in a hepatic porcine model. Radiology 2005; 236:132-9
13. Omae K, Hiraki T, et al. Long Term Survival after Radiofrequency Ablation of Lung Oligometastases from Five Types of Primary Lesions: A Retrospective Evaluation. J Vasc Interv Radiol 2016; 27:1362-70
14. Timmerman R, McGarry R, et al. Excessive toxicity when treating central tumors in a phase II study of stereotactic body radiation therapy for medically inoperable early-stage lung cancer. J Clin Oncol 2006; 24(30):4833-4839
15. Bezjak A, Paulus R, et al. Efficacy and toxicity analysis of NRG Oncology/RTOG 0813 trial of stereotactic body radiation therapy for centrally located non-small cell lung cancer (NSCLC). Int J Radiat Oncol Biol Phys 2016; 96(2):S8
16. Chang JY, Li QQ, et al. Stereotactic ablative radiation therapy for centrally located early stage or isolated parenchymal recurrences of non-small cell lung cancer:how to fly in a "no fly zone". Int J Radiat Oncol Biol Phys 2014;88(5):1120-28

17. Ettinger DS, Wood DE, et al. Non-small cell lung cancer, version 1. 2020: Featured updates to the NCCN guidelines. JNCCN 2019; 17: 1464-72.
18. Welch BT, Brinjijki W, et al. A national analysis of the complications, cost, and mortlity of percutaneous lung ablation. J Vasc Interv Radiol 2015;26:787-91
19. Kashima M, Yamakado K, et al. Complications of 1000 lung radiofrequency ablation sessions in 420 patients: a single center's experiences AJR Am J Roentgenol 2011; 197:W576-80
20. Cannella M, Cornelis F, et al. Bronchopleural fistula after radiofrequency ablation of lung tumours. Cardiovasc Intervent Radiol 2011;34: Suppl 2:S171-4
21. Zheng A, Yang X, et al. Bronchopleural fistula after lung ablation: Experience in two cases and literature review. Indian J of Cancer 2015; 52(6): 41-46.
22. Bilal H, Mahmood S, et al. Is radiofrequency ablation more effective than stereotactic ablative radiotherapy in patients with early stage non-small cell lung cancer: A National Cancer Data Base study. J Thorac Cardiovasc Surg 2020; 160: 1350-7. e11.
23. Fonck M, Pers JT, et al. Pulmonary Thermal Ablation Enables Long Chemotherapy-Free Survival in Metastatic Colorectal Cancer Patients. Cardiovasc Interv Radiol 2018; 41: 1727-1734
24. Delpla A, de Baere, et al. Role of Thermal Ablation in Colorectal Cancer Lung Metastases. Cancers 2021; 13:908
25. Chehab M, Thakor A, et al. Adult and Pediatric Antibiotic Prophylaxis during Vascular and IR Procedures: A Society of Interventional Radiology Practice Parameter Update Endorsed by the Cardiovascular and Interventional Radiological Society of Europe and the Canadian Association for Interventional Radiology. J Vasc Interv Radiol 2018; 29:1483-1501
26. Araujo-Filho J, Alves Menezes R, et al. Lung Radiofrequency ablation: Post-procedure imaging patterns and late follow-up. Eur J Radiol Open. 2020; 7:100276

CHAPTER 15

NEUROINTERVENTIONAL ONCOLOGY

JOHN MADARANG MD, AARON BRAKE MS IV, ADIP BHARGAV MD, FRANK DESTEFANO DO, JOSEPH DOMINO MD

Introduction

Cancer treatment is evolving with the development of less invasive options and the use of biologic therapies such as immunotherapy and small molecule kinase inhibitors. Intraarterial (IA) delivery of chemotherapeutic agents has gained renewed interest due to improved delivery devices and novel therapeutics. IA delivery may be advantageous because it can deliver chemotherapy directly to the tumor bed, optimize drug doses, reduce off-target effects and toxicities, and improve patient compliance, especially for immunotherapies. IA delivery of chemotherapy has several pharmacokinetic considerations that must be taken into account when administering the drug. The dose, concentration, volume of distribution, rate, and frequency of administration may need to be independently established based on the specific drug and the intended therapeutic effect. One primary focus of pharmacokinetics in IA delivery is maximizing drug uptake into tumors, particularly in central nervous system (CNS) tumors where the drug must pass through the blood-brain barrier. The following chapter presents an overview of the current treatment options for intracranial tumors and retinoblastoma using intra-arterial delivery of chemotherapeutics. We will discuss the strategies and developments in this field, with the aim of highlighting the promising future of this relatively new area of therapy. It is important to note that this chapter serves as a primer on the subject and that we anticipate significant advancements and new developments in the near future that may change the landscape of this field.

Advantages of Intra-arterial Chemotherapy in the Central Nervous System

Investigations of intra-arterial chemotherapy (IAC) for solid cancers can be traced back as early as the 1950s with an initial report describing the propitious infusion of nitrogen mustard into the brachial artery of a patient with Hodgkin's lymphoma.[11,27,34] These early experiences led to the study of IAC applications for various systemic cancers as well as cancers of the CNS including gliomas initially. Interest in intra-arterial delivery stemmed from theoretical toxicity and pharmacokinetics/pharmacodynamics considerations compared to (IV) administration which was corroborated by initial studies in hepatocellular cancer, lymphoma, gastric cancer, melanoma, and pancreatic cancer, among others.[11,34,57] Wilson adapted this approach to malignant glioma in the 1960s where he attempted continuous arterial infusion of nitrogen mustard in patients suffering from this disease with mixed results.[57] Though enthusiasm for IAC in brain tumors and CNS disease diminished due to concerns of brain toxicity from these early studies, there has been renewed interest in recent years with the advent of state-of-the-art endovascular technology and novel chemotherapeutics that have begun to realize the advantages of intra-arterial administration of therapeutic agents.

The fundamental advantages of IAC in the CNS remain the same as for systemic cancers. Intravenous administration of cytotoxic chemotherapy is limited by first-pass metabolism by the liver in the majority of cases and by systemic toxicity of the chemotherapy at off-target sites.[34,53] As a result, this has implications for dose maximums and achieving an acceptable therapeutic window that may potentially hinder the efficacy of the chemotherapy. With IAC, the therapeutic agent can theoretically be selectively targeted to the tumor or region of interest by navigating tissue- or tumor-specific arterial beds and thereby minimize off-target chemotherapy exposure.[53,56] Local delivery of chemotherapy with this method may also permit higher doses of chemotherapy to be delivered and improved response to therapy. Initial investigations of IAC with nitrosourea agents, the chemotherapy of choice at the time, were disappointing in brain tumors with unacceptable toxicity to normal brain parenchyma and surrounding structures.[11,34,46,53,56] The nature of the chemotherapy used in these studies as well as the lack of current selective catheterization approaches contributed to the toxicity seen in these studies despite intra-arterial administration.[11,21,53,56]

The development of microcatheter technology and methods for super-selective catheterization in the CNS have begun to enable the purported advantages of IAC. The ability to select smaller caliber vessels, such as the ophthalmic artery in the context of retinoblastoma for example, have minimized brain toxicity and off-target effects seen in early studies.[11,53] Similarly, recent studies of IAC for gliomas have demonstrated promising safety profiles and early indications of potential therapeutic benefit compared to IV administration, though this remains an area of active study.[11,34,53,56] The discovery of new therapeutic agents beyond cytotoxic chemotherapy has also increased the feasibility and versatility of IA administration. Unlike nitrosourea agents, monoclonal antibodies such as Bevacizumab and other novel therapies including cellular and immunotherapies that are amenable to IA administration tend to be more inherently targeted resulting in less severe off-target toxicity.[11,56] Investigation of IA administration of the latter therapies is still in its infancy but hold promise for future clinical application given favorable safety profiles.

Challenges and Pitfalls of Intra-arterial Chemotherapy in the Central Nervous System

The growing use of IAC administration for CNS tumors has not come without substantial challenges and limitations. Since its inception, delineating optimal dosing strategies for IA administration has been of concern. While almost all data pertaining to chemotherapy dosing efficacy is based on conventional IV administration, it is difficult to extrapolate this literature for IA administration when considering drug pharmacodynamics, tumor uptake metabolism, and overall systemic toxicity. The RADPLAT protocol for IA administration of cisplatin in squamous cell carcinoma of the head and neck may suggest that higher drug concentrations are achievable without significantly elevated risk for systemic toxicity.[30,44,45] In this protocol, concomitant administration of platinum-binding molecules, like sodium thiosulfate, are capable of binding cisplatin before entering systemic circulation.[13] While this may provide a foundation for future advancements, current literature reciprocating similar findings specific for CNS tumors is limited.[38] Other earlier areas of focus seeking to limit systemic toxicity include the use of pulsatile administration and reducing the infusion speed, although neither have shown improved benefit.[5,17]

Attempts in the past for IA administration using conventional dosing methodology like weight and body-surface area were met with complications including vascular and neurologic toxicity including vision loss, stroke, and leukoencephalopathy.[39,40] These findings suggested a need to better estimate the perfusion volume of brain tissue susceptible to drug delivery to provide super-selective IA administration. Chen et al sought to better understand this by proposing a mechanism that overlays 3-dimensional angiography with MRI to provide a perfusion map for targeted, super-selective delivery of IAC.[10] While novel, this method requires the use of invasive studies like diagnostic cerebral angiography. This consideration is more reasonable for tumors of the lung, liver, and colon. However, intracranial catheterization carries substantially higher risk in comparison to other organs.

The ability to refine and sophisticate IA modalities allow for better targeting of CNS tumors locally while limiting the risk of both toxicity to adjacent healthy brain parenchyma and systemic toxicity. It is important to note that the push for less systemic administration also raises concern for not adequately treating unknown metastatic disease. This is less of a concern for primary brain tumors that do not historically metastasize. However, this may prove disadvantageous in high-grade glioma shown to have micro-seeding behavior and medulloblastoma with characteristic propensity to metastasize to distant areas of the CNS.

Unique to CNS tumors lies the necessity for crossing the blood-brain barrier (BBB) with IA chemotherapies to improve tumor uptake. Efforts to surpass or temporarily disable the BBB have been studied extensively to improve chemotherapy bioavailability in IV administration. These same limitations are present with IA administration. Previous studies have demonstrated success with overcoming the BBB during IA administration utilizing hyperosmolar agents, such as mannitol.[7,16,19] Other modalities including laser interstitial thermotherapy (LITT) and focused ultrasound have been described. These modalities, while promising, provide time constraints for delivery of IAC as well as special considerations for interactions related to disrupting the BBB. The combined use of IAC and BBB disrupting agents have been shown to be well tolerated by patients, although, reports of toxicity-related side effects have been noted.[36,51] Currently, the use of BBB disruption during IAC is offered in very limited sites across the world.

Although not unique to neuro-oncology, general procedural risks of IAC administration are important to note. IA treatment is inherently more invasive in comparison to standard IV methods which may result in complications. The use of heparin during the procedure may substantially increase the risk of inadvertent bleeding in select patients. Other risks inherent to the procedure include hematoma, infection, local vascular injury, pseudoaneurysm, stroke, and death. It is important that clinicians continually weigh the potential benefit of IAC with the procedural risk inherent to each unique patient.[55]

Intra-arterial Chemotherapy in Retinoblastoma

Retinoblastoma, an eye cancer affecting young children, has approximately 8,000 new global cases each year.[14,34,26] While retinoblastoma is a curable disease if detected early and treated aggressively, traditional treatments like enucleation and IV chemotherapy can have significant side effects.[8,20,37,48] This form of chemotherapy, initially used as an adjuvant to external beam radiation therapy in the 1950s, has since become a stand-alone treatment and is now considered part of the standard care for retinoblastoma.[23,25,43]

The treatment involves super-selective micro-catheterization of the ophthalmic artery and direct injection of therapeutic agent using a while the patient is under general anesthesia.[25] The procedure is primarily an outpatient procedure with recurrent doses spaced out over the course of a few months. Topical corticosteroids, short-acting mydriatics, and oral aspirin are used to reduce the risk of complications. A combination of Topotecan and Carboplatin are the most frequently used chemotherapeutic agents.[2,18] The dosing and drug selection depend on the tumor stage, laterality, and recurrence status. Despite a lack of published clinical trials to prove it's efficacy and safety, the available studies support IAC as an effective therapeutic.[34]

Overall, IAC has been reported to be more effective at treating advanced retinoblastoma,[12,33,47] and preventing local tumor recurrence.[49] It is also useful for bilateral retinoblastoma.[2] All this while also avoiding many of the significant clinical side effects associated with systemic chemotherapy.[1,9] Current guidelines advocate for IAC as a primary treatment for unilateral retinoblastoma in moderate to severe tumor burden and for bilateral advanced retinoblastoma and as secondary therapy for cases of recurrent tumor, persistent tumor, or in the setting of subretinal seeding.[33]

There are risks and drawbacks of using IAC delivery, including self-resolving side effects such as periocular edema and hyperemia, ptosis, focal madarosis as well as more serious side effect is 3rd and 6th cranial nerve palsies, optic atrophy.[35,33] Although stroke or retinal ischemia is rare, there is always a risk of intracranial vascular events when performing intracranial catheter manipulation.[33] The super-selective nature of IAC delivery also limits the systemic therapeutic benefits as described in the above section. Therefore, careful patient selection is critical when considering this treatment. Despite these limitations, retinoblastoma represents one of the first mainstream uses of interventional neuro-oncology and exemplifies that the benefits of IAC appear to outweigh the risks when used with caution by experienced practitioners. Clinical trials are underway to evaluate its safety and efficacy and it is possible we will begin to see the demand for this treatment increase in the future.

Intra-arterial Chemotherapy in Primary Brain Malignancies

CNS tumors, specifically glioblastoma, continue to be a significant challenge to successfully treat through best medical management and surgical resection. As discussed above, although IAC has seen recent promising results in other areas, CNS lesions are still one of the most unexplored areas for this modality of treatment due to its unique nature. However, with significant advancement in catheter technology and our understanding of the BBB and how it can be temporarily disrupted, new treatments are beginning to be explored for this technique.

Glioblastoma still accounts for roughly half of all malignant brain tumors and continues to have an abysmal 1-year survival rate of 40% and 17% at 2-years.[34] The current standard of care, the Stupp protocol, is a combination of safe surgical resection without new neurological deficits, radiation therapy over a 6-week period, and chemotherapy over an extended period.[54] Due to the BBB, however, chemotherapy is very limited as most chemotherapeutic agents are unable to penetrate the BB and therefore cannot reach sufficient concentration to assist in treatment. Initially, IA cisplatin was explored but ultimately unsuccessful.[41] However, a combination of IA cisplatin and etoposide administered to the tumor bed prior to radiotherapy has demonstrated some benefit due to the postulated disruption of the BBB by etoposide.[32] In this trial, the first group received IAC every 3 weeks followed by WBRT, and the second group received IAC during WBRT. The first group had a significant survival advantage, with a median survival of 20 months versus 7 months for glioblastoma and 45 months versus 12 months for anaplastic astrocytoma. Both groups had minimal side effects and were given steroids in the same regimen to assist with cerebral edema. It is theorized that this effect is that the concomitant WBRT disrupts the vasculature supply, therefore the IAC is not as effective.[31] Many other studies have been done comparing IA versus IV nimustine for newly diagnosed GBM, however they have shown that there is no benefit.[22,28,50] Another chemotherapy recently explored with some promise is bevacizumab. Patek et al explored IAC bevacizumab in newly diagnosed patients after performing a disruption of the BBB on a small non-matched cohort which demonstrated a significant improvement in both progression free survival (47.4% at 12 months) and overall survival (23.1 months median overall survival).[42] Recently, Chen et al have explored the use of perfusion guidance to enhance the precision of IAC. For this method, a pre-angiographic MRI brain w/ is performed and then fused with intraprocedural angiography to delineate a super-selective catheterization target vessel or vessels to be treated with IAC. Chen et al postulate that this advancement in technology, as demonstrated with some illustrative cases, can be used for precise intracranial IAC for glioblastoma and that this method should be used for further exploration and advancement of IAC treatment modalities.[10]

Additionally, a few studies have explored IAC for recurrent GBM. In these studies, IA bevacizumab was explored after a disruption of the BBB by mannitol infusion. These studies demonstrated a statistically significant decrease in tumor enhancement at 1 month as well as increase in progression free survival of 10 months,[6,7] as compared to IV treatment of the same modality with significantly lower progression free survival rates.[15,29]

Another pathology explored for IAC has been with Primary central nervous system lymphoma (PCNSL). PCSNL accounts for roughly 2% of CNS malignancies.[34] With current treatment modalities, 5-year survival is estimated to be around 30%.[58] Classically, PCNSL is treated with radiation therapy as well as IV methotrexate, although with significant toxicity related side effects.[4] Sonoda et al investigated IAC as a way to help with the significant toxicity complications associated with this treatment regimen. Following the same radiation guidelines, Sonoda et al administered IA ACNU in conjunction with the radiation treatments. Overall survival rates were comparable to slightly improved to the IV methotrexate regimen and overall treatment response was 100%.[52] A significant toxicity was noted in individuals over the age of 60 whom demonstrated a late neurotoxicity similar to the patients receiving high-does methotrexate, and therefore, Sonoda et al recommended this regimen for those under 60 and an alternative one for those over 60 to avoid this toxicity. Further studies have been conducted exploring IA methotrexate with the disruption of the BBB. In this study, mannitol and etoposide were used to disrupt the BBB and in conjunction with an IA methotrexate regimen they achieved an overall response rate of 81.9% and concluded that their results were comparable or possible superior to high dose IV methotrexate without the significant risk of neurotoxicity,[3] which was also seen in a similar smaller study coming to the same conclusions.[24]

Overall, IAC is a promising relatively new and vastly unexplored treatment modality for CNS lesions. Although few reports and trials have been completed for this modality, it is apparent that as catheter and imaging technology has advanced, IAC is becoming more and more viable every day. At the least of IAC's possibilities and demonstrated in multiple studies above, it has the potential to provide patients with the same benefits of IV chemotherapy without the toxic side effects common with traditional IV methods or even the neurotoxic side effects as super-selective methods advance, providing patients with a better quality of life throughout their treatment. At its best, as illustrated in early studies above, IAC may even provide an increase in progression free and overall survival rates for malignancies currently known to be death sentences with current best medical management. IAC continues to be an area that requires significant more research to become the standard of care, but great strides in the last decade have been made to further its course. As more research is conducted, it is clear that IAC in conjunction with advancements in imaging technologies as adjuncts will be crucial in the future of CNS malignancy treatment regimens.

References

1. Abramson DH, Francis JH, Dunkel IJ, Marr BP, Brodie SE, Gobin YP: Ophthalmic artery chemosurgery for retinoblastoma prevents new intraocular tumors. **Ophthalmology 120:**560-565, 2013
2. Abramson DH, Marr BP, Francis JH, Dunkel IJ, Fabius AW, Brodie SE, et al: Simultaneous Bilateral Ophthalmic Artery Chemosurgery for Bilateral Retinoblastoma (Tandem Therapy). **PLoS One 11:**e0156806, 2016
3. Angelov L, Doolittle ND, Kraemer DF, Siegal T, Barnett GH, Peereboom DM, et al: Blood-brain barrier disruption and intra-arterial methotrexate-based therapy for newly diagnosed primary CNS lymphoma: a multi-institutional experience. **J Clin Oncol 27:**3503-3509, 2009
4. Batchelor TT: Primary central nervous system lymphoma: A curable disease. **Hematol Oncol 37 Suppl 1:**15-18, 2019
5. Blacklock JB, Wright DC, Dedrick RL, Blasberg RG, Lutz RJ, Doppman JL, et al: Drug streaming during intra-arterial chemotherapy. **J Neurosurg 64:**284-291, 1986

6. Boockvar JA, Tsiouris AJ, Hofstetter CP, Kovanlikaya I, Fralin S, Kesavabhotla K, et al: Safety and maximum tolerated dose of superselective intraarterial cerebral infusion of bevacizumab after osmotic blood-brain barrier disruption for recurrent malignant glioma. Clinical article. **J Neurosurg 114:**624-632, 2011
7. Burkhardt J-K, Riina H, Shin BJ, Christos P, Kesavabhotla K, Hofstetter CP, et al: Intra-arterial delivery of bevacizumab after blood-brain barrier disruption for the treatment of recurrent glioblastoma: progression-free survival and overall survival. **World neurosurgery 77:**130-134, 2012
8. Chan HS, Gallie BL, Munier FL, Beck Popovic M: Chemotherapy for retinoblastoma. **Ophthalmol Clin North Am 18:**55-63, viii, 2005
9. Chen Q, Zhang B, Dong Y, Mo X, Zhang L, Huang W, et al: Comparison between intravenous chemotherapy and intra-arterial chemotherapy for retinoblastoma: a meta-analysis. **BMC cancer 18:**1-11, 2018
10. Chen SR, Chen MM, Ene C, Lang FF, Kan P: Perfusion-guided endovascular super-selective intra-arterial infusion for treatment of malignant brain tumors. **J Neurointerv Surg 14:**533-538, 2022
11. D'Amico RS, Khatri D, Reichman N, Patel NV, Wong T, Fralin SR, et al: Super selective intra-arterial cerebral infusion of modern chemotherapeutics after blood-brain barrier disruption: where are we now, and where we are going. **J Neurooncol 147:**261-278, 2020
12. Dalvin LA, Kumari M, Essuman VA, Shohelly Shipa S, Ancona-Lezama D, Lucio-Alvarez JA, et al: Primary Intra-Arterial Chemotherapy for Retinoblastoma in the Intravitreal Chemotherapy Era: Five Years of Experience. **Ocul Oncol Pathol 5:**139-146, 2019
13. Elferink F, van der Vijgh WJ, Klein I, Pinedo HM: Interaction of cisplatin and carboplatin with sodium thiosulfate: reaction rates and protein binding. **Clin Chem 32:**641-645, 1986
14. Fabian ID, Sagoo MS: Understanding retinoblastoma: epidemiology and genetics. **Community Eye Health 31:**7, 2018
15. Friedman HS, Prados MD, Wen PY, Mikkelsen T, Schiff D, Abrey LE, et al: Bevacizumab alone and in combination with irinotecan in recurrent glioblastoma. **J Clin Oncol 27:**4733-4740, 2009
16. Gerber NU, Mynarek M, von Hoff K, Friedrich C, Resch A, Rutkowski S: Recent developments and current concepts in medulloblastoma. **Cancer Treat Rev 40:**356-365, 2014
17. Gobin YP, Cloughesy TF, Chow KL, Duckwiler GR, Sayre JW, Milanese K, et al: Intraarterial chemotherapy for brain tumors by using

a spatial dose fractionation algorithm and pulsatile delivery. **Radiology 218:**724-732, 2001
18. Gobin YP, Dunkel IJ, Marr BP, Brodie SE, Abramson DH: Intra-arterial chemotherapy for the management of retinoblastoma: four-year experience. **Arch Ophthalmol 129:**732-737, 2011
19. Guillaume DJ, Doolittle ND, Gahramanov S, Hedrick NA, Delashaw JB, Neuwelt EA: Intra-arterial chemotherapy with osmotic blood-brain barrier disruption for aggressive oligodendroglial tumors: results of a phase I study. **Neurosurgery 66:**48-58; discussion 58, 2010
20. Houston SK, Murray TG, Wolfe SQ, Fernandes CE: Current update on retinoblastoma. **Int Ophthalmol Clin 51:**77-91, 2011
21. Huang R, Boltze J, Li S: Strategies for Improved Intra-arterial Treatments Targeting Brain Tumors: a Systematic Review. **Front Oncol 10:**1443, 2020
22. Imbesi F, Marchioni E, Benericetti E, Zappoli F, Galli A, Corato M, et al: A randomized phase III study: comparison between intravenous and intraarterial ACNU administration in newly diagnosed primary glioblastomas. **Anticancer research 26:**553-558, 2006
23. Inomata M, Kaneko A: Chemosensitivity profiles of primary and cultured human retinoblastoma cells in a human tumor clonogenic assay. **Jpn J Cancer Res 78:**858-868, 1987
24. Iorio-Morin C, Gahide G, Morin C, Vanderweyen D, Roy MA, St-Pierre I, et al: Management of Primary Central Nervous System Lymphoma Using Intra-Arterial Chemotherapy With Osmotic Blood-Brain Barrier Disruption: Retrospective Analysis of the Sherbrooke Cohort. **Front Oncol 10:**543648, 2020
25. Kaneko A, Suzuki S: Eye-preservation treatment of retinoblastoma with vitreous seeding. **Jpn J Clin Oncol 33:**601-607, 2003
26. Kim JY, Park Y: Treatment of Retinoblastoma: The Role of External Beam Radiotherapy. **Yonsei Med J 56:**1478-1491, 2015
27. Klopp CT, Alford TC, Bateman J, Berry GN, Winship T: Fractionated intra-arterial cancer; chemotherapy with methyl bis amine hydrochloride; a preliminary report. **Ann Surg 132:**811-832, 1950
28. Kochi M, Kitamura I, Goto T, Nishi T, Takeshima H, Saito Y, et al: Randomized comparison of intra-arterial versus intravenous infusion of ACNU for newly diagnosed patients with glioblastoma. **Journal of neuro-oncology 49:**63-70, 2000
29. Kreisl TN, Kim L, Moore K, Duic P, Royce C, Stroud I, et al: Phase II trial of single-agent bevacizumab followed by bevacizumab plus irinotecan at tumor progression in recurrent glioblastoma. **Journal of clinical oncology 27:**740, 2009

30. Kumar P, Robbins KT: Treatment of advanced head and neck cancer with intra-arterial cisplatin and concurrent radiation therapy: the 'RADPLAT' protocol. **Curr Oncol Rep 3:**59-65, 2001
31. Madajewicz S, Chowhan N, Iliya A, Roque C, Beaton R, Davis R, et al: Intracarotid chemotherapy with etoposide and cisplatin for malignant brain tumors. **Cancer 67:**2844-2849, 1991
32. Madajewicz S, Chowhan N, Tfayli A, Roque C, Meek A, Davis R, et al: Therapy for patients with high grade astrocytoma using intraarterial chemotherapy and radiation therapy. **Cancer 88:**2350-2356, 2000
33. Manjandavida FP, Stathopoulos C, Zhang J, Honavar SG, Shields CL: Intra-arterial chemotherapy in retinoblastoma - A paradigm change. **Indian J Ophthalmol 67:**740-754, 2019
34. Mott BT, Iyer A, Smith E, Fargen K, Brown P, Wolfe SQ: Current Indications for Intraarterial Chemotherapy in Neurointerventional Surgery. **Stroke: Vascular and Interventional Neurology 0:**e000425, 2022
35. Muen WJ, Kingston JE, Robertson F, Brew S, Sagoo MS, Reddy MA: Efficacy and complications of super-selective intra-ophthalmic artery melphalan for the treatment of refractory retinoblastoma. **Ophthalmology 119:**611-616, 2012
36. Muldoon LL, Pagel MA, Netto JP, Neuwelt EA: Intra-arterial administration improves temozolomide delivery and efficacy in a model of intracerebral metastasis, but has unexpected brain toxicity. **Journal of neuro-oncology 126:**447-454, 2016
37. Murphree AL, Villablanca JG, Deegan WF, 3rd, Sato JK, Malogolowkin M, Fisher A, et al: Chemotherapy plus local treatment in the management of intraocular retinoblastoma. **Arch Ophthalmol 114:**1348-1356, 1996
38. Neuwelt EA, Gilmer-Knight K, Lacy C, Nicholson HS, Kraemer DF, Doolittle ND, et al: Toxicity profile of delayed high dose sodium thiosulfate in children treated with carboplatin in conjunction with blood-brain-barrier disruption. **Pediatr Blood Cancer 47:**174-182, 2006
39. Newton HB: Intra-arterial chemotherapy of primary brain tumors. **Curr Treat Options Oncol 6:**519-530, 2005
40. Newton HB: Neurological complications of chemotherapy to the central nervous system. **Handb Clin Neurol 105:**903-916, 2012
41. Newton HB, Page MA, Junck L, Greenberg HS: Intra-arterial cisplatin for the treatment of malignant gliomas. **J Neurooncol 7:**39-45, 1989
42. Patel NV, Wong T, Fralin SR, Li M, McKeown A, Gruber D, et al: Repeated superselective intraarterial bevacizumab after blood brain

barrier disruption for newly diagnosed glioblastoma: a phase I/II clinical trial. **J Neurooncol 155:**117-124, 2021
43. Reese AB, Hyman GA, Tapley ND, Forrest AW: The treatment of retinoblastoma by x-ray and triethylene melamine. **AMA Arch Ophthalmol 60:**897-906, 1958
44. Robbins KT, Hoffman RM: "Decadose" effects of cisplatin on squamous cell carcinoma of the upper aerodigestive tract. I. Histoculture experiments. **Laryngoscope 106:**32-36, 1996
45. Robbins KT, Storniolo AM, Hryniuk WM, Howell SB: "Decadose" effects of cisplatin on squamous cell carcinoma of the upper aerodigestive tract. II. Clinical studies. **Laryngoscope 106:**37-42, 1996
46. Shapiro WR: Current therapy for brain tumors: back to the future. **Arch Neurol 56:**429-432, 1999
47. Shields CL, Alset AE, Say EA, Caywood E, Jabbour P, Shields JA: Retinoblastoma Control With Primary Intra-arterial Chemotherapy: Outcomes Before and During the Intravitreal Chemotherapy Era. **J Pediatr Ophthalmol Strabismus 53:**275-284, 2016
48. Shields CL, De Potter P, Himelstein BP, Shields JA, Meadows AT, Maris JM: Chemoreduction in the initial management of intraocular retinoblastoma. **Arch Ophthalmol 114:**1330-1338, 1996
49. Shields CL, Say EA, Pointdujour-Lim R, Cao C, Jabbour PM, Shields JA: Rescue intra-arterial chemotherapy following retinoblastoma recurrence after initial intra-arterial chemotherapy. **J Fr Ophtalmol 38:**542-549, 2015
50. Silvani A, Eoli M, Salmaggi A, Erbetta A, Fariselli L, Boiardi A: Intra-arterial ACNU and carboplatin versus intravenous chemotherapy with cisplatin and BCNU in newly diagnosed patients with glioblastoma. **Neurol Sci 23:**219-224, 2002
51. Simonett JM, Skalet AH, Lujan BJ, Neuwelt EA, Ambady P, Lin P: Risk Factors and Disease Course for Blood-Brain Barrier Disruption-Associated Maculopathy. **JAMA Ophthalmol 139:**143-149, 2021
52. Sonoda Y, Matsumoto K, Kakuto Y, Nishino Y, Kumabe T, Tominaga T, et al: Primary CNS lymphoma treated with combined intra-arterial ACNU and radiotherapy. **Acta Neurochir (Wien) 149:**1183-1189; discussion 1189, 2007
53. Srinivasan VM, Lang FF, Chen SR, Chen MM, Gumin J, Johnson J, et al: Advances in endovascular neuro-oncology: endovascular selective intra-arterial (ESIA) infusion of targeted biologic therapy for brain tumors. **J Neurointerv Surg 12:**197-203, 2020
54. Stupp R, Mason W: Bent MJ van den et al. on behalf of the European Organisation for Research and Treatment of Cancer (EORTC) Brain

Tumor and Radiotherapy Groups and National Cancer Institute of Canada Clinical Trials Group (NCIC CTG) (2005) Radiotherapy plus concomitant and adjuvant temozolomide for patients with newly diagnosed glioblastoma. **N Engl J Med 352:**987-996

55. Tavakol M, Ashraf S, Brener SJ: Risks and complications of coronary angiography: a comprehensive review. **Glob J Health Sci 4:**65-93, 2012
56. van Solinge TS, Nieland L, Chiocca EA, Broekman MLD: Advances in local therapy for glioblastoma - taking the fight to the tumour. **Nat Rev Neurol 18:**221-236, 2022
57. Wilson CB: Chemotherapy of Brain Tumors by Continuous Arterial Infusion. **Surgery 55:**640-653, 1964
58. Yang XL, Liu YB: Advances in Pathobiology of Primary Central Nervous System Lymphoma. **Chin Med J (Engl) 130:**1973-1979, 2017

CHAPTER 16

PRE-OPERATIVE EMBOLIZATION FOR HEAD AND NECK PATHOLOGY

JOHN MADARANG MD, ZACHARY NICEK MD, NICK HANNA MD, ADRIEN CAYE MS IV

Pre-operative embolization is commonly used to aid in the successful resection of intracranial and spinal tumors. The goal of pre-operative embolization is to minimize blood loss, decrease operating time and improve visualization of the surgical field by devascularizing the tumor. Additionally, neuroendovascular embolization can be used as the sole treatment modality for non-operable patients. Many factors impact the decision to undergo pre-operative embolization including tumor location, tumor blood supply, experience of the interventionist, ease of resection and preference of the surgeon (1).

Pre-operative embolization is most often used as an adjunct to surgical resection of a tumor. The primary goals of pre-operative embolization are to reduce blood loss during surgical resection, soften the tumor, and decrease operating time. Pre-operative embolization is indicated for large or highly vascular tumors, tumors with arterial supply from the external carotid artery, or a blood supply originating opposite of the surgical approach (1-3). Pre-operative embolization is commonly indicated for meningiomas, glomus jugulare, juvenile nasopharyngeal angiofibroma, and metastatic lesions (1). Pre-operative embolization is also indicated for tumors composed of multiple, independent vascular compartments and those in close proximity to cranial nerves or vascular structures (3). Additionally, embolization may be used to reduce the size of tumors for palliation purposes in non-operable patients (1).

There are several factors that warrant caution when considering the use of pre-operative embolization. Tumors that share blood supply with non-target tissues or the presence of extracranial to intracranial anastomotic connections confer greater risk of complications (4). Tumors with blood supply derived from the ICA, its small branches, or the ophthalmic artery pose significant risks that may not be outweighed by the benefits (4, 5). Caution should be taken to ensure that embolic material does not reflux into the parent vessel and cause unintended embolization of non-target tissues (4). Additionally, the risk of thromboembolic stroke and arterial perforation are increased when embolization is performed through pial vessels due to their fragility (4). Patients with significant peripheral vascular disease or history of stroke have increased risks of complications and may not be suitable candidates for embolization (6).

Pre-operative imaging is important for evaluation of the tumor and its relationship with neurological and vascular structures. The choice of pre-embolization imaging modalities is based on the information sought by the surgeon or interventionalist. Tumors often display a characteristic appearance on CT or MRI imaging modalities and can help predict the origin of blood supply (1, 7). For example, paragangliomas are nearly always supplied by the ascending pharyngeal artery, while meningiomas are most commonly supplied by the middle meningeal artery (1, 7). Computed Tomography (CT) scans can reveal the size and location of the tumor as well as any bone erosion.

Magnetic Resonance Imaging (MRI) allows for visualization of anatomical relationships and involvement of brain parenchyma or dura. Post-embolization changes on MRI may show decreased enhancement and reduced diffusion of devascularized portions of the tumor. However, assessment of embolization utilizing MRI may be complicated by contrast leakage, hemorrhage, necrosis and different grades of recanalization. MRI images based on cerebral blood volume or cerebrospinal fluid may not reveal the full efficacy of embolization due to compensatory vasodilation. T2-weighted MRI allows examination of tumor hypoxia due to decreased blood flow and is evidenced by areas of decreased T2 signal. MR perfusion with intraarterial injections has been reported to be helpful in analyzing the efficacy of embolization. Intraarterial MR perfusion can be used to image an area of interest and assess the perfusion status post-embolization, thus allowing the interventionalists to determine whether the embolization was successful and guide therapeutics (7).

Angiography may be used to visualize vascular structures encased by the tumor as well as anastomotic connections and collateral flow. Digital subtraction angiography (DSA) can be used to assess tumor vascularity and its connections to surrounding vessels (7). Selective catheterization of the carotid arteries and distal branches is required to characterize the blood supply (1). Carotid balloon occlusion test may be indicated to determine the risk of arterial sacrifice prior to or during surgery (3). Superselective catheterization can reveal intracranial anastomoses that may complicate embolization and require caution during embolization. Finally, tumor blush should be measured both pre- and post-embolization to quantify the efficacy of embolization. It is important to evaluate the contralateral carotid branches to exclude contribution to tumor blush. The goal of embolization is a reduction in the amount of tumor blush by 80% or more (1).

Timing of the Surgery: The effects of embolization may be transient depending on the material used and degree of devascularization. Early resection (<24 hours) after embolization does not allow sufficient time for devascularization and tumor necrosis to occur. Thrombus formation and multinucleated giant cell reaction have been found to occur within 7 days of embolization. Recanalization and partial revascularization can begin after 7 days in up to 30% of vessels. Tumor softening and ease of resection were found to be greatest at 7 to 9 days post-embolization. Thus, surgical resection should occur within 1 to 8 days after embolization. Longer time intervals between embolization and surgical resection allow for more tumor necrosis and tumor softening but have been associated with increased risk of tumor hemorrhage and collateral revascularization. Earlier resection can avoid the delayed edema and mass effects in the days following embolization but may not allow sufficient time for devascularization. This can result in longer operating times, increased blood loss and decreased tumor necrosis. Steroids may be given for large tumors or tumors at risk of mass effect from post-embolization edema if surgery is to be delayed (1). Highly vascular tumors are at great risk of tumor infarction, swelling and herniation and should undergo embolization just prior to surgery (1). The benefits and risks should be assessed on a case-by-case basis to determine optimal timing of post-embolization surgical resection (1, 7).

Embolic Material: Which embolic material to use is an important factor to consider in pre-operative embolization. Embolic materials are divided into particles, powders, and liquid embolic agents. Each type of material has advantages and disadvantages that must be considered on a case-by-case basis. An ideal embolic agent is one that causes permanent distal vascular occlusion and resultant tumor necrosis (1, 7).

Particulate embolic agents vary in size and shape, with the most commonly used embolic agent being polyvinyl alcohol (PVA) particles. PVA particles are composed of a solid, sponge-like material that expands in aqueous solution. PVA particles are commonly used in a solution of non-heparinized saline mixed with non-ionic contrast medium. They are an efficacious embolic material because they produce an inflammatory response that aids in thrombosis and occlusion of vessels. PVA particles range in size from small (50 to 150 microns) to larger particles (150-250 microns). Smaller particles can penetrate deeper into tumor capillary beds but are associated with an increased risk of injury to the vasa nervorum and entering intracranial circulation. Larger particles are less likely to over-penetrate and cause cranial nerve palsies or enter intracranial circulation but may lead to large-vessel occlusion or predispose to particle aggregation and result in hemorrhage (1-3, 7). Distal coil embolization can be used to prevent non-target embolization of distal structures. Once embolization has been completed, the feeding vessel may be coiled more proximally, thereby reducing the risk of recanalization (8).

Embolization with PVA particles begins with diagnostic angiography to establish the main vascular supply of the tumor. Using a transfemoral route, a microcatheter system is placed in the feeding vessels as close as possible to the tumor. Under fluoroscopic guidance, PVA particles are injected, and embolization is ended when near stasis is observed in the main feeding vessels or when reflux of emboli into non-target vessels is observed. Post-embolization DSA can then be used to quantify the reduction in tumor blush and extent of tumor devascularization (3, 7).

Microspheres are another competing particulate embolic agent that are generally larger (400 microns) than PVA particles (50-250 microns). Microspheres are flexible, compressible, and suspended in contrast material. Microspheres are compressible by up to 33%, allowing them to pass through the catheter and then return to their original diameter upon deployment. This allows them to be easily utilized without worry of catheter blockage. Trisacryl gelatin microspheres are associated with significantly less blood loss than PVA particles and have similar complication rates. Microspheres have been found to have better distal penetration than PVA particles, because of their propensity to form chains in small vessels, as opposed to PVA particles, which form clusters. Use of microspheres and large PVA particles (150-250 microns) is generally considered safer than smaller PVA particles and results in fewer incidents of hemorrhage (2, 7).

Glue emboli are associated with lower complication rates than particulate embolic agents. N-butyl cyanoacrylate (NBCA) is a commonly used glue which has rapid effects, completely fills vessels, and forms an adherent cast.

NBCA, has been shown to have decreased rates of hemorrhagic and ischemic complications when compared to particulate emboli. NBCA also has the advantage of usage in a broader range of microcatheters, thus allowing for improved distal navigation compared to particle emboli. NBCA is able to simultaneously enter both intratumoral vessels and feeders, thus reducing the risk of intratumoral bleeding. NBCA can be used with lower injection pressures, thus reducing the risk of intratumoral hemorrhage, a common complication of particles. One injection technique uses concurrent 5% dextrose in water solution through the catheter to help NBCA penetrate deeper into the target vessels. Caution must be taken when using NBCA to prevent adherence of the microcatheter to the vessel wall and requires withdrawal of the microcatheter after each injection to prevent entrapment. If the microcatheter cannot be advanced close enough to the tumor, there is a risk the NBCA may obstruct the vessel proximally and lead to reflux of NBCA into non-target vessels (2, 8).

Embolization using NBCA typically begins with insertion of a catheter beyond the carotid bifurcation. A microcatheter is then introduced and navigated through the feeding artery as close to the tumor as possible. Injection of 4ml of .4% lidocaine is administered via the microcatheter, followed by 5% glucose solution. Then a 17-25% mixture of NBCA and lipiodol is warmed to reduce viscosity and injected into the target vessel. The mixture of NBCA and lipiodol is radiopaque, which allows easier identification of embolic material in non-target vessels. Injection of NBCA into dural vessels causes pain, and thus injection of lidocaine can significantly reduce associated pain. Once injected, NBCA forms a hard cast that can entrap the microcatheter tip, thus requiring complete withdrawal after each injection. A microcatheter with a detachable distal tip can be used thereby decreasing risk of vasospasm, stroke or hemorrhage due to excessive traction on blood vessels (2,8).

Liquid embolic agents have a lower risk of hemorrhage when compared to solid particles and are used when the microcatheter can be navigated close to the tumor (7). Concurrent use of coils and balloons helps prevent entry of liquid embolic agents into unintended vessels. Onyx (MEDTRONIC), an Ethylene vinyl alcohol (EVOH) copolymer, is a commonly used liquid embolic agent that has many benefits over traditional PVA particles (2). ONYX precipitates in a radial fashion forming a cast, allowing for a slow and controlled injection with deeper penetration into the tumor capillary bed (9). Onyx is available in 3 formulations, 18, 20, and 34, with varying concentrations of EVOH (6%, 6.5%, 8%, respectively) (13). Additionally, Onyx does not initially adhere to the vessel wall or reflux into the catheter and thus does not require withdrawal after each injection like NBCA. The slow precipitation rate of Onyx and its easy intraoperative visualization allows for its administration to be intermittently stopped to monitor nontarget embolization (2, 9). Onyx is capable of deeply penetrating tumor vascular beds and vascular pedicles with decreased risk of catheter entrapment. Onyx must be injected slowly, as it is dissolved in dimethyl sulfoxide (DMSO), which is toxic and can lead to vasospasm and necrosis of vessels (10). Additionally, all catheters and syringes must be compatible with DMSO use. Surgeons must use caution with monopolar cautery as Onyx embolized vessels can combust.

The embolization technique using Onyx typically begins with obtaining femoral access and systematic heparinization of the patient. The vascular supply is characterized with diagnostic angiography of the feeding vessel and any anastomoses are identified. A microcatheter is then navigated over a microwire to the target vessel as close to the tumor as possible. Superselective microcatheter angiography is then performed to rule out distal vascular supply to non-target tissues. Embolization is then performed through the microcatheter. Typical Onyx embolization requires the "plug and push" technique, which involves the creation of a plug around the microcatheter tip to prevent reflux proximally. Small volumes of Onyx are injected, followed by small periods of waiting (typically 2 minutes), to allow the plug to form immediately proximal to the microcatheter tip. The plug and push technique reduces the risk of reflux proximally to the catheter tip but prolongs operative time and increases exposure to radiation for the patient and interventionist. Use of a dual-lumen balloon catheter has been shown to promote deep penetration into the tumor vascular bed without the need for proximal microcatheter plug. The balloon catheter can be advanced to the target vessel where the balloon is then inflated for proximal occlusion, rather than forming a plug proximally to the microcatheter tip. Prevention of distal, non-target embolization can be accomplished with the use of coil embolization prior to Onyx injection. Post-embolization angiography can be used to monitor for non-targeted embolization and to evaluate the degree of devascularization (10, 11).

SQUID

SQUID is another EVOH copolymer that has recently been used in the embolization of intracranial tumors. SQUID is composed of micronized Tantalum powder suspended in EVOH and dimethyl-sulfoxide (DMSO). SQUID is available in four compositions, depending on the desired viscosity and concentration of tantalum. SQUID 18 is similar to Onyx 18 in its characteristics, while SQUID 12 is more fluid with a lower viscosity. The lower viscosity of SQUID 12 provides superior penetration into tumor capillary beds including areas that may be difficult to reach for a surgeon. SQUID is radiopaque and its formulary with lower tantalum concentration helps visualize structures behind dense embolic casts under fluoroscopy. (12,13)

SQUID is injected in a similar fashion as Onyx. A microcatheter is navigated to the target vessel in similar fashion. Prior to injection of Squid, the microcatheter tip is flushed with 5ml of saline solution and then .35 ml of DMSO is used to fill the dead space. SQUID is then injected slowly to allow a plug formation around the microcatheter tip. Once a plug is formed, distal penetration of Squid can begin, with pauses in administration every 2 to 3 minutes to monitor for unintended embolization of non-target vessels and to reset the fluoroscopic roadmap guidance (13).

Route of Embolization: Pre-operative embolization may proceed via the traditional trans-arterial approach or via direct puncture of the tumor. Trans-arterial embolization is performed with superselective catheterization and embolization of feeding pedicles and is the preferred method for embolization of intracranial tumors (1). Trans-arterial approaches offer the benefit of being able to target tumors located deep in the brain parenchyma without the need for craniotomy (4, 14). Trans-arterial approaches may be performed with any of the embolic agents previously outlined, with slight variations in each technique depending on the agent used. Trans-arterial approaches can be limited by tortuous vessels, dangerous extracranial to intracranial anastomoses and unfavorable origin of blood supply (12).

The percutaneous direct puncture involves directly penetrating the tumor capillary bed with a needle and injecting a liquid embolic agent such as Onyx or Squid. Percutaneous direct puncture is performed on extra-cranial tumors, or intracranial tumors endonasally, intraorally or after a craniotomy. To perform this technique, diagnostic angiography is typically used to assess the extent of tumor blush, feeding and draining vessels and to identify any extracranial to intracranial anastomoses. The needle is then inserted under direct vision into the center of the tumor under roadmap guidance with care not to puncture any non-target vessels. An intratumoral angiogram is then performed to confirm that the needle is appropriately placed in the tumor, and to detect any anastomotic connections. The microcatheter tip dead space is then filled with DMSO prior to injection of the EVOH copolymer (Onyx, Squid). EVOH copolymer is then injected into each vascular compartment until filled with intermittent trans-arterial angiograms to assess tumor devascularization. A balloon microcatheter via femoral access can be used to prevent reflux from into proximal arteries such as the external carotid artery. A postembolization trans-arterial angiogram is used to measure the degree of tumor devascularization and reduction in tumor blush (12, 14).

The percutaneous direct puncture technique offers several advantages over the trans-arterial technique. One such advantage of the direct puncture technique is that it is able to more completely fill the tumor microvascular bed and creates a distinctive tumoral cast that is likely to result in complete and irreversible occlusion of the target vessels when compared to the trans-arterial approach. Trans-arterial approaches are more likely to result in inadequate devascularization due to decreased penetration of embolic material. Additionally, percutaneous allows for easier access to the tumor vascular bed and is less likely to cause inadvertent embolization through anastomotic connections, as the embolic material must traverse the tumor parenchyma before reaching the feeding pedicles. Direct puncture also avoids the challenges of navigating tortuous vessels or those arising from difficult angles. Direct puncture also results in shorter fluoroscopy time and likely decreased intraoperative blood loss (12, 14).

Complications: Pre-operative embolization is a useful neoadjuvant therapy for the surgical resection of tumors, however, it is not without complications. The most common major complication associated with pre-operative embolization is cranial nerve damage. Other major complications include ischemic or hemorrhagic events, edema causing mass effect, hydrocephalus, seizures, and hemiparesis. The overall complication rate ranges from 0 to 9 %, depending on the location of the tumor, origin of blood supply, anastomotic connections and which embolic agent was used (2, 7). When focusing on feeding vessels arising solely from the internal carotid artery, the overall complication rate rose to 21% with a 9% risk of permanent neurological complications (6, 16). This increased risk has led many to avoid or significantly limit the amount of embolization performed on ICA derived vessels (2, 5, 6, 7). There are relatively few comparisons of different embolic agents and most of the literature consists of case series. A systematic review of literature regarding pre-operative embolization of skull based meningiomas with PVA, NBCA, and Onyx found an overall complication rate of 12%, major complication rate of 6%, and mortality rate of .2% (15). Liquid embolic agents are associated with a lower risk of hemorrhage than particle embolic agents (2).

Common tumors: Meningiomas are pathologically benign, enhancing, dural based tumors that are divided into two groups: convexity/parasagittal and skull based meningiomas (4, 7, 17). Convex meningiomas located in the cranial vault are supplied by meningeal, superficial temporal, and temporal arteries. The most common blood supply for convex meningiomas is the middle meningeal artery, which is ultimately supplied by the external carotid artery (7). Because their blood supply is usually superficial and easily accessed, convexity meningiomas don't often require pre-operative embolization. On the other hand, large convexity meningiomas with multidirectional blood supplies are good embolization candidates due to their increased risk of blood loss during surgical resection. The most common location for a skull-based meningioma is the sphenoid ridge, followed by the anterior fossa, tentorium, and petroclivus. Because of their location, skull based meningiomas are often found adjacent to cranial nerve and supplied by deep, higher risk vessels (6, 17). Skull based meningiomas receive their blood supply from the internal carotid artery, external carotid artery and branches of the vertebrobasilar circulation (6, 7). Embolization of meningiomas in the anterior fossa can lead to unintended occlusion of the ophthalmic artery, leading to blindness or retrograde flow via the ophthalmic artery to the ICA, leading to a stroke. Embolization of meningiomas is often complicated due to dual blood supply arising from both the ECA and the ICA. Posterior fossa meningiomas are typically supplied by the ICA, ascending pharyngeal artery and vertebral arteries, all of which are considered high risk vessels (2, 17).

Hemangioblastomas are benign, hypervascular that are most commonly located in the posterior fossa, followed by the spinal cord. Cerebellar hemangioblastomas are usually supplied by branches of the anterior-inferior, posterior-inferior, and superior cerebellar arteries. Due to their location near vital neurological structures and hypervascularity, treatment of hemangioblastomas is complicated and requires a higher threshold for embolization. Treatment is often reserved for large tumors whose blood supply is deep and inaccessible until late in the surgical resection. Due to the confined space of the posterior fossa, there is an increased risk of post-embolization peritumoral edema that can lead to brainstem compression or herniation (17, 18).

Glomus jugulare tumors are neuroendocrine tumors (paragangliomas) that arise in the jugular foramen. They often present in the middle ear with hearing loss, tinnitus, or lower cranial nerve compression symptoms. Rarely, they can present with catecholamine hypersecretion and have a distinctive salt-and-pepper appearance on MRI. Glomus Jugulare tumors are commonly supplied by the ascending pharyngeal artery, but may also be supplied by the ICA, middle meningeal artery, or occipital artery (17).

Carotid body tumors are the most common paraganglioma tumors found in the head and neck. They arise from the carotid body and present as palpable, pulsatile neck masses that can cause pain, hoarseness or dysphagia. They have a characteristic appearance on angiography in which there is hypervascular blush that splays between the carotid bifurcation. The tumor is usually fed by the ascending pharyngeal artery, which ascends posteriorly and supplies the tumor superiorly, but may also be supplied by branches of the external carotid artery. The tumor may lie between the internal and external carotid arteries, may adhere to either artery, or encase 1 or both. Direct tumor puncture is the preferred technique for embolization of carotid body tumors. This technique provides greater devascularization, avoids navigation of tortuous small feeding vessels, and reduces the risk of unintentional embolization of the distal ascending pharyngeal artery. Pre-operative embolization of carotid body tumors was found to be safe and effective, with a decrease in intraoperative blood loss and operative time (17, 19).

Juvenile nasal angiofibromas (JNA) are highly vascular and locally aggressive tumors. They are considered benign tumors that present with nasal obstruction and recurrent epistaxis. They are the most common primary tumor of the nasopharynx and occur most often in adolescent males. JNA tumors are usually supplied by the internal maxillary artery or ascending pharyngeal artery but may receive additional blood supply from branches of the external and internal carotid arteries (18, 20). Bilateral carotid angiography is necessary to delineate the vascular supply, as JNAs can be supplied by both external carotid arteries. Complications from embolization of JNA tumors includes unintentional occlusion of superficial branches feeding the skin of the face, and occlusion of the central retinal artery (17, 20).

Common spinal tumors amenable to preoperative embolization include hemangioblastoma, hemangioma, giant cell tumor, osteoblastoma, and metastases (renal cell, thyroid, hepatocellular carcinoma). Prior to embolization, it is important to perform angiography of vessels both two levels above and two levels below the tumor to adequately delineate the vascular supply. It is important to visualize the vertebral arteries, external carotid arteries, intercostal arteries and iliac arteries, depending on the level of the tumor (17, 21). A microangiogram should be performed to identify intratumoral arteriovenous shunting or any anastomoses to the spinal cord vasculature (8).

Practical Considerations: The following are a set of guidelines proposed by Waldron et al to guide neurointerventionalists in avoiding complications. First, careful microcatheter angiograms must be performed prior to embolization of any vessel. This is to ensure that there are no unanticipated branches of normal vasculature or anastomotic connections that could be occluded along with the blood supply to the tumor. It is also important to understand where normal anastomoses are located to avoid unintentional reflux of embolic material into non-target vessels. Use of small particle PVA or liquid embolic agents requires extra caution to avoid embolizing arteries supplying cranial nerves. Next, the microcatheter must be well seated in the target vessel to prevent it from becoming dislodged from the force of injection and leading to unintended embolization of a non-target vessel. Finally, always use high quality DSA imaging for the embolization procedure (6, 7).

Liquid embolic embolization requires that the microcatheter be positioned as close to the target vessel as possible to achieve maximum intratumoral penetration. If there is insufficient distance proximally for a plug to form, or if there is a risk that distal penetration of Onyx may embolize non-target vessels, then NBCA is preferred. Coils may be used on tumors with rapid arteriovenous shunting to partially devascularize the tumor and make it safer to use the desired liquid embolic agent. Additionally, it is important to consider the tumor vascular anatomy when choosing an embolic material. If distal selective catheterization of tumor vasculature is not possible, then PVA particles are preferred over liquid embolic agents (10, 17). Care must be taken to choose the correct particle size and to identify any risky collateral flow. Direct tumor puncture offers better tumor penetration than trans-arterial technique and avoids the challenges of navigating difficult arterial anatomy, however, there is in increased risk of unintentional embolization of venous structures (14, 17). Complete devascularization of the tumor results in significantly less risk of requiring intraoperative transfusions than partial devascularization. However, it is important to balance the benefit of complete devascularization with the risk of a more aggressive approach (2).

References

1. Duffis, E., Gandhi, C,, Prestigiacomo, C., Abruzzo., et al. Head, Neck, and brain tumor embolization guidelines. J NeuroIntervent Surg 2012;4:251-255. doi:10.1136/neurointsurg-2012-010350
2. Yoon, N., Shah, A., Couldwell, W., Kalani, Y., Park, M. Preoperative embolization of skull base meningiomas: current indications, techniques, and pearls for complication avoidance
3. Gruber, A., Bavinzski, G., Killer, M., Richling, B. Preoperative Embolization of Hypervascular Skull Base Tumors. Minim Invas Neurosurg 2000; 43: 62-71.
4. Sekhar, L., Biswas, A., Hallam, D., Kim, L., Douglas, J., Ghodke, B. Neuroendovascular Management of Tumors and Vascular Malformations of the Head and Neck. Neurosurg Clin N Am 20(2009) 453-485. DOI:10.1016/j.nec.2009.07.007
5. Carli, D., Sluzewski, M., Beute, G., van Rooij, W. Complications of Particle Embolization of Meningiomas: Frequency, Risk Factors, and Outcome. Am J Neuroradiol. 2010 Jan;31(1):152-4. DOI:10.3174/ajnr.A1754
6. Waldron, J., Sughrue, M., Hetts, S., Mills, S., et al. Embolization of Skull Base Meningiomas and Feeding Vessels Arising From the Internal Carotid Circulation. Neurosurgery. 2011 Jan;68(1):162-9. DOI:10.1227/NEU.0b013e318fe2de9
7. Shah, A., Choudhri, O., Jung, H., Li, G. Preoperative endovascular embolization of meningiomas: update on therapeutic options. Neurosurg Focus 38 (3):E7,1-8. 2015 DOI:10.3171/2014.12.FOCUS14728
8. Omid-Fard, N., Fisher, C., Heran, M., The evolution of pre-operative spine tumour embolization. Br J Radiol 2019; 92: 20180899. DOI:10.1259/bjr.20180899
9. Rangel-Castilla, L., Shah, A., Klucznik, R., Diaz, O., Preoperative Onyx embolization of hypervascular head, neck, and spinal tumors. Experience with 100 consecutive cases from a single tertiary center. NeuroIntervent Surg 2014;6:51-56 DOI:10.1136/neurintsurg-2012-010542
10. Przybylowski, C., Baranoski, J., See, A., Flores, B., et al. Preoperative embolization of skull base meningiomas: Outcomes in the Onyx era. World Neurosurg. 2018;116:e371-e379. DOI:10.1016/j.wneu.2018.04.208

11. Ladner, T., Lakomkin, N., Davis, B., Cheng, J., Devin, C., Mocco, J. Minimizing bleeding complications in spinal tumor surgery with preoperative Onyx embolization via dual-lumen balloon catheter. J NeuroIntervent Surg 2016;8:210-215. DOI:10.1136/neurintsurg-2014-011505
Carli, D., Sluzewski, M., Beute, G., van Rooij, W. Complications of Particle Embolization of Meningiomas: Frequency, Risk Factors, and Outcome. Am J Neuroradiol. 2010 Jan;31(1):152-4. DOI:10.3174/ajnr.A1754
12. Pedicelli, A., Lozupone, E., Valente, I., et al. Pre-operative direct puncture embolization of head and neck hypervascular tumors using SQUID 12. Interv Neuroradiol. 2020 Jun;26(3) 346-353. DOI:10.1177/1591019919895882
13. Akmangit, I., Daglioglu, E., Kaya, T., Alagoz, F., et al. Preliminary Experience with Squid: A New Liquid Embolizing Agent for AVM, AV Fistulas and Tumors. Turk Neurosurg.2014;24(4):565-70. DOI:10.5137/1019-5149.JTN.11179-14.0
14. Elhammady, M., Peterson, E., Johnson, J., Aziz-Sultan, M., Preoperative Onyx Embolization of Vascular Head and Neck Tumors by Direct Puncture. World Neurosurg. (2012) 77, 5/6:725-730. DOI: 10.1016/j.wneu.2011.02.033
15. Ilyas, A., Przybylowski, C., Chen, C., Ding, D., et al. Preoperative embolization of skull base meningiomas: A systematic review.
16. Rosen CL, Ammerman JM, Sekhar LN, Bank WO. Outcome analysis of preoperative embolization in cranial base surgery. Acta Neurochir (Wien). 2002;144(11):1157-1164.
17. Ashour, R., Aziz-Sultan, A. Preoperative Tumor Embolization. Neurosurg Clin N Am 25 (2014) 607-617. DOI:10.1016/j.nec.2014.04.015
18. Ampie, L., Choy, W., Lamano, J., Kesavabhotla, K., et al. Safety and outcomes of preoperative embolization of intracranial hemangioblastomas: A systematic review. Clin Neurol Neurosurg. 2016 Nov;150:143-151. DOI:10.1016/j.clineuro.2016.09.008
19. Jackson, R., Myhill, J., Padhya, T., McCaffrey, J., et al. The Effects of Preoperative Embolization on Carotid Boyd Paraganglioma Surgery: A Systematic Review and Meta-Analysis. Otolaryngol Head Neck Surg. 2015 Dec;153(6):943-50. DOI:10.1177/0194599815605323
20. Lopez, F., Triantafyllou, A., Snyderman, C., Hunt, J., et al. Nasal juvenile angiofibroma: Current perspectives with emphasis on management. Head Neck 2017 May;39(5):1033-1045. DOI:10.1002/hed.24696

21. Facchini, G., Parmeggiani, A., Peta, G., Martella, C., et al. The role of percutaneous transarterial embolization in the management of spinal bone tumors: a literature review. Eur Spine J. 2021 Oct;30(10):2839-2851. DOI:10.1007/s00586-021-06963-5

CHAPTER 17

SPINE PATHOLOGY ABLATION

ALAN REEVES MD, JOHN GAO MD,
ADRIEN CAYE MS IV, ROBERT TURNER MS IV,
JOSEPH DOMINO MD, FRANK STEFANO DO,
ADIP BHARGAV MD

Percutaneous image-guided ablation techniques are minimally invasive, safe and effective treatments for patients with benign and metastatic spinal tumors. Tumors of the spine can lead to deformity, fractures, spinal cord compression, and chronic pain. Radiation therapy has long been the standard of care for local control and palliation of pain for vertebral metastasis. Radiation therapy is not effective in all types of tumors and is limited by the cumulative tolerance of the spinal cord. Additionally, radiation therapy can exclude patients from some systemic chemotherapy trials. Surgery is often limited by its morbidity, poor functional status of the patient, and shortened life expectancy (1).

Percutaneous ablation has recently emerged as an efficacious treatment for local tumor control and palliation of symptoms. There are several different and unique ablation techniques, each with its own advantages and disadvantages. These different techniques allow for a tailored treatment plan depending on the size, location and histology of the tumor. The following discussion will explore these different techniques, protective measures used to prevent neurological injury, and some of the tumors commonly found in and around the spinal cord.

Radiofrequency Ablation (RFA): RFA is one of several emerging minimally invasive ablative interventions for the treatment of metastatic tumors of the spinal column (2, 3). Indications for the clinical use of RFA currently encompass curative therapy for benign bone tumors, such as osteoid osteomas, and palliative therapy for metastatic tumors of the spine (3-5).

This technique enables targeted ablation of mass lesions with minimal off-target thermal energy dissipation. Multiple platforms are available for commercial use that employ a variety of electrode probes including unipolar and bipolar systems to generate high-frequency oscillating current at the target site. The thermal energy induces coagulative necrosis through local frictional heat (3, 6, 7). Using fluoroscopic guidance, the pedicle is cannulated with the electrode probe at the junction of the transverse process and superior articulating facet. The probe is then advanced into the vertebral body with a margin of approximately 1 cm between the osseous lesion and surrounding neural structures to minimize risk of off-target injury. However, recent iterations of this technology have further refined the accuracy of the ablative zone. A recent platform currently undergoing study in a prospective clinical trial utilizes an optional thermocouple in combination with a closed-loop water-cooling system to monitor the temperature changes in the ablative zone at the exposed tip of the electrode probe and to automatically adjust the radiofrequency parameters to achieve the desired ablation (3, 6, 7) The closed-loop water-cooling system ensures minimal heat dissipation, charring effect, and thermal sink effect outside the ablative zone (3, 6, 7).

Cryoablation is usually performed on large spinal metastases with soft tissue involvement, or large tumors associated with the posterior vertebral components. Cryoablation uses liquid argon to rapidly drop the temperature at the cryoprobe tip and create an enlarging ice ball. The ice ball of tissue is then thawed, most commonly with helium, which results in an osmotic gradient across the cell membranes. Intracellular freezing and ice crystal formation damages cell organelles. Extracellular freezing creates a relative imbalance between intracellular and extracellular electrolyte concentrations, thereby leading to an extracellular water shift. This extracellular water shift leads to increased intracellular electrolyte concentrations which damages the cell membrane and enzymes. Complete cell death is achieved with a temperature of -40°C or lower. Additionally, focal cellular ischemia is achieved. Typically, cryoablation is performed using at least 1 freeze, active thaw, and freeze cycle, usually lasting 10 minutes, 5 minutes, and 10 minutes, respectively (1, 8-10).

The procedure begins by placing the patient in the supine position. A CT scan is performed to assess for any evolution of the tumor since the most recent imaging. This allows for re-evaluation of the planned procedure, technical changes or even abortion of the procedure if it is deemed too risky. Trans-osseous access should be performed with precision to avoid neurovascular complications. Due to the variable origin of the Adamkiewicz's artery, extrapedicular coaxial bone access is strongly discouraged. Caution should be taken to avoid iatrogenic injury to vascular or neurological structures while positioning any protective measures. When accessing the anterior epidural space trans-foraminally, the needle should be precisely placed through Kambin's triangle to avoid neurovascular structures. A 3D volumetric image should be obtained prior to the ablation to verify the position of all devices. This allows modification of the parameters regulating the ablation probes. Any protective measures should be constantly monitored during the ablation procedure. All devices are withdrawn upon completion of the ablation procedure. Vertebral augmentation may be considered in cases of large malignant tumors located in vertebral body (3).

Cryoablation procedures are performed under general anesthesia with the use of CT or MRI guidance. Argon gas based cryoablation systems allow for use of multiple probes per generator (1, 8, 9). 14-17 gauge internally tunneled cryoprobes are placed directly into the tumor. Argon-gas is then circulated inside of the cryoprobe and expands at the tip. This expansion causes rapid cooling of the surrounding tissue through the Joule-Thomson effect. Cryoprobes typically range from 1.2mm to 2.4 mm diameter shafts, which are able to produce predictable ablation zones. Multiple probes can be placed within 1-2cm of one another and 1 cm from the tumor margin, thus creating overlapping zones of ablation and ensuring complete tumor coverage. The temperature at the ice ball transition zone is 0°C, and thus not sufficient to cause permanent cell death. Complete cell death is achieved at 3mm margin from the transition zone, thus necessitating that the ice ball extends beyond the tumor margins. CT imaging is performed every few minutes to monitor the size and location of the ice ball. Ice ball formation is visible as hypoattenuation in soft tissues on CT and a signal void area on MRI. It should be noted that intraosseous ice balls may not be visible on CT, especially with osteoblastic lesions. Several cycles of freezing and then thawing are performed, with the final thaw performed with helium gas. MRI-compatible cryoprobes offer an alternative to CT guided cryoablation. MRI guidance advantages include high tissue contrast resolution, improved visualization of intraosseous ice balls, real-time temperature monitoring, and avoids ionizing radiation (1, 8, 10).

Laser Interstitial thermotherapy (LITT), also known as stereotactic laser ablation, is used to target soft tissues in the vertebral body and epidural space (11). This technique uses real-time MRI temperature monitoring and laser energy to produce rapid temperature increases in the target tissue. This rapid heating of tissue leads to protein denaturation and tissue necrosis (10,

12). Immediate post procedural imaging will reveal tissue destruction and coagulative necrosis via lack of contrast enhancement (11).

The procedure begins with imaging of the target lesion in 3 planes. T2-weighted imaging is obtained to localize the tumor. The patient is placed in the prone position and one or more guide needles are inserted into the tumor under MRI guidance. The guide needle is advanced incrementally under intermittent or real-time image guidance, which allows for adjustments in the trajectory. Applicators are inserted into the guide needle in a coaxial fashion. The guide needles are then pulled back to expose laser fiber tip. The laser is then activated at low power (3 or 4 W) and MRI thermometry is performed to ensure the laser tip is in the desired location. The laser fiber should be placed approximately 6 mm from the thecal sac, as the area of ablation produced by a laser fiber is roughly 5mm on either side. A workstation monitors the magnitude and phase changes of the MRI scans in real time. Phase subtraction from the base line is used to map the temperature and predict regions of tissue destruction. Control points can be placed on the images and used to enhance the safety of the procedure prior to the delivery of any therapeutic doses. Once the laser fiber's position has been confirmed, a therapeutic dose is delivered. If temperatures reach a critical level, the system will deactivate, thus protecting the spinal cord or other important structures from thermal damage. Each laser fiber is operated at 15 W for a maximum of 90 seconds while MRI thermometry monitors the extent of ablation in real time. Use of multiple laser fibers from different entry points may be necessary depending on the size of the tumor. Post-procedural T1-weighted images, with and without contrast, are obtained to confirm the area of tissue damage. Patients are typically admitted for an observation period of two days, and discharged once pain is controlled. Patients are usually able to ambulate without assistance. Following a LITT procedure, patients may undergo a spinal stereotactic radiosurgery to cover the gross tumor volume (11-13).

A major advantage of cryoablation is the ability to monitor in real-time the formation of the ice ball, thus ensuring the entire tumor is covered and sparing other nearby structures (10). Cryoablation is effective at reducing pain with decreased likelihood of producing post-ablation edema and pain rebound. Additionally, the analgesic effects may be related to the cooling mechanism of cryoablation which can provide an anesthetic effect on the treated area and nerves. Cement augmentation can also provide analgesic effects and may be synergistic when combined with cryoablation. Local tumor control was achieved with success rates of 60% to 100%, depending on follow-up time points. In general, cryoablation was well tolerated with an overall complication rate of 8.1%. Commonly used protective measures include injection of warmed 5% dextrose solution to displace the spinal cord, cutaneous protection with application of warm saline, and intraprocedural motor-evoked potential monitoring (14).

Microwave Ablation (MWA) is a technique which uses one or multiple antennae to deliver electromagnetic energy to the target tissue. The electromagnetic microwaves cause polar molecules in the target tissue to continuously realign with the oscillating electromagnetic field. This leads to agitation of ionic molecules, frictional heating, and causes coagulative necrosis in the tumor (15). MWA results in higher intratumoral temperatures, shorter procedural times, and larger, more uniform ablation zones due to less perfusion-mediated tissue cooling and less influence by variable tissue impedance (1, 16).

MWA is performed under CT guidance with light conscious sedation (16, 17). Intratumoral injections of anesthetic agents can be used throughout the procedure for local anesthetic effect. For osseous osteosclerotic lesions and osteolytic lesions, a 10-13 gauge bone needle is inserted into the center of the lesion under CT guidance. The microwave antenna, ranging in size from 14 gauge to 11 gauge, is then inserted coaxially into the bone needles. Once the MWA antenna is in place, the coaxial introducer is retracted to prevent any interference with the microwave emissions from the probe tip. For lesions larger than 4 cm, the microwave antenna can be repositioned between ablation cycles to create a larger ablation zone. The MWA power is set between 30 W and 70 W and applied for 1 to 8 minutes depending on the tumor size. Thermocouple needles can be inserted in cases involving lesions close to neural structures to monitor in real-time temperature variations. Additionally, lower-limb neurological exams (motor, sensory) are performed in between ablation cycles to monitor for complications. To prevent complications, MWA was discontinued if the temperature exceeded 42°C. Post-procedural CT images are immediately obtained to identify any complications. Cementoplasty can be combined with MWA in patients at high risk for fracture (16, 17).

MWA was found to significantly improve pain in patients, especially when combined with cement augmentation. Local tumor control was also achieved with a high rate of success. MWA is generally well tolerated, with transient paresthesias and skin burns being the most commonly reported complications. An important consideration when using MWA on spinal lesions is its ability to rapidly deliver high amounts of energy to large ablation zones, which could damage neural structures. Still, MWA is preferrable to radiofrequency ablation due to MWA's ability to provide more effective heating and deeper penetration, especially in osteosclerotic lesions (1, 15, 16)

Magnetic Resonance-guided focused ultrasound: High-Intensity Focused Ultrasound is a non-invasive technique that uses high-energy ultrasound waves to ablate tissue within a small volume. HIFU is used for lesions that are at least 10 mm below the skin surface and not obscured by structures with high absorption or reflective properties, such as air-filled organs, non-target bone or metallic implants. HIFU is typically combined with MRI to deliver energy and rapidly increase tissue temperatures up to 90°C leading to coagulative necrosis. Additional effects of HIFU energy are cavitation, microstreaming, and radiation force which cause mechanical stress on cellular membranes. HIFU has also been associated with stimulating the host immune response against the tumor and enhancing the therapeutic effect of chemotherapy and radiation therapy (18, 19). The use of HIFU is mainly indicated in extra-spinal lesions such as osteoid osteoma or bone metastasis (9, 10).

HIFU can be performed as a single session or multi-session outpatient procedure. The procedure may be performed under general anesthesia if the procedure calls for continuous high-intensity ultrasound waves or conscious sedation if low-intensity, pulse-wave focused ultrasound will be used. The patient is placed supine on the table and an optimal acoustic window is obtained between the transducer and target region. It is important to ensure that there is no scar or air-fluid interface in the acoustic window which can interfere with the acoustic field and lead to complications. An initial set of images is obtained, either T1 or T2 weighted sequences, with or without fat saturation. Once the MR images are obtained, the operator outlines the skin and bone, identifies the treatment region, and any areas where ultrasound energy must be limited. An anatomic fiducial marker is placed to monitor any movement of the patient during the procedure. A series of low power sonications are performed to calibrate the area of transducer focus. Treatment is then initiated with full power sonications and ablation is achieved with target tissue temperatures ranging between 60°C to 80°C. MR thermometry is used to monitor increases in temperature during the procedure. Post-procedural T-1 weighted images with gadolinium are obtained and hypointense non-enhancing areas reveal ablated volumes (18).

HIFU is generally well tolerated with low complication rates. The most common complication was sonication pain, followed by third-degree skin burns or fractures. Pain relief following treatment is fast and durable, and reported to be effective in 60 to 100% of patients. HIFU is contraindicated in patients with high risk of fracture of the targeted area and a history of prior stabilization with metallic hardware. MR guided HIFU has several advantages for the treatment of pain from bone metastases, including a good safety profile, no limitations on the type of bone lesion, and no limit to the number of treatment sessions. Additionally, concurrent chemotherapy does not need to be stopped in order to receive HIFU treatment (18, 20).

Protective measures: Due to the proximity of the ablation zone to vital neurological structures, there is an inherent risk of permanent injury when performing thermal ablation in the spine. Several factors influence the risk of neurological injury, including duration of thermal effect, distance from the ablation zone, presence of intact vertebral cortex, absolute temperature, and type of nerve fiber. Thermal insulation, temperature and neurophysiologic monitoring are used to minimize potential thermal injury during spinal ablation procedures. Thermal insulation involves the use of hydrodissection and instillation of warm or cool liquid to displace the structure at risk. Use of hydrodissection during radiofrequency ablation should be performed without saline solutions due to their high electric conductivity. Continuous temperature monitoring can be performed by placing thermocouples close to the at-risk structures, usually within the neuroforamina or epidural space. Neurophysiologic monitoring and nerve electrostimulation can be used to monitor for impending neurologic deficit. Skin injury is another potential complication that can be avoided with active thermoprotection, such as surface application of warm saline in a glove or gauze (1, 3, 10).

References

1. Tomasian, A., Jennings, J., Hot and Cold Spine Tumor Ablations. Neuroimaging Clin N Am. 2019 Nov;29(4):529-538. DOI:10.1016/j.nic.2019.07.001
2. Hadzipasic, M., Giantini-Larsen, A. M., Tatsui, C. E. & Shin, J. H. Emerging Percutaneous Ablative and Radiosurgical Techniques for Treatment of Spinal Metastases. *Neurosurg Clin N Am* 31, 141-150, DOI:10.1016/j.nec.2019.08.017 (2020).
3. Cazzato, R., Auloge, P., De Marini, P., Boatta, E., et al. Spinal Tumor Ablation: Indications, Techniques, and Clinical Management. Tech Vasc Interv Radiol. 2020 Jun;23(2):100677. DOI:10.1016/j.tvir.2020.100677
4. Levy, J. *et al.* Radiofrequency Ablation for the Palliative Treatment of Bone Metastases: Outcomes from the Multicenter OsteoCool Tumor

Ablation Post-Market Study (OPuS One Study) in 100 Patients. *J Vasc Interv Radiol* 31, 1745-1752, doi:10.1016/j.jvir.2020.07.014 (2020).
5. De Filippo, M. *et al.* Radiofrequency ablation of osteoid osteoma. *Acta Biomed* 89, 175-185, doi:10.23750/abm.v89i1-S.7021 (2018).
6. Angileri, S. A. *et al.* Cooled radiofrequency ablation technology for painful bone tumors. *Acta Biomed* 91, e2020007, doi:10.23750/abm.v91i10-S.10271 (2020).
7. Medtronic. (2019).
8. McMenomy, B., Kurup, N., Johnson, G., Carter, R., et al. Percutaneous Cryoablation of Musculoskeletal Oligometastatic Disease for Complete Remission. J Vasc Interv Radiol 2013;24:207-231. DOI:10.1016/j.jvir.2012.10.019 (2013).
9. Sgalambro, F., Zugaro, L., Bruno, F., Palumbo, P., et al. Interventional Radiology in the Management of Metastases and Bone Tumors. J Clin Med 2022 Jun; 11(12):3265.
10. Tsoumakidou, G., Koch, G., Caudrelier, J., Garnon, J., et al. Image-Guided Spinal Ablation: A Review. Cardiovasc Intervent Radiol (2016) 39:1229-1238. DOI: 10.1007/s00270-016-1402-6 (2016).
11. Vega, R., Ghia, A., Tatsui, C., Percutaneous Hybrid Therapy for Spinal Metastatic Disease: Laser Interstitial Thermal Therapy and Spinal Stereotactic Radiosurgery. Neurosurg Clin N Am 2020 Apr;31(2):211-219. DOI:10.1016/j.nec.2019.11.006 (2020).
12. Ahrar, K., Stafford, J., Magnetic Resonance Imaging-Guided Laser Ablation of Bone Tumors. Tech Vasc Interv Radiol. 2011 Sep;14(3):177-82. DOI:10.1053/j.tvir.2011.02.010 (2011).
13. Chen, C., Lee, I., Tatsui, C., Elder, T., Sloan, A. Laser interstitial thermotherapy (LITT) for the treatment of tumors of the brain and spine: a brief review. J Neurooncol 151, 429-442 (2021). DOI:10.1007/s11060-020-03652-z (2021).
14. Sagoo, N., Haider, A., Ozair, A., Vannabouathong, C. Percutaneous image-guided cryoablation of spinal metastases: A systematic Review. J Clin Neurosci. 2022 Feb;96:120-126. DOI:10.1016/j.jocn.2021.11.088 (2022).
15. Sagoo, N., Haider, A., Rowe, S., Haider, M., et al. Microwave Ablation as a Treatment for Spinal Metastatic Tumors: A Systematic Review. World Neurosurg. 2021 Apr;148:15-23. DOI:10.1016/j.wneu.2020.12.162 (2021).
16. Kastler, A., Alnassan, H., Aubry, S., Kastler, B. Microwave thermal ablation of spinal metastatic bone tumors. J Vasc Interv Radiol. 2014 Sep;25(9):1470-5. DOI:10.1016/j.jvir.2014.06.007 (2014).

17. Pusceddu, C., Sotgia, B., Fele, R.M., Melis, L. Treatment of Bone Metastases with Microwave Thermal Ablation. J Vasc Interv Radiol 2013; 24:229-233. DOI:10.1016/j.jvir.2012.10.009 (2013).
18. Dababou, S., Marrocchio, C., Scipione, R., Erasmus, H. High-Intensity Focused Ultrasound for Pain Management in Patients with Cancer. Radiographics. 2018 Mar-Apr;38(2):603-623. DOI:10.1148/rg.2018170129 (2018).
19. Tsukamoto, S., Kido, A., Tanaka, Y., Facchini, G. Current Overview of Treatment for Metastatic Bone Disease. Curr Oncol. 2021 Oct; 28(5):3347-3372. DOI: 10.3390/curroncol28050290 (2021).
20. Gennaro, N., Sconfienza, L., Ambrogi, F., Boveri, S., Lanza, E. Thermal ablation to relieve pain from metastatic bone disease: A systematic review. Skeletal Radiol. 2019 Aug;48(8):1161-1169. DOI:10.1007/s00256-018-3140-0 (2019).

CHAPTER 18

THYROID RADIOFREQUENCY ABLATION (RFA)

ALAN REEVES MD, NICOLETTE DUMAS MD

Radiofrequency ablation (RFA) has been utilized as a treatment for multiple different tumors found throughout the body, most commonly in the lungs, liver, bone, and kidneys since the early 2000s. Since that time, multiple different probes and procedures have been developed to refine the technique. This technology is commonly used and well developed outside of the United States for treatment of benign, symptomatic thyroid nodules. In the United States, RFA is an emerging, minimally invasive treatment for symptomatic benign thyroid nodules, which includes autonomously functioning thyroid nodules. Classically, surgery has been the preferred treatment option for benign and malignant thyroid tumors; however, it has several drawbacks, such as scarring, the need for general anesthesia, and the risk of inducing hypothyroidism. RFA provides an alternative for those who do not wish to undergo surgery, wish to eliminate the risks of surgery, and an alternative for those who are not surgical candidates. (1, 2, 3, 4, 5)

Indications

Most thyroid nodules are benign and only require serial observation without intervention. Some nodules can grow to be quite large and can lead to compressive symptoms, such as dysphagia (most common), neck fullness, choking, foreign body sensation, and dyspnea. These large nodules can also lead to cosmetic concerns, especially in those with thin or small necks. (1, 6, 7) To be considered for radiofrequency ablation, the patient must be symptomatic with evidence of enlarging thyroid nodules. Most institutions include symptom and cosmetic questionnaires in the pre-procedure work up and post-procedure evaluations. (1,6) It is important to note that while RFA of thyroid nodules has become a preferred treatment in other countries, at the time of this writing, the American Thyroid Association does not have a treatment guideline for RFA. Pioneering institutions are creating their own guidelines utilizing published literature from other countries.

In terms of nodule size or volume, there have been no definite criteria developed for thyroid RFA. The need for treatment of thyroid nodules depends on each patient's cosmetic problems and/or symptoms, which vary accordingly due to location of the thyroid nodule to critical structures and the circumference of the neck. (6) Smaller nodules are easier to fully treat and have a decreased incidence of recurrence and need for re-treatment. (7)

Imaging

Ultrasound (US) evaluation of the thyroid nodules to be treated is extremely important. This elucidates the composition of the nodules (solid, mixed cystic and solid, cystic) and will help determine whether RFA is indicated. RFA is most beneficial for patients with cosmetic or compressive symptoms who have predominately solid or cystic and solid thyroid nodules. (4) Purely cystic nodules are not well treated with RFA. (3,5) Also, thyroid nodules with heavy calcifications because the probe is difficult to visualize as the risks of non-target RFA or under treatment are present. (7) US imaging also shows location of the nodules within the thyroid and their proximity to any important adjacent structures, such as the carotid artery, recurrent laryngeal nerve, vagus nerve, esophagus, and trachea. US can also show any enlarged feeding vessels which may complicate the RFA procedure. If there are any suspicious imaging features, such as extra-thyroid extension or indeterminate enlarged lymph nodes, then further work up, including biopsy of those areas of concern, should be performed. (6,7)

Biopsy

To qualify for RFA, these nodules should be proved benign by either fine needle aspiration and/or core biopsies. Most require two benign biopsy results or a single benign biopsy result with imaging highly suggestive of benign nodules. (6)

Previously Treated Nodules

RFA re-treatment can be performed in previously treated nodules with marginal regrowth, a nodule with volume reduction of <50%, or an incomplete resolution or recurrence of compressive symptoms or cosmetic problems.

Laboratory

Most institutions require pre-procedure blood work, usually including a CBC and PT/INR. All patients should have a pre-procedure TSH, T3, and free T4 drawn to determine baseline levels. (7)

Procedure

In the United States, there are a several pioneering institutions performing RFA of thyroid nodules. These institutions vary in whether the procedure is performed under local anesthesia only, local anesthesia plus intravenous sedation, or general anesthesia. It should be noted that those who perform RFA outside of the United States overwhelmingly perform the procedure with local anesthesia only and only resort to sedation or general anesthesia under special circumstances. (2, 3, 6, 7, 8) Some institutions prefer intravenous sedation or general anesthesia so there is no unwanted patient movement during the procedure. Each institution will need to establish their own protocol for how best to proceed for thyroid RFA procedure.

Understanding the anatomy of the thyroid and important adjacent structures, such as the jugular vein, carotid artery, vagus nerve, recurrently laryngeal nerve, trachea, and esophagus is essential to successfully performing this procedure and minimizing any complications. (7, 9, 10)

There are two basic techniques used for performing the RFA procedure: transisthmic approach and moving shot technique.

Transisthmic Approach

The probe is inserted into the isthmus from medial to lateral, into the nodule, with the ultrasound probe held in the transverse position. With this approach, the electrode and whole ablation course can be monitored by the transverse ultrasound view. This technique is favored because the probe tip is positioned away from the recurrent laryngeal nerve, electrode position remains stable even when the patient coughs or swallows and prevents leakage of hot fluids into the peri-thyroid tissues. (1, 3, 5, 6, 7, 8, 9)

Moving Shot Technique

This technique consists of subdividing the thyroid nodules into multiple small conceptual ablation units. The conceptual units are smaller at the periphery of a nodule and larger in the center of a nodule or in regions remote from critical structures. The electrode tip is initially positioned in the deepest and most remote portion of the nodule, with subsequent retraction to the most superficial portion of the nodule. The electrode tip moves slowly but continuously to prevent the RF ablation cutoff phenomenon. Then, when an echogenic area is detected at the tip of the electrode, the electrode tip is retracted slowly. Finally, the electrode tip is superficially repositioned in the long axis of the electrode and pulled along it again. This technique has some disadvantages including multiple insertion points. (3, 5, 6, 7, 8, 9)

Modified Moving Shot Technique

This technique is the same as the moving shot technique except that the probe is not removed from the skin and instead redirected while the probe remains under the skin and back into the nodule. (5)

Hydrodissection

If the thyroid nodule is adjacent to critical structures, such as the recurrent laryngeal nerve, vagal nerve, carotid artery, trachea, or esophagus, then hydrodissection can be utilized to ensure safety of the surrounding structures. (5, 6, 7, 9) A solution of 5% dextrose is injected between the target tumor and the adjacent critical structure. Due the neck anatomy, the fluid may disperse rapidly and may need to be injected continuously throughout the procedure. It is imperative to not use normal saline to hydrodissect as it is an ionic solution which can conduct electricity and this could lead to burns of these adjacent structures when the RFA probe is turned on. (6, 7, 9)

Post-procedure

RFA of thyroid nodules is typically an outpatient procedure. The patient's neck is expected to be mildly painful for several days. (1) The pain can be managed with ice and over the counter oral analgesics. There may be mild bruising of the skin due to lidocaine injection or where the probe entered the skin. The nodules should decrease in size with corresponding decrease in symptoms over the next 1-3 months. Follow up TSH, T3 and free T4 should be performed and compared to baseline labs, especially in autonomously functioning thyroid nodules. Symptom and cosmetic scores should be compared to pre-procedure evaluations. (6) Ultrasound should be performed to evaluate the ablated nodules with pre-procedure size comparison and to guide whether any further procedures are needed. (3, 6, 7)

Complications

RFA has excellent outcomes and low complication rate, especially compared to surgical complications. The most feared complication post thyroid RFA procedure is damage to either the vagal or recurrent laryngeal nerves. (3) Permanent voice changes can be caused by thermal damage to the recurrent laryngeal nerve. Other complications include transient dysphonia, local pain, hematoma, fever, skin infections, mild burns, thyrotoxicosis, hypothyroidism, Horner syndrome. (10)

Outcomes

RFA has excellent outcomes. Recent studies have shown that thyroid nodules decrease in volume approximately 85-95% one year post procedure. There are also significant improvements in compressive symptoms and cosmetic issues. RFA has shown similar efficacy to surgery with a significantly lower complication rate. It has been shown to have better results with smaller thyroid nodules. Larger nodules may require more than one treatment to attain desired cosmetic or compressive symptom relief. RFA returns 40-50% of patients with autonomously functioning thyroid nodules to a euthyroid state. (1,2,3)

References

1. Hamidi, Oksana, et al. "Outcomes of Radiofrequency Ablation Therapy for Large Benign Thyroid Nodules: A Mayo Clinic Case Series." *Mayo Clinic Proceedings*, vol. 93, no. 8, 2018, pp. 1018–1025. *PubMed*, https://doi.org/10.1016/j.mayocp.2017.12.011. Accessed 23 Jan. 2022.
2. Haugen, Bryan R et al. "2015 American Thyroid Association Management Guidelines for Adult Patients with Thyroid Nodules and Differentiated Thyroid Cancer: The American Thyroid Association Guidelines Task Force on Thyroid Nodules and Differentiated Thyroid

Cancer." *Thyroid : official journal of the American Thyroid Association* vol. 26,1 (2016): 1-133. doi:10.1089/thy.2015.0020

3. Lee, Minkyoung, et al. "Clinical Practice Guidelines for Radiofrequency Ablation of Benign Thyroid Nodules: A Systematic Review." *Ultrasonography*, vol. 40, no. 2, 2021, pp. 256–264. *PubMed*, https://doi.org/10.14366/usg.20015. Accessed 24 Jan. 2022.
4. Mauri, Giovanni, et al. "Laser and Radiofrequency Ablations for Benign and Malignant Thyroid Tumors." *International Journal of Hyperthermia*, vol. 36, no. 2, 2019, pp. 13–20. *PubMed*, https://doi.org/10.1080/02656736.2019.1622795. Accessed 24 Jan. 2022.
5. Kim, Ji-hoon, et al. "2017 Thyroid Radiofrequency Ablation Guideline: Korean Society of Thyroid Radiology." *Korean Journal of Radiology*, vol. 19, no. 4, 2018, p. 632. *PubMed*, https://doi.org/10.3348/kjr.2018.19.4.632. Accessed 24 Jan. 2022.
6. Park, Hye Sun, et al. "Thyroid Radiofrequency Ablation: Updates on Innovative Devices and Techniques." *Korean Journal of Radiology*, vol. 18, no. 4, 2017, p. 615. *PubMed*, https://doi.org/10.3348/kjr.2017.18.4.615. Accessed 24 Jan. 2022.
7. Lee, Ming-Tsang, and Chih-Yuan Wang. "Radiofrequency Ablation in Nodular Thyroid Diseases." *Journal of Medical Ultrasound*, vol. 21, no. 2, June 2013, pp. 62–70. *PubMed*, https://doi.org/10.1016/j.jmu.2013.04.006. Accessed 24 Jan. 2022
8. Zhu, Yaqiong, et al. "Solid Benign Thyroid Nodules (>10 ML): A Retrospective Study on the Efficacy and Safety of Sonographically Guided Ethanol Ablation Combined with Radiofrequency Ablation." *International Journal of Hyperthermia*, vol. 37, no. 1, 2020, pp. 157–167. *PubMed*, https://doi.org/10.1080/02656736.2020.1717647. Accessed 24 Jan. 2022.
9. Cervelli, Rosa, et al. "Radiofrequency Ablation in the Treatment of Benign Thyroid Nodules: An Efficient and Safe Alternative to Surgery." *Journal of Vascular and Interventional Radiology*, vol. 28, no. 10, 24 Aug. 2017, pp. 1400–1408. *PubMed*, https://doi.org/10.1016/j.jvir.2017.07.009.
10. Vahab, Fatourechi. "Thyroid and Parathyroid Office Based Ultrasonography- Review Article." *Iranian Journal of Public Health*, vol. 43, 2014, pp. 11–18. *PubMed*, Accessed 24 Jan. 2022.

CHAPTER 19

CONCLUSION/OUTLOOK

AARON ROHR MD, MS

The core make-up of interventional oncology (IO) is fundamentally described, yet always evolving. Regardless of organ system, there is a constant demand and response for new innovative approaches to treat neoplasms. This textbook describes a great deal of evolutional changes throughout the realm of IO, yet omits a vast array of new treatment processes, approaches, therapies, etc., due to sheer volume of their existence. While this text does describe new innovations and therapies, only time will tell what new revolutionary breakthroughs will be adapted for future IO practices. Regardless, understanding the essentials and foundation of IO is pertinent for its further development. Our group of physicians believe that not only is this one of the most exciting fields of medicine to practice, but also one of the most rewarding.